Trauma

and

Recovery

on War's

Border

Trauma and Recovery on War's Border

A GUIDE FOR GLOBAL HEALTH WORKERS

Kathleen Allden, MD,

and

Nancy Murakami, LCSW,

editors

DARTMOUTH COLLEGE PRESS

Hanover, New Hampshire

DARTMOUTH COLLEGE PRESS
An imprint of University Press of New England
www.upne.com
© 2015 Trustees of Dartmouth College
All rights reserved
Manufactured in the United States of America
Typeset in Minion and Franklin Gothic by
Westchester Publishing Services

For permission to reproduce any of the material in this book, contact
Permissions, University Press of New England, One Court Street, Suite 250,
Lebanon NH 03766; or visit www.upne.com

Library of Congress Cataloging-in-Publication Data

Trauma and recovery on war's border : a guide for global health workers / Kathleen
Allden and Nancy Murakami, editors.
    p. ; cm.
   Includes bibliographical references and index.
   ISBN 978-1-61168-694-4 (cloth : alk. paper)—ISBN 978-1-61168-695-1 (pbk. : alk.
paper)—ISBN 978-1-61168-696-8 (ebook)
   I. Allden, Kathleen, editor. II. Murakami, Nancy, editor.
   [DNLM: 1. Mental Health—ethnology—Myanmar. 2. Refugees—psychology—
Myanmar. 3. Mental Disorders—therapy—Myanmar. 4. Vulnerable Populations—
psychology—Myanmar. 5. War—Myanmar. 6. Wounds and Injuries—psychology—
Myanmar. WA 305 JB8]
RA790.5
362.19689—dc23   2014031691

5 4 3 2 1

Contents

Foreword

More than ever before, people along the Thai-Burma border are openly discussing the impact of human rights violations on mental health. There has been a significant transformation in understanding mental health issues, the sociocultural intricacies of these issues, and the awareness that we cannot solve our most pressing social issues without addressing the stigma associated with mental health. This is particularly true for the most marginalized members of our community. Inside Burma, community leaders have a general understanding of mental health, but issues such as HIV and AIDS, political imprisonment, amputation, gender-based violence, and rape are still so stigmatized and thought of as personal issues that people are not openly discussing them or their psychosocial effects. From experience, however, we know that changing this attitude is difficult but possible.

For decades, populations of Burma have been moving back and forth across state and national boundaries. People have been migrating to neighboring and distant countries. The populations that manage to establish themselves along Burma's borders are diverse and complex, but we are bound together by the experiences of flight and struggle. We have been displaced so many times that we have had to develop a range of coping skills and systems of support to survive. It is in our monasteries, schools, and hospitals that we have come together and shared our experiences and sought comfort and care.

With unprecedented international attention focused on creating a lasting peace process in Burma today, our ability to rebuild our society will hinge on whether we can emerge with the openness to cope with our past, even while dealing with the uncertainty of the future. The cease-fire process has begun in Burma, but we have not yet seen community rebuilding. If we fail to highlight and deal with the psychosocial issues, trust-building and peace-building cannot be done with confidence. Furthermore, without exploring these issues at multiple levels—community, program, and policy—there will not be effective rebuilding.

Organizations along the border manage many important health programs, such as those for HIV and malaria, but we now want to see more programs and targeted funding for mental health, and we want to hear organizations, leaders, and politicians talking about mental health. We need more opportunities for health workers, religious leaders, teachers, social workers, and community leaders to work together on solving psychosocial issues in nonhierarchical ways. In addition to individuals who need mental health assistance, groups such as former political prisoners, women, abandoned children, and amputees also have specific and unique needs that must be addressed.

From our experiences at Mae Tao Clinic, we believe that access to mental health care is integral to the healing process. It is important for moving beyond the cycle of violence that has affected many of us. In our nearly fifteen-year collaboration with Burma Border Projects, through increased training and capacity for providing mental health care, we have witnessed the transformative power that access to such support enables. For the first time, we are successfully helping our communities address issues of gender-based violence, mental illness, and child development following decades of trauma. We have a structure and a language that empowers us to help people. Different members of the community have come forward to be a part of this movement. I believe that all people who can access these services have the opportunity to rebuild their lives, and that is why people at all levels of society—politicians, soldiers, teachers, students, and even those who commit violence against others—should be entitled to care.

We believe mental health is a basic human right. At this critical stage of reconciliation, it must be prioritized at a national level. It is essential to restoring power to individuals and communities that will in turn participate in shaping our future, allowing many to return from the periphery. Mental health care is empowering the people, so we must speak up, get involved, and organize to promote this right for all.

This book is a collaborative effort, consolidating the best of what we have learned from working on mental health issues for the people most affected by decades of oppression in Burma. I hope that people coming to Burma or the Burma border will identify our strengths and our already existing resources and programs. The community needs technical support, but there must be awareness of the existing local culture, knowledge, and expertise. Mental health is a sensitive and stigmatized topic, but it can also be empowering when addressed appropriately. Under the government of Burma, so many topics are sensitive, so we must take on the responsibility of challenging oppression, stigma, isolation, and fear in order to address the mental health issues of both victim and perpetrator.

DR. CYNTHIA MAUNG
Cofounder, Mae Tao Clinic, Mae Sot, Thailand

Acknowledgments

The editors would like to thank all current and past staff and board members of Burma Border Projects (BBP), especially founder and executive director Michael Forhan. Michael's steadfast dedication to the people of Burma has kept BBP alive and growing for sixteen years and allows us to look forward to BBP's new initiatives inside Myanmar.

We would also like to thank Lucinda Lai, our extraordinarily talented editorial assistant. Lucinda was awarded a Haas Service Fellowship from Stanford University to live at the Burma border for one year to help us organize and launch this project. Lucinda continued to work with us to complete this volume as she earned a master's degree as a Gates Cambridge Scholar and then as a medical student at Harvard.

For her patient leadership and guidance and her inspirational vision for the future, the editors dedicate this book with gratitude to Dr. Cynthia Maung, founder and director of Mae Tao Clinic.

We also extend our gratitude to our Burmese friends and colleagues at the Burma border, inside Myanmar, and in various countries around the world for their welcoming partnership, for their trust, and for all that they have taught us.

Myanmar (Burma)

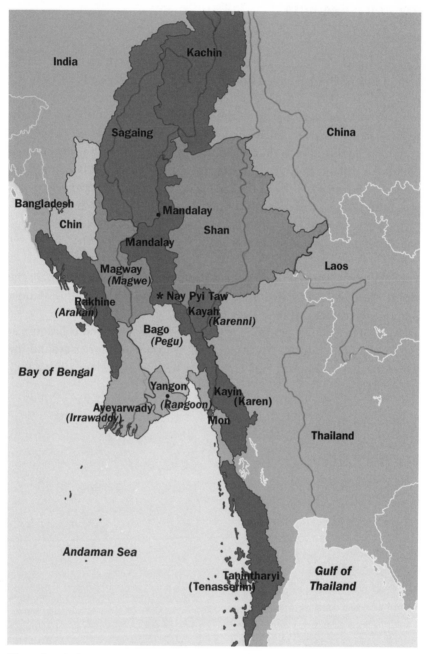

When a location's name has changed over time, the older version is shown in parentheses.

Refugee camps in Thailand at the Burma border and nearby cities/towns

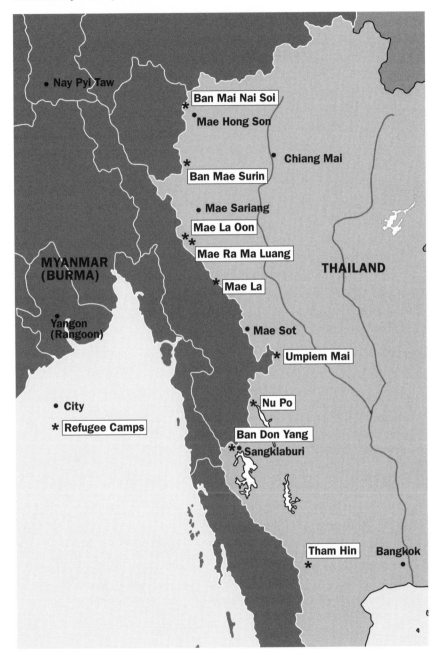

Part I.

Introduction

Chapter 1

Global Mental Health in

War-Affected Communities

Kathleen Allden

For many, psychological suffering can be the most enduring consequence of war, human rights violations, torture, and natural or human-generated disaster. Such suffering can significantly affect a person's ability to function and return to a meaningful, productive life within his or her family and community. As a result, societies highly affected by war and violence can have sizable percentages of their population unable to participate effectively in rebuilding the society unless they heal. Fortunately, the human spirit is profoundly capable of emerging with great resilience from war, violence, and grief. The severity of violence, the types of losses, the level of disruption, and the meaning given to the experiences will shape a person's reaction. Counterbalancing a person's traumatic experiences are the supports that remain intact, the degree to which a person feels empowered, and the extent to which he or she finds a purpose to life going forward.[1] When those supports are damaged or destroyed, humanitarian initiatives can strengthen or help restore them.

For decades, large numbers of Burmese citizens have fled to neighboring countries, particularly Thailand, seeking safety from war and the many forms of violence inside Myanmar perpetrated by the repressive military regime in control of that country. Finally, after decades of violence and oppression, there are signs of hope and reform. This book describes efforts among the "helping professions" to contribute to the process of healing, postconflict reconstruction, and peace-building through mental health interventions and psychosocial assistance. The authors describe their efforts, along with the respective theoretical underpinnings of intervention drawn from an expanding academic and scientific literature on best practices in humanitarian assistance and global mental health. Emphasizing partnership and the importance of cross-cultural understanding, each chapter addresses a different challenge and is a collaborative effort between international and Burmese actors.

In 1989, the military regime changed Burma's official name to Myanmar. This politicized the country's name. The region along the border has traditionally been referred to as the Burma border by prodemocracy and humanitarian actors. Recently, with signs that the country is opening up and is more engaged in democratic changes and respectful of human rights, the name Myanmar is increasingly used. The authors in this volume use the terms interchangeably, mostly using the term "Burma border" for activities outside Myanmar and the country name Myanmar for activities inside the country.

Providing mental health and psychosocial support for societies in developing countries affected by war, natural disaster, and political instability presents a complex nexus of problems requiring unique solutions tailored to each context. Solutions, in turn, require creative input from multiple disciplines ranging from medicine, nursing, psychology, social work, and public health to anthropology, social sciences, and political activism. An increasing number of students and professionals at various levels of their careers are entering complicated postconflict locations such as the Burma border and Myanmar, usually with good intentions but too often with little or no experience in international mental health or humanitarian assistance. Before taking any action in the field, they need to understand and appreciate the importance of the cultural, historical, and political context, and how best to apply their academic knowledge to develop services that will do no harm, that are based on good theory and evidence, and that recognize and honor the strengths, knowledge, and resources of the communities and individuals with whom they are working. The goal of this edited volume is to orient these students and professionals and provide guidance as they embark on their work in the field. Although this book focuses on the Burma border and Myanmar, the experiences and lessons learned by the contributing authors will be helpful to humanitarians working in other resource-poor, postconflict regions around the world.

War and Violence in Myanmar

For decades, Myanmar's population of approximately 50 million has struggled for democracy and human rights against a brutal military regime. Years of war and oppression forced large numbers to flee their homes. Although recently there have been signs of political improvements in Myanmar, Human Rights Watch stated in *World Report 2013* that "Burma's human rights situation remained poor."[2] With over one hundred ethnic groups, Myanmar is purported to have the richest ethnic diversity in Asia. The majority of the population, estimated at 50 to 75 percent, is ethnic Burman; most live in the central region of the country. Ethnic minority groups typically live in the mountainous frontier regions. The largest minorities are the Shan (9 percent) and the Karen (7 percent); the Mon, Rakhaine,

Karenni, Kachin, Chin, Akha, Lahu, Wa, Kayan, Danu, Naga, Kokang, Palaoung, Pa-O, Rohingya, Tavoyan, Chinese, and Indian make up about 5 percent. Minority group demands for autonomy and self-determination within their respective regions of the country, often in the form of militant insurgency, have been brutally suppressed by the Burmese military. Civilians in these ethnic areas suffer the harshest treatment; thousands have been forcibly relocated and their land confiscated.[3] Christina Fink, in her chapter "Burmese Sanctuary-Seekers and Migrants in Thailand," provides the reader with further historical and political details and a contextualized discussion of political oppression and violence perpetrated by the Burmese government against its own people.

Refugees and Displaced Persons

According to the 1951 United Nations Refugee Convention, a refugee is someone who fled his or her home and country owing to "a well-founded fear of persecution because of his/her race, religion, nationality, membership in a particular social group, or political opinion."[4] In *Mid-Year Trends 2013*, the UN High Commissioner for Refugees reports that the total number of "persons of concern" reached an all-time high of 38.7 million. The report cites 11.1 million refugees; 987,500 asylum seekers; 20.8 million internally displaced persons (people who have not crossed an international border but have moved to a different region within their own country); 3.5 million stateless persons; and 1.4 million other persons of concern. It also reports that Myanmar remained one of the top ten source countries for refugees.[5]

The UN's 2013 "Country Operations Profile—Myanmar" reports that there are 415,343 refugees and 25,621 asylum seekers outside the country and that inside Myanmar there are 430,400 internally displaced persons and 808,075 stateless persons (mostly Muslims from Rakhine State).[6] Thailand, which has a long history of hosting refugees within its boundaries, is not a signatory to the 1951 UN Refugee Convention. The UN's 2013 "Country Operations Profile—Thailand" reports that there are 84,900 registered and an estimated 62,000 unregistered refugees from Myanmar living in nine camps along the border. The number of unregistered refugees and asylum seekers from Myanmar continues to grow inside and outside refugee camps. These people are regarded as illegal migrants under Thai immigration law and are subject to arrest, detention, and deportation. Since resettlement to third countries was initiated in 2005, more than 80,000 registered refugees have left the camps for Western countries. Nevertheless, growing numbers of unregistered people in the camps have caused camp populations to remain steady. The report goes on to point out that refugees began arriving in Thai

camps during the 1980s and that now this "constitutes one of the most protracted displacement situations in the world. The prolonged confinement
of these refugees in camps has created many social, psychological and protection concerns. It has also resulted in a dependency among the refugees
on assistance."[7]

Additionally, over 1 million migrant workers from Burma are registered
through Thailand's National Verification Program. For a number of reasons, however, many migrants cross the border illegally, leading to a much
higher estimate of up to 3 million. Many of these migrants face harsh conditions working in garment factories and fish-processing factories or spray-
ing crops and doing other high-risk, dangerous jobs paying as little as US$2
per day.[8]

Psychological and Psychosocial Consequences of War Trauma and Forced Relocation

Civilian populations, especially in unstable parts of the world, are increasingly affected by war. During the first half of the twentieth century, the
majority of war casualties around the globe were soldiers. The nature of
war changed, however, and by the mid-twentieth century civilians were increasingly becoming the targets of armed conflict. Since the end of the
Cold War, the world has seen the decline of interstate conflict and the rise
of intrastate conflict as internal dissent and ethnic conflicts erupted in
multiple locations; Myanmar is a tragic example of this phenomenon. Now,
at the beginning of the twenty-first century, the International Committee
of the Red Cross reports that while the number of deaths caused by actual
military engagement during battle is declining, the numbers of people killed
because of war remains high.[9] Given these changing trends and growing
numbers of war-affected civilians, the psychological and psychosocial effect of war on civilians has become an area of intense study.

Since the Vietnam War and Khmer Rouge genocide in Cambodia, a
burgeoning literature, far beyond the scope of this chapter to review, has
grown concerning the psychological, neuropsychiatric, and psychosocial
consequences of war, refugee displacement, and human rights abuse among
adults and children. For more than three decades, researchers in mental
health have been documenting the effects of war and forced migration in
conflict-affected regions of the world. Their work reveals that while not
everyone exposed develops mental health problems, with increased exposure
to war trauma, atrocities, and forced displacement, significant percentages
of affected populations experience increasing symptoms of depression,
posttraumatic stress disorder (PTSD), and symptoms of other disorders,

such as generalized anxiety and somatoform disorder.[10] This research also indicates that these symptoms can seriously compromise a traumatized individual's ability to function.[11] The connection between psychological symptomatology and diminished functioning is important because of the implications for people's ability to deal with adversity, to care for themselves and their family members during conflict and during forced relocation, and to contribute to reconstruction of their society postconflict. Although there are few studies on the effects of war and human rights violations among Burmese people, the studies that exist suggest effects similar to populations in other highly affected conflict and postconflict regions. These studies document Burmese people's high exposure to trauma and also, where measured, significant rates of depression and anxiety among Burmese refugee populations in Thailand inside and outside refugee camps and in war-affected eastern Myanmar.[12]

A number of factors that cut across socioeconomic class and cultural identity place war-affected individuals at heightened risk of developing mental problems, while other factors may be protective. Risk factors that increase the likelihood that a person is at risk for mental health problems and mental illness include but are not limited to poor physical health, head injury, being female, poor educational level, poverty, unemployment, overcrowding, poor sanitation, collapse of social structures and loss of social supports, perceived lack of control over traumatic events, and preexisting history of psychiatric illness. Fortunately and importantly, there are factors that protect people, contribute to their resilience, and enhance their chances for coping and recovering meaningful productive lives. Protective factors include a caring nuclear or extended family, social supports, sharing with others, engaging in self-help groups that empower, the possibility to work or generate income, the ability to participate in cultural ceremonies or religious rituals, the availability of recreation or leisure activities, political or religious inspiration as a source of meaning and comfort, and preexisting coping skills.[13]

When protective factors break down or prove insufficient, an individual will have a diminished capacity to care for him- or herself and family or to participate in rebuilding the war-damaged or displaced community and society. This fact draws attention to the importance of mental health and psychosocial support as critical to many individuals' survival and to a society's human capital: the knowledge, expertise, proficiencies, skills, and creativity required for people to work and contribute to socioeconomic stability and progress.

Overview of Global Mental Health

To further recognize the significance of mental health disorders in war-affected areas, one should consider the global burden of disease. Since 1990, the World Health Organization (WHO) has been measuring the global burden of disease with metrics known as disability-adjusted life years or DALYs and years lived with disability or YLDs. DALYs combine the sum of years of potential life lost to premature death with years of productive life lost to disability.[14] Mental disorders can, of course, be fatal and thereby contribute to the mortality rate. According to WHO estimates in 2005, neuropsychiatric disorders accounted for between 1 and 3 million deaths per year and between 1 and 4 percent of all years of life lost. Most of these deaths were caused by dementia, epilepsy, and Parkinson's disease, but 40,000 deaths were attributed to mental disorders such as unipolar and bipolar depression, schizophrenia, and PTSD, and 182,000 deaths to alcohol and drug abuse.[15] Nevertheless, mental disorders usually cause disability, not death. Using DALYs, WHO reported in its recent update on the global burden of disease that neuropsychiatric conditions account for up to one-quarter of all disability-adjusted life years and up to one-third of all years lived with disability. In low- and middle-income countries, where most war-affected communities are, four of the top ten causes of years lost to disability are mental disorders: depression, substance and alcohol use disorders, schizophrenia, and bipolar disorder.[16] Additionally, armed conflict, a major cause of death and injury worldwide, is seen as a significant factor contributing to the global burden of disease.[17] The authors of the first article in the landmark series on global mental health in the *Lancet* in 2007 draw attention to factors that make this scenario even worse. Depression can forecast the onset and progression of physical and social disabilities. Similarly, being disabled is a risk factor for developing depression, which in turn influences the course of physical health conditions. Hence the title "No Health without Mental Health."[18]

Now one can begin to grasp why mental health is a critical topic in war-affected and refugee communities. These communities are typically poor, and the burden of disease due to mental disorders is high; this, in turn, leads to significant levels of disability in the population. Yet, at the same time, human capital is vital to coping and postconflict reconstruction. In spite of the high need, resources for addressing mental health are scarce and always underfunded. Indeed, nearly one-third of countries worldwide do not even have a public budget for mental health. In Africa and Asia, most countries spend less than 1 percent of their small health budgets on mental health services.[19] The sad reality is that resources to address mental disorders are woefully lacking around the world, especially in low-income countries such as Myanmar, and those services that are available in these countries are inequitably distributed, with wealthy citizens getting care and the poor none.[20]

One should not draw attention to mental health without underscoring the problem of stigma. Certainly, there have been some advances in the treatment of the mentally ill in developed countries. Yet even in a rich country such as the United States, one sees homeless mentally ill men and women on the streets of all major cities, and large numbers of mentally ill people are held in jails instead of being sent to treatment programs. In poor countries the situation is worse. The mentally ill are abused, marginalized, feared, and ridiculed. They might be chained to their beds, locked in shacks behind the family home, or worse, and too often denied basic human rights. The renowned psychiatrist and anthropologist Arthur Kleinman calls attention to the plight of countless mentally ill people around the world exposed to "the horrors of being shunned, isolated, [and] deprived of the most basic of human rights" when he writes: "The fundamental truth of global mental health is moral: individuals with mental illness exist under the worst of moral conditions. The widespread stigma of mental illness, which prevails in countries as disparate as China, India, Kenya, Romania, Egypt, and the USA, marks individuals with severe psychiatric disorders as virtually non-human." He advises that "any effective change in global mental health will have to prioritize moral transformation as the foundation for reform of global mental health, much as it was for the reform that spurred HIV/AIDS treatment in Africa and Asia."[21]

Social and Cultural Dimensions

Whenever approaching mental health or psychosocial interventions in a country or society other than one's own, there are countless cross-cultural considerations. Every society struggles with questions about the meaning of suffering, illness (including mental illness), and death. Every culture has developed bodies of knowledge to help people understand and cope with these issues, as well as healers to provide various modes of therapeutic intervention aimed at providing relief.[22] Indeed, all aspects of the way illness is experienced are shaped by the cultural framework of the sufferer and those to whom he or she turns for help. At the same time, a society's economic and political structures play critical roles in determining health and mental health risks and treatment resources.[23] The field of medical anthropology explores how "sicknesses" are "culturally constructed" by asking how a society's understandings of and responses to disease are shaped by their cultural assumptions about the meaning of life, the functioning of the human body, and the causes of ill health and misfortune.[24] Medical anthropology also takes on the question of health inequities by exposing processes by which people are victimized or constrained by "structural violence" inflicted by politically and economically repressive regimes against the poor and marginalized.[25] Structural violence is a term that describes "the social—economic, political, legal, religious, and cultural—structures that stop individuals, groups, and societies from reaching their full potential . . . which lowers the actual degree to which someone is able to meet their needs."[26] The violence behind the suffering of the Burmese people is clearly derived not only from war but also from "structural violence" perpetrated at many levels by a repressive regime in Myanmar as well as inadequate responses from the international community to assist refugee populations trapped outside their home country.

An understanding of social and cultural dimensions of health and mental health requires global mental health workers to grasp the concepts of cultural idioms of distress and suffering within the culture in which they are working. To do so, one needs to appreciate that every culture attributes its own meaning to symptoms and illness. Every culture has its own model of disease and a unique way to find healing and restoration of well-being. It is not possible for a global health or mental health worker to know all this information about every culture that he or she will encounter during a career. However, global mental health workers can develop and maintain awareness of these topics with each cultural group by asking probing questions and learning to recognize how the particular cultural group conceptualizes health and illness and the words that groups use to describe these issues. To assist in this process, Kleinman and others at Harvard University developed a list of eight questions a clinician can ask in order to understand an illness from a patient's point of view, which take into consideration the patient's beliefs about his or her illness: (1) What do you think caused the problem? (2) Why do you think it happened when it did? (3) What do you think your sickness does to you? (4) How severe is your sickness? (5) What kind of treatment do you think you should receive? (6) What are the most important results you hope to receive from this treatment? (7) What are the chief problems your sickness has caused for you? and (8) What do you fear most about your sickness?[27]

These topics are at the heart of medical anthropology. While a review of this major academic area of the social sciences is beyond the scope of this chapter, several points can be made that serve as building blocks for developing a competent cross-cultural approach to evaluation and intervention at an individual clinical level or community-based psychosocial support level. To work effectively as a global mental health worker, one needs to recognize biases and perspectives that are based on one's personal, cultural, and social background. It is often difficult to step back and recognize these factors, but a grasp of these matters will help prevent global mental health workers from making errors in judgment and imposing diagnoses that are inaccurate, wrong, and stigmatizing, and treatments that are ineffective, unnecessary, and potentially harmful. This type of self-reflection is rarely encouraged or fostered during conventional medical and psychiatric training in the West, with its emphasis on a biomedical paradigm. There may be some exposure to this process in training programs for psychologists and social workers. Peer supervision, staff meetings, and group discussion among international staff can help raise and maintain awareness of biases and prejudices.

Collaboration with members of the affected cultural group will provide invaluable guidance on cultural understanding. Typically, collaboration requires building a cross-cultural team with representatives of the affected community working side by side with international global mental health workers. Also, whenever possible, global mental health workers should reach out to engage and collaborate with traditional healers. The role of local traditional healers and healing practices should not be underestimated, because people in developing countries usually turn to traditional healers first.

Principles of Mental Health and Psychosocial Support

Because research is hard to conduct in war-affected and postconflict regions, the evidence base for mental health and psychosocial supports that would help humanitarian assistance providers develop and offer effective services in those regions is still in relatively early development. Nevertheless, using data that do exist in multiple disciplines, along with consensus and intelligent collaboration between experienced humanitarian professionals, scholars from academia, and policy makers, progress has indeed been made that has facilitated the development of many practical resources and guidelines. Three basic resources with which a global mental health worker should be familiar are the Sphere Project *Humanitarian Charter and Minimum Standards of Humanitarian Response*, the Inter-Agency Standing Committee *Guidelines on Mental Health and Psychosocial Support*, and WHO's Mental Health Gap Action Programme. These three resources can serve as the foundation for further study to refine one's skills and expertise. Again, there is an intersection between humanitarian assistance for war-affected communities and global mental health. To be effective, one must be familiar with overlapping strategies.

The Sphere Project was established in 1997 as a global network of nongovernmental agencies and the International Red Cross and Red Crescent Movement with the goal of improving the quality of assistance during response to disasters. The project's work is based on two core beliefs: "first, that those affected by disaster or conflict have a right to life with dignity and, therefore, a right to assistance; and second, that all possible steps should be taken to alleviate human suffering arising out of disaster or conflict."[28] In 2000, in what has become the gold standard for humanitarian assistance, the Sphere Project published the *Humanitarian Charter and Minimum Standards of Humanitarian Response* (also knows as the *Sphere Handbook*, updated most recently in 2011) to codify ethical convictions about the role of humanitarian agencies, guiding principles, and duties. The minimum standards are evidence-based and represent sector-wide consensus on best practice in humanitarian response. The authors identify minimum standards for four critical lifesaving sectors. These standards are set out in the *Sphere Handbook*'s four technical chapters: water supply, sanitation, and hygiene promotion; food security and nutrition; shelter, settlement, and nonfood items; and health action.[29] While no one can dispute the significance of this landmark charter and these standards, the handbook provides only cursory guidance on the topic of mental health and psychosocial support. The fact that these large agencies all agreed that mental health and psychosocial support must be included among the minimum standards is momentous. Nevertheless, only three of the handbook's 393 pages are devoted to this topic.[30]

The Inter-Agency Standing Committee (IASC) is a committee of executive heads of United Nations agencies, intergovernmental organizations, Red Cross and Red Crescent agencies, and nongovernmental organizations responsible for global humanitarian policy. In 2005, the IASC established a task force to develop guidelines on mental health and psychosocial support in emergencies. The task force completed its work, and IASC published the *Guidelines on Mental Health and Psychosocial Support* in 2007. The term "mental health and psychosocial support" refers to various types of assistance that aim to prevent or treat mental disorders or protect or promote psychosocial well-being. Although "mental health" and "psychosocial support" are related and overlapping terms, they are often used by humanitarian assistance providers and policy makers to indicate different and sometimes even competing approaches. In fields outside the health sector— for example, in education or protection—assistance providers tend to speak of supporting psychosocial well-being. Health agencies and assistance programs more often use the term "mental health," but they also use the terms "psychosocial rehabilitation" and "psychosocial treatment" to describe nonbiological interventions for people with mental disorders. The IASC sought to highlight the critical need for multisectoral action by bringing various perspectives and approaches to bear in a set of unified guidelines to foster collaboration among this broad group of providers and to communicate the importance of complementary approaches.[31]

The goal of the IASC guidelines is articulated in the introduction: "The primary purpose of these guidelines is to enable humanitarian actors and communities to plan, establish and coordinate a set of minimum multisectoral responses to protect and improve people's mental health and psychosocial well-being in the midst of an emergency." However, the guidelines go beyond initial minimum responses, which are seen as the first steps to laying "the foundation for more comprehensive efforts." The guidelines also provide strategies for mental health and psychosocial support for all phases of an emergency. They describe strategies for preparedness before an emergency, comprehensive steps that can be taken during the acute emergency phase, and then steps for the postacute stabilization phase and on into reconstruction. All the strategies are based on six core principles, summarized as follows:

1. Human rights and equity: Promote human rights for all those affected and protect those at heightened risk for human rights violations.
2. Participation: Maximize participation of the local affected population, enable local people to retain or resume control over decisions that affect their lives, and build local ownership that is important for program quality, equity, and sustainability.
3. Do no harm: Because this field lacks extensive scientific evidence regarding outcomes efficacy, and because this field deals with highly sensitive issues, work in this field has the potential to cause harm. To reduce risk, providers should obtain sufficient information, develop cultural sensitivity and competence, stay updated, coordinate and learn from others, and understand power relations between outsiders and the community affected by the emergency.
4. Build on available resources and capacities: All affected groups have assets and resources; therefore, support self-help and strengthen resources already present in the population.
5. Integrated support systems: Stand-alone programs that have a single focus such as response to rape or to PTSD can fragment care and

increase stigma. It is better to integrate mental health and psychosocial support into wider, more sustainable systems such as schools, health services, general mental health services, or social services.

6. Multilayered supports: During humanitarian emergencies, people are affected in many different ways requiring different types of responses. The IASC guidelines provide a schematic way to envision how to develop a layered system of supports to meet the needs of different groups—"the intervention pyramid."[32] The framework set out by the IASC intervention pyramid will be used by authors in subsequent chapters to present various models of intervention implemented at the Burma border and inside Myanmar.

The "intervention pyramid for mental health and psychosocial support" consists of four layers: specialized services at the tip, focused nonspecialized supports in the upper middle, community and family supports in the lower middle, and basic services and security at the bottom. The pyramidal shape reflects the proportion of the population that will need each particular level of services.

All people affected by the emergency will need to be protected and receive basic services such as food, water, and shelter; hence the large base of the pyramid reflects the needs of virtually the entire affected population. The lower-middle layer of the pyramid is smaller than the base, reflecting a smaller but still significant proportion of the affected population. These are individuals and families who, if they receive help, will be able to cope and maintain their mental health despite experiencing major losses, deaths of loved ones, and/or disruptions of family and community networks. The interventions they may require include, for example, family tracing and reunification and participation in healing ceremonies, parenting programs, educational activities, women's groups, youth groups, and other activities to strengthen coping.

The upper-middle layer of the pyramid, a still smaller segment of the affected community, includes survivors of rape and gender-based violence, torture, and atrocities, and former child soldiers, land mine victims, and others highly affected by violence and loss. This segment may need interventions such as focused, nonspecialized support from trained and supervised workers. These workers may not need years of specialized training to provide support. They may be community workers trained to provide emotional or vocational support. These interventions also include basic mental health care provided by primary health care services and "psychological first aid," a form of intervention that promotes an environment of safety, calm, connectedness, self-efficacy, empowerment, and hope. Without support, this sizable segment of the population is at risk of developing mental disorders and resultant social disabilities.

At the tip of the pyramid is the most vulnerable group in the affected population. This group, though the smallest, consists of thousands of people who continue to suffer and experience difficulties in daily functioning, despite receiving the support already described. These people may be suicidal or psychotic; they may have mental illnesses, developmental disabilities, head injuries, or epilepsy. Traumatic experiences inevitably worsen mental illness for those already suffering. War usually damages or destroys the health care and mental health care infrastructure, making it hard or impossible to obtain mental health treatment. In resource-poor countries, there may have been no community-based mental health services even before the violence began. These people need individualized and specialized psychological and psychiatric interventions. They can be referred to specialized services, if such programs exist, or initiation of programs for longer-term training and supervision of general or primary health care providers may be required.[33]

In light of its studies on the global burden of disease, WHO recognized that mental, neurological, and substance use disorders are common all over the world, that they contribute significantly to the global burden of disease, and that 75 percent of those affected are in low-income countries with virtually no access to treatment. Therefore, to respond to this critical need for treatment, WHO launched the Mental Health Gap Action Programme (mhGAP). mhGAP is based on the premise that even in low-income countries, with proper care that includes psychosocial assistance and medication, countless suicides could be prevented and millions of people could be treated and return to normal, productive lives.[34] In 2010, with the aim of scaling up services for mental, neurological, and substance use disorders in countries with scarce resources, WHO published the *mhGAP Intervention Guide for Mental, Neurological and Substance Use Disorders in Non-specialized Health Settings*. The *Intervention Guide* sets out general principles for communicating with the people seeking help and the people who care for them at home, and for assessing, treating and monitoring, mobilizing and providing social support, protecting human rights, and attending to overall well-being. It focuses on the following high-priority disorders and provides decision trees for evaluation and treatment for each: depression, bipolar disorder, psychosis, epilepsy/seizures, developmental disorders (in children and adolescents), behavioral disorders (in children and adolescents), dementia (in older people), alcohol use disorders, drug use disorders, and self-harm/suicide.[35] Although the discussion of treatments and interventions is not as lengthy or detailed as specialized mental health programs would need, the *Intervention Guide* provides the framework necessary to begin to address mental disorders in a primary health care setting in a low-resource area. This is far more than is usually available to primary care providers in remote war-affected, low-income regions. Although the interventions are not specific to war-affected individuals, the methods for assessment and treatment outlined in the guide are basic ones that apply everywhere and that can be adapted for clinics in refugee camps, health programs serving displaced people and migrants, and other settings serving people affected by human rights abuse, political violence, or war. For example, the decision tree concerning suicide and self-harm includes instruction on how to assess whether the person has committed a serious act of self-harm, how to assess whether there is imminent risk of suicide and what to do if there is; advises the provider to determine whether the person has a concomitant medical, mental, or neurological illness or substance use problem; and then gives advice about how to address the suicidal person's need for protection and treatment.[36] These steps are necessary in any setting and would be useful and relevant inside Myanmar at remote health outposts or could be used by "backpack medics" who travel from village to village providing care. They would be useful in any health program in any town along the Burma border crowded with migrants, refugees, and marginalized minority groups.

Overview

Trauma and Recovery on War's Border: A Guide for Global Health Workers is a resource for best practices and provides a detailed case study of how these practices have been utilized. For students and professionals entering or already working in the area of humanitarian assistance, this book provides basic principles of global mental health and psychosocial assistance and examples of how theory is applied, at times by trial and error, in a region deeply scarred by war and violence. The reader will also see in some of the examples how programs can develop and expand organically within the affected community. In these cases, community members work together to devise solutions to challenges identified as priorities by their community, often without the benefit of manuals and theoretical guidelines, which are typically published in English, not in local languages. Those who are setting out to work in Myanmar or at the Burma border will find this an important resource to orient them to the context, culture, and challenges of working in that region. The content is grounded in principles of sustainable humanitarian aid, cultural competence, and empowerment.

Coeditors Kathleen Allden and Nancy Murakami developed the idea for this book from their long-term involvement with Burma Border Projects (BBP), since 1999 a pioneering organization on the Thai-Burma border (and now inside Myanmar) with a primary mission to provide mental health resources, training, and support to strengthen the skills of local community-based organizations and individuals. Contributing authors are local and international experts representing academia, nongovernmental organizations, and community-based organizations and health care centers. All authors have firsthand experience at the Burma border and/or in Myanmar.

The book is divided into five parts. Part I provides this introductory chapter on global mental health in war-affected communities and a chapter on the historical and political background of conflict in Myanmar and the current situation for Burmese living in exile in Thailand.

In Part II, authors cover mental health and psychosocial assessment and intervention with an emphasis on a community-based and "strengths-based" approach, with case examples of programs inside and outside refugee camps. Part III, on vulnerable groups and challenges, includes chapters covering a variety of topics, such as children, gender-based violence, drug and alcohol abuse, former political prisoners, torture survivors, land mine victims, and people with HIV and other chronic illnesses. Part IV deals with managing, supervising, and evaluating programs. This part contains chapters on vicarious traumatization and resilience among health workers, staff training and supervision, and research and program evaluation. Part V looks toward the future of the people of Myanmar with a chapter that focuses on empowerment and transformation for a country recovering from decades of psychological trauma and oppression.

Notes

1 Neil Boothby and Alison Strang, *A World Turned Upside Down: Social Ecological Approaches to Children in War Zones* (Bloomfield, CT: Kumarian Press, 2006), 5–6.

2 Human Rights Watch, *World Report 2013: Burma* (Human Rights Watch, 2013), http://www.hrw.org/world-report/2013/country-chapters/burma.

3 Chizom Ekeh and Martin Smith, "Minorities in Burma," *Minority Rights Group International* (2007), http://www.minorityrights.org/?lid=3546.

4 United Nations General Assembly, *Convention Relating to the Status of Refugees*, Treaty Series, vol. 189 (July 28, 1951), 16, http://unhcr.org.au/unhcr/images/convention%20and%20protocol.pdf.

5   United Nations High Commissioner for Refugees, *Mid-Year Trends 2013* (United Nations High Commissioner for Refugees, 2013), http://www.unhcr.org/52af08d26.html.

6   United Nations High Commissioner for Refugees, "2013 UNHCR Country Operations Profile—Myanmar," 2013, http://unhcr.org/cgi-bin/texis/vtx/page?page=49e4877d6&submit=GO.

7   United Nations High Commissioner for Refugees, "2013 UNHCR Country Operations Profile—Thailand," 2013, http://www.unhcr.org/pages/49e489646.html.

8   "Burmese Migrant Workers in Thailand: Myanmar's Overflow," *Economist*, March 19, 2009, http://www.economist.com/node/13334070.

9   Andreas Wenger and Simon JA Mason, "The Civilianization of Armed Conflict: Trends and Implications," *International Review of the Red Cross* 90, no. 872 (2008): 837–838, doi:10.1017/S1816383109000277.

10 Richard F Mollica, Grace Wyshak, and James Lavelle, "The Psychosocial Impact of War Trauma and Torture on Southeast Asian Refugees," *American Journal of Psychiatry* 144, no. 12 (December 1987): 1567–1572; Joop TVM de Jong et al., "Lifetime Events and Posttraumatic Stress Disorder in 4 Postconflict Settings," *JAMA: Journal of the American Medical Association* 286, no. 5 (August 1, 2001): 555–562; Joop TVM de Jong, Ivan H Komproe, and Mark Van Ommeren, "Common Mental Disorders in Postconflict Settings," *Lancet* 361, no. 9375 (June 21, 2003): 2128–2130, doi:10.1016/S0140-6736(03)13692-6; Richard F Mollica et al., "The Effect of Trauma and Confinement on Functional Health and Mental Health Status of Cambodians Living in Thailand-Cambodia Border Camps," *JAMA: Journal of the American Medical Association* 270, no. 5 (August 4, 1993): 581–586.

11 Richard F Mollica et al., "Disability Associated with Psychiatric Comorbidity and Health Status in Bosnian Refugees Living in Croatia," *JAMA: Journal of the American Medical Association* 282, no. 5 (August 4, 1999): 433–439; Richard F Mollica et al., "Longitudinal Study of Psychiatric Symptoms, Disability, Mortality, and Emigration among Bosnian Refugees," *JAMA: Journal of the American Medical Association* 286, no. 5 (August 1, 2001): 546–554; Richard F Mollica, Charles Poole, and Svang Tor, "Symptoms, Functioning, and Health Problems in a Massively Traumatized Population: The Legacy of the Cambodian Tragedy," in *Adversity, Stress, and Psychopathology*, ed. Bruce P Dohrenwend (New York: Oxford University Press, 1998), 34–51; Ronald C Kessler, "Posttraumatic Stress Disorder: The Burden to the Individual and to Society," *Journal of Clinical Psychiatry* 61 suppl. 5 (2000): 4–12; discussion, 13–14.

12 Barbara Lopes Cardozo et al., "Karenni Refugees Living in Thai-Burmese Border Camps: Traumatic Experiences, Mental Health Outcomes, and Social Functioning," *Social Science & Medicine (1982)* 58, no. 12 (June 2004): 2637–2644,

doi:10.1016/j.socscimed.2003.09.024; Kathleen Allden et al., "Burmese Political Dissidents in Thailand: Trauma and Survival among Young Adults in Exile," *American Journal of Public Health* 86, no. 11 (November 1996): 1561–1569; Luke C. Mullany et al., "Population-Based Survey Methods to Quantify Associations between Human Rights Violations and Health Outcomes among Internally Displaced Persons in Eastern Burma," *Journal of Epidemiology and Community Health* 61, no. 10 (October 1, 2007): 908–914, doi:10.1136/jech.2006.055087.

13 Joop de Jong, "Public Mental Health, Traumatic Stress and Human Rights Violations in Low-Income Countries," in *Trauma, War, and Violence: Public Mental Health in Socio-Cultural Context*, ed. Joop de Jong, Springer Series in Social/Clinical Psychology (Boston Springer US, 2002), 6–7, http://link.springer.com/chapter/10.1007/0-306-47675-4_1.

14 World Health Organization, "DALYs Definition," *World Health Organization*, May 11, 2001, http://www.who.int/mental_health/management/depression/daly/en/.

15 Colin D Mathers and Dejan Loncar, "Projections of Global Mortality and Burden of Disease from 2002 to 2030," *PLoS Med* 3, no. 11 (November 28, 2006): e442, doi:10.1371/journal.pmed.0030442.

16 World Health Organization, *The Global Burden of Disease: 2004 Update* (Geneva: World Health Organization, 2008), 35–36, http://www.who.int/healthinfo/global_burden_disease/2004_report_update/en/.

17 Christopher JL Murray, "Armed Conflict as a Public Health Problem," *BMJ* 324, no. 7333 (February 9, 2002): 346–349, doi:10.1136/bmj.324.7333.346.

18 Martin Prince et al., "No Health without Mental Health," *Lancet* 370, no. 9590 (September 2007): 859–877, doi:10.1016/S0140-6736(07)61238-0.

19 World Health Organization, "Project Atlas: Resources for Mental Health," 2013, http://www.who.int/mental_health/evidence/atlas/en/.

20 Shekhar Saxena et al., "Resources for Mental Health: Scarcity, Inequity, and Inefficiency," *Lancet* 370, no. 9590 (September 8, 2007): 878–889, doi:10.1016/S0140-6736(07)61239-2.

21 Arthur Kleinman, "Global Mental Health: A Failure of Humanity," *Lancet* 374, no. 9690 (August 2009): 603–604, doi:10.1016/S0140-6736(09)61510-5.

22 Byron Good et al., eds., "Introduction," in *A Reader in Medical Anthropology: Theoretical Trajectories, Emergent Realities* (West Sussex, UK: Wiley-Blackwell, 2010), 1.

23 Donald Joralemon, *Exploring Medical Anthropology* (Upper Saddle River, NJ: Prentice Hall, 2010), ix.

24 Ibid., 9.

25 Craig Janes and Kitty Corbett, "Anthropology and Global Health," in *A Reader in Medical Anthropology: Theoretical Trajectories, Emergent Realities*, ed. Byron Good et al. (West Sussex, UK: Wiley-Blackwell, 2010), 405–407.

26 Paul E Farmer et al., "Structural Violence and Clinical Medicine," *PLoS Med* 3, no. 10 (October 24, 2006): e449, doi:10.1371/journal.pmed.0030449.

27 A Kleinman, L Eisenberg, and B Good, "Culture, Illness, and Care: Clinical Lessons from Anthropologic and Cross-Cultural Research," *Annals of Internal Medicine* 88, no. 2 (February 1978): 251–258.

28 The Sphere Project, *Humanitarian Charter and Minimum Standards in Disaster Response* (Geneva: The Sphere Project, 2004).

29 Ibid.

30 Ibid., 333–336.

31 Mark van Ommeren and Mike Wessells, "Inter-Agency Agreement on Mental Health and Psychosocial Support in Emergency Settings," *Bulletin of the World Health Organization* 85, no. 11 (November 2007): 822, doi:10.2471/BLT.07.047894.

32 Inter-Agency Standing Committee, *IASC Guidelines on Mental Health and Psychosocial Support in Emergency Settings* (Geneva: Inter-Agency Standing Committee, 2007), 5–10.

33 Ibid., 11–13.

34 World Health Organization, "WHO Mental Health Gap Action Programme (mhGAP)," http://www.who.int/mental_health/mhgap/en/.

35 World Health Organization and Mental Health Gap Action Programme, *mhGAP Intervention Guide for Mental, Neurological and Substance Use Disorders in Non-specialized Health Settings* (Geneva: World Health Organization, 2010), 6–8.

36 Ibid., 73–78.

Bibliography

Allden, Kathleen, Charles Poole, Sapang Chantavanich, Khin Ohmar, Nyi Nyi Aung, and Richard F Mollica. "Burmese Political Dissidents in Thailand: Trauma and Survival among Young Adults in Exile." *American Journal of Public Health* 86, no. 11 (November 1996): 1561–1569.

Boothby, Neil, and Alison Strang. *A World Turned Upside Down: Social Ecological Approaches to Children in War Zones*. Bloomfield, CT: Kumarian Press, 2006.

"Burmese Migrant Workers in Thailand: Myanmar's Overflow." *Economist*, March 19, 2009. http://www.economist.com/node/13334070.

de Jong, Joop. "Public Mental Health, Traumatic Stress and Human Rights Violations in Low-Income Countries." In *Trauma, War, and Violence: Public Mental Health in Socio-Cultural Context*, edited by Joop de Jong, 1–91. Springer Series in Social/

Clinical Psychology. Boston: Springer US, 2002.
http://link.springer.com/chapter/10.1007/0-306-47675-4_1.

de Jong, Joop TVM, Ivan H Komproe, and Mark Van Ommeren. "Common Mental Disorders in Postconflict Settings." *Lancet* 361, no. 9375 (June 21, 2003): 2128–2130. doi:10.1016/S0140-6736(03)13692-6.

de Jong, Joop TVM, Ivan H Komproe, Mark Van Ommeren, Mustafa El Masri, Mesfin Araya, Noureddine Khaled, Willem van De Put, and Daya Somasundaram. "Lifetime Events and Posttraumatic Stress Disorder in 4 Postconflict Settings." *JAMA: Journal of the American Medical Association* 286, no. 5 (August 1, 2001): 555–562.

Ekeh, Chizom, and Martin Smith. "Minorities in Burma." *Minority Rights Group International* (2007). http://www.minorityrights.org/?lid=3546.

Farmer, Paul E, Bruce Nizeye, Sara Stulac, and Salmaan Keshavjee. "Structural Violence and Clinical Medicine." *PLoS Med* 3, no. 10 (October 24, 2006): e449. doi:10.1371/journal.pmed.0030449.

Good, Byron, Michael MJ Fischer, Sarah S Willen, and Mary-Jo DelVecchio Good, eds. "Introduction." In *A Reader in Medical Anthropology: Theoretical Trajectories, Emergent Realities*, 1–6. West Sussex, UK: Wiley-Blackwell, 2010.

Human Rights Watch. *World Report 2013: Burma*. Human Rights Watch, 2013. http://www.hrw.org/world-report/2013/country-chapters/burma.

Inter-Agency Standing Committee. *IASC Guidelines on Mental Health and Psychosocial Support in Emergency Settings*. Geneva: Inter-Agency Standing Committee (IASC), 2007.

Janes, Craig, and Kitty Corbett. "Anthropology and Global Health." In *A Reader in Medical Anthropology: Theoretical Trajectories, Emergent Realities*, edited by Byron Good, Michael MJ Fischer, Sarah S Willen, and Mary-Jo DelVecchio Good, 405–407. West Sussex, UK: Wiley-Blackwell, 2010.

Joralemon, Donald. *Exploring Medical Anthropology*. Upper Saddle River, NJ: Prentice Hall, 2010.

Kessler, Ronald C. "Posttraumatic Stress Disorder: The Burden to the Individual and to Society." *Journal of Clinical Psychiatry* 61, suppl. 5 (2000): 4–12; discussion 13–14.

Kleinman, A, L Eisenberg, and B Good. "Culture, Illness, and Care: Clinical Lessons from Anthropologic and Cross-Cultural Research." *Annals of Internal Medicine* 88, no. 2 (February 1978): 251–258.

Kleinman, Arthur. "Global Mental Health: A Failure of Humanity." *Lancet* 374, no. 9690 (August 2009): 603–604. doi:10.1016/S0140-6736(09)61510-5.

Lopes Cardozo, Barbara, Leisel Talley, Ann Burton, and Carol Crawford. "Karenni Refugees Living in Thai-Burmese Border Camps: Traumatic Experiences, Mental Health Outcomes, and Social Functioning." *Social Science & Medicine (1982)* 58, no. 12 (June 2004): 2637–2644. doi:10.1016/j.socscimed.2003.09.024.

Mathers, Colin D, and Dejan Loncar. "Projections of Global Mortality and Burden of Disease from 2002 to 2030." *PLoS Med* 3, no. 11 (November 28, 2006): e442. doi:10.1371/journal.pmed.0030442.

Mollica, Richard F, Karen Donelan, Svang Tor, James Lavelle, Christopher Elias, Martin Frankel, and Robert J Blendon. "The Effect of Trauma and Confinement on Functional Health and Mental Health Status of Cambodians Living in Thailand-Cambodia Border Camps." *JAMA: Journal of the American Medical Association* 270, no. 5 (August 4, 1993): 581–586.

Mollica, Richard F, Keith McInnes, Narcisa Sarajlić, James Lavelle, Iris Sarajlić, and Michael P Massagli. "Disability Associated with Psychiatric Comorbidity and Health Status in Bosnian Refugees Living in Croatia." *JAMA: Journal of the American Medical Association* 282, no. 5 (August 4, 1999): 433–439.

Mollica, Richard F, Charles Poole, and Svang Tor. "Symptoms, Functioning, and Health Problems in a Massively Traumatized Population: The Legacy of the Cambodian Tragedy." In *Adversity, Stress, and Psychopathology*, edited by Bruce P Dohrenwend, 34–51. New York: Oxford University Press, 1998.

Mollica, Richard F, Narcisa Sarajlic, Miriam Chernoff, James Lavelle, Iris S Vukovic, and Michael P Massagli. "Longitudinal Study of Psychiatric Symptoms, Disability, Mortality, and Emigration among Bosnian Refugees." *JAMA: Journal of the American Medical Association* 286, no. 5 (August 1, 2001): 546–554.

Mollica, Richard F, Grace Wyshak, and James Lavelle. "The Psychosocial Impact of War Trauma and Torture on Southeast Asian Refugees." *American Journal of Psychiatry* 144, no. 12 (December 1987): 1567–1572.

Mullany, Luke C, Adam K Richards, Catherine I Lee, Voravit Suwanvanichkij, Cynthia Maung, Mahn Mahn, Chris Beyrer, and Thomas J Lee. "Population-Based Survey Methods to Quantify Associations between Human Rights Violations and Health Outcomes among Internally Displaced Persons in Eastern Burma." *Journal of Epidemiology and Community Health* 61, no. 10 (October 1, 2007): 908–914. doi:10.1136/jech.2006.055087.

Murray, Christopher JL. "Armed Conflict as a Public Health Problem." *BMJ* 324, no. 7333 (February 9, 2002): 346–349. doi:10.1136/bmj.324.7333.346.

Prince, Martin, Vikram Patel, Shekhar Saxena, Mario Maj, Joanna Maselko, Michael R Phillips, and Atif Rahman. "No Health Without Mental Health." *Lancet* 370, no. 9590 (September 2007): 859–877. doi:10.1016/S0140-6736(07)61238-0.

Saxena, Shekhar, Graham Thornicroft, Martin Knapp, and Harvey Whiteford. "Resources for Mental Health: Scarcity, Inequity, and Inefficiency." *Lancet* 370, no. 9590 (September 8, 2007): 878–889. doi:10.1016/S0140-6736(07)61239-2.

The Sphere Project. *Humanitarian Charter and Minimum Standards in Disaster Response.* Geneva: The Sphere Project, 2004.

United Nations General Assembly. *Convention Relating to the Status of Refugees.* Treaty Series, vol. 189, July 28, 1951. http://unhcr.org.au/unhcr/images/convention%20and%20protocol.pdf.

United Nations High Commissioner for Refugees. *Mid-Year Trends 2013.* United Nations High Commissioner for Refugees, 2012. http://www.unhcr.org/52af08d26.html.

———. "2013 UNHCR Country Operations Profile—Myanmar," 2013. http://unhcr.org/cgi-bin/texis/vtx/page?page=49e4877d6&submit=GO.

———. "2013 UNHCR Country Operations Profile—Thailand," 2013. http://www.unhcr.org/pages/49e489646.html.

Van Ommeren, Mark, and Mike Wessells. "Inter-agency Agreement on Mental Health and Psychosocial Support in Emergency Settings." *Bulletin of the World Health Organization* 85, no. 11 (November 2007): 822. doi:10.2471/BLT.07.047894.

Wenger, Andreas, and Simon JA Mason. "The Civilianization of Armed Conflict: Trends and Implications." *International Review of the Red Cross* 90, no. 872 (2008): 835–852. doi:10.1017/S1816383109000277.

World Health Organization. "DALYs Definition." *World Health Organization.* May 11, 2011. http://www.who.int/mental_health/management/depression/daly/en/.

———. *The Global Burden of Disease: 2004 Update.* Geneva: World Health Organization, 2008. http://www.who.int/healthinfo/global_burden_disease/2004_report_update/en/.

———. "Project Atlas: Resources for Mental Health," 2013. http://www.who.int/mental_health/evidence/atlas/en/.

———. "WHO Mental Health Gap Action Programme (mhGAP)." 2. http://www.who.int/mental_health/mhgap/en/.

World Health Organization and Mental Health Gap Action Programme. *mhGAP Intervention Guide for Mental, Neurological and Substance Use Disorders in Non-specialized Health Settings.* Geneva: World Health Organization, 2010.

Chapter 2

Burmese Sanctuary-Seekers and Migrants in Thailand

Policies, Experiences, and Prospects

Christina Fink

Decades of military rule in Myanmar, which is also called Burma, deeply affected large segments of the country's population in terms of rights, livelihoods, and psychological well-being.[1] Successive governments' suppression of ethnic minority demands for autonomy and the use of counterinsurgency operations rather than negotiations to resolve ethnic conflicts resulted in decades of civil war and widespread suffering. In central Myanmar, the regimes' extensive use of intimidation and force to stifle dissent and protect their rule created a culture of unease and mistrust. Economic mismanagement, extortion, and the frequent demands for forced labor in rural areas also affected people's livelihoods, adding stress and increasing families' and communities' insecurity.

Between 1988 and 2010, more than 2 million Burmese entered Thailand to eke out a living while well over 150,000 sought sanctuary, either in refugee camps or in towns and cities. Given the large numbers, the Thai government was reluctant to provide permanent residence or official recognition of their right to stay, but in practice, accommodations were made. Many Burmese in Thailand faced financial difficulties, security concerns, and abuse, and large numbers were living with the trauma they had experienced in Myanmar. Nevertheless, they sought to cope with their challenges and restore their spirits through various means, including prayer and meditation, seeking out comfort and support from family, friends, and fellow survivors, and, in some cases, through accessing more formal mental health services.

Significant numbers of migrants and displaced people from Myanmar have also ended up in China, India, and Bangladesh; however, it is beyond the scope of this chapter to discuss the policies of those governments. Suffice it to say that Burmese there have also lived in challenging and insecure circumstances but have sought to manage their situations as best they can.

In the first part of this chapter, I briefly examine the social, political, and economic landscape in Myanmar since independence and discuss the particular stresses experienced by politically active individuals and communities in various parts of the country. In the second part, I address

Thai policies toward Burmese activists, refugees, and migrant workers in Thailand and consider their effects. The chapter concludes with a brief discussion of how trauma is being managed and how the prospect of peace in Myanmar may allow for a more holistic healing process to begin.

The Historical Context

Myanmar has a population of approximately 55 million, of which about two-thirds are ethnic Burmans. The rest of the population comprises a number of other ethnicities and people of mixed ethnicity. The seven ethnic states that ring the central plains are named after the largest non-Burman ethnic groups: Arakan, Chin, Kachin, Karen, Karenni, Mon, and Shan, and there are several other smaller ethnic groups as well, each with its own language and cultural traditions. In addition, people of Chinese and Indian descent live around the country; in many cases, their ancestors arrived during the colonial period. Most Burmese profess Buddhism as their faith, while smaller numbers of people identify as Christians, Muslims, and Hindus. Animism, or the worship of ancestral and natural spirits, is practiced in various forms, both on its own and in combination with Buddhism.

Prior to British colonization in the 1800s, the borders that delineate Myanmar today did not exist. Kings in the plains sought tribute from the peoples living in the surrounding mountains but exerted little to no administrative control over them. Under British rule, a Burman nationalist movement developed in the plains, where the British ruled directly. In the hills, loyal princes and chiefs of various ethnicities were allowed to continue to govern. During World War II, people in many parts of the country suffered from the battles between the Japanese and the Allies, as well as from the hostilities that emerged between Burmans, who initially allied themselves with the Japanese, and people of other ethnicities, who remained loyal to the British. However, after the war, the former university student leader and head of the Burma National Army, General Aung San, was able to broaden the independence movement and persuade several key ethnic leaders to support the idea of establishing a democratic federal union based on the principle of equality.

Burma gained independence in 1948, but the jubilation was tempered by the fact that General Aung San and many members of his cabinet had been assassinated by a political rival in mid-1947, and the country was awash in guns. In the late 1940s and early 1950s, Communist and ethnic nationalist groups took up arms against the government to advance their political interests, and local militias organized by politicians, government departments, and others were active in many locales. Meanwhile, the newly formed *tatmadaw*, or armed forces, began growing in size and strength as the army leadership sought to quell the insurgencies by military means. Many of the people who were now considered "ethnic minorities" in a Burmese nation-state were disappointed that the ethnic state governments had little real autonomy in practice. In addition, the central government did not provide much financial or development assistance, because its focus was on restoring peace in central Burma first.

In the capital, a stalemate between the two main parties in parliament provided the opportunity for General Ne Win, the commander of the army, to assume political power as the head of a caretaker government from 1958 to 1960. In 1962, as some prominent ethnic politicians were calling for greater autonomy in the ethnic states, General Ne Win staged a coup. He asserted that Burma was in danger of disintegrating and only the army could hold the country together. This contention, together with the claim that the military alone could be counted on to work for the good of the country, was used as the primary rationale for continued military rule for almost fifty years.[2]

Military Rule: 1962–2011

The period of military rule was characterized by intolerance for criticism, Burmanization (although implemented unevenly), and the elevation of the military over the rest of society. In 1962, General Ne Win and the military regime sought to consolidate their power by abolishing the parliament, centralizing control over the ethnic states, eliminating the private media, and shutting down or taking control of most independent associations. While many people had initially welcomed the idea of a brief period of military governance, assuming it would lead to the restoration of order and peace, a climate of fear was instilled instead. A number of prominent Burman and non-Burman politicians were imprisoned, and when university students organized protests over new regulations on campus, the army blew up the student union. Many Burmese could not help but ruefully recall a traditional saying referring to government as one of the five enemies, along with fire, water (floods and storms), thieves, and malevolent people.

From 1962 to 2011, there were some differences in the structure of administration and the economic policies of the various military-led or military-backed governments, but the repression of all forms of political dissent and the refusal to negotiate a political settlement with the ethnic nationalist groups remained constant throughout. From 1962 to 1974, the military ruled as a revolutionary council and private businesses were nationalized. People of South Asian and Chinese descent, many of whom were business owners, were encouraged to leave the country. In 1974, Burma became a one-party state in name, with the Burma Socialist Programme Party fronting for the military, but General Ne Win remained in charge. The military leadership felt that only the military could hold the country together, and that one important way to build national unity was to Burmanize the indigenous ethnic minorities. Policies included the teaching of a standardized curriculum emphasizing the history of Burman-led kingdoms and Burman heroes, forbidding the teaching of ethnic minority languages in schools, promoting Burman-style practices of Buddhism, and at times impeding the practice of other religions. Successive governments insisted on a unitary state, asserting that if federalism were reintroduced, the ethnic minority leaders in the ethnic states would not be satisfied and would go on to demand outright independence.

In early August 1988, nationwide prodemocracy protests broke out and the military temporarily retreated to its barracks. However, in mid-September, the military reestablished control. The generals organized a multiparty election in 1990 and allowed the National League for Democracy, led by Aung San Suu Kyi, General Aung San's daughter, and a number of other parties to run. As the National League for Democracy began to gain support, the military put Aung San Suu Kyi under house arrest in 1989 and arrested many members of her party during the campaign period. Still, her party trounced the military-backed party, so the military government annulled the results and continued to rule, first as the State Law and Order Restoration Council, and then, from 1997 to 2011, as the State Peace and Development Council.

The military regimes in power from 1988 to 2011 solicited foreign investment, but the continued civil war in northern and eastern Myanmar, poor infrastructure, and the difficulties of doing business with the generals scared most businesspeople off. Economic sanctions imposed by the United States and some other Western countries in response to the grave human rights situation in the country also deterred investors.

In the 1990s, the military government began talking about a road map to democracy, but demonstrated little commitment to following through on it. A constitution-drafting convention met periodically from 1993 to 2007, but a new constitution was not finalized until after the 2007 protests, when monks took to the streets chanting verses of compassion in an effort to compel the military leadership to be more responsive to the economic suffering of the people. Nervous that this could lead to larger political protests, the military beat the monks and hauled them away to detention centers, an act that embittered many civilians against the army.

Attention to these events was somewhat diverted when General Than Shwe, the head of the regime, oversaw a referendum on the constitution in 2008 and an election for a new government in 2010. However, both events involved intimidation and fraud, and the constitution enshrined the principle of the military taking a leading role in politics through a number of provisions. These included the reservation of 25 percent of the seats for military personnel in all elected bodies and the requirement that the president have a military background.

Hopes were not high that much would change after the election, given that President Thein Sein, a military general who had served as the prime minister previously, had been handpicked by General Than Shwe. However, he began to take steps to open up the political arena and to initiate economic reforms. Nobel Peace Laureate Aung San Suu Kyi, who had spent most of the past twenty-one years under house arrest, was released, and hundreds of political prisoners were freed in early 2012. In April 2012, Aung San Suu Kyi and members of her party were able to run for seats in a by-election and take their seats in parliament. Since then, parliamentarians from various parties have worked to develop the role of the parliament as an active legislative body responsive to the interests of constituents.

In a bid to restore the country's international legitimacy and jumpstart the economy, President Thein Sein's government reestablished friendly relations with Western countries and introduced economic reforms. The government also established a peace-making committee, which was charged with initiating talks with over a dozen armed ethnic groups and the prodemocracy groups in exile. By mid-2012, all but one ethnic armed group had made a ceasefire agreement with government negotiators. Although skirmishes between the tatmadaw and ethnic armed groups continued to break out and fighting intensified in Kachin State, there was hope that a lasting peace might be reached. In early 2013, the government's peace team and the ethnic armed groups began discussing how to proceed to political talks, which could potentially include parliamentarians and relevant civil society groups as well. However, the tatmadaw leadership had been involved only minimally in the peace process, raising concerns about what kind of political settlement the tatmadaw would be willing to accept. Meanwhile, various international agencies and refugees began thinking about what conditions would need to be in place for voluntary repatriation, including guarantees of physical safety, livelihood opportunities, and land rights.

Despite the continuing uncertainties, for those who had sought sanctuary in Thailand or elsewhere, returning home finally became a possibility. In considering what to do, Burmese abroad had to reassess all they had been through and consider how they might go about reconstructing their lives and reintegrating into their communities if they returned. As the next section of this chapter will make clear, many had experienced extraordinary suffering, for agonizingly long periods of time, but at the same time, people from Myanmar have made great efforts to cope and to make the best of their lives.

Expressing Dissent, Enduring Prison, and Returning to the World beyond Bars

From 1962 to 2011, any form of public criticism of the government, the armed forces, or state institutions, whether expressed through protests, interviews with foreign journalists, music, or art, was dealt with harshly. Those who were caught or identified by others were sent to interrogation centers where they were physically and mentally tortured to elicit information about their activities and to break their spirits. Publications by former political prisoners and Amnesty International (see, for instance, Amnesty International 2000a, 2000b, 2005; Assistance Association for Political Prisoners 2001; Aye 1999) reveal how the interrogators sought to humiliate and violate their captives, many of whom were high school and university students.[3] As Bo Kyi, a former political prisoner, explains,

> Various physical torture methods are being used, including systematic beatings (aimed at inflicting permanent injury), unsystematic beatings (using rifle butts, truncheons, etc.), electric torture (applying electrodes to sensitive parts of the body, such as the gums, ears, fingertips, and sexual organs), and "moe dewa," or water torture (drops of water fall onto the victim's head until, after a number of hours, they feel like a pounding hammer). Another common practice is burning victims with cigarettes.[4]

Many survivors also talk of the "helicopter," in which prisoners were tied by their wrists to a hook in the ceiling and spun around, and the "motorcycle" in which they had to stand in a half-squat on the tips of their toes and pretend to ride a motorcycle, complete with making "vroom vroom" sounds. While in the interrogation center, detainees were held in solitary confinement when not being interrogated and were denied sleep, food, and drink, at least during the first days, in order to disorient and weaken them.[5]

After enduring several days or longer in an interrogation center, the arrested person would be charged and a perfunctory trial held in a closed court or a court inside a prison. Prison sentences of five to twenty years were common in the early 1990s, and after 1997, many political prisoners were sentenced to decades of imprisonment in order to silence them and terrify other would-be activists. Although exact figures are not available for the number of individuals who were incarcerated for nonviolent political acts, and various organizations define political prisoners differently, several thousand individuals were political prisoners during this period, with some experiencing more than one incarceration. Many thousands more were detained and interrogated at police stations and temporary detention facilities and then released within a period of days, but these incidents were frightening enough to cause trauma for some detainees.

For many, one of the most psychologically damaging aspects of prison life was not being recognized as political prisoners. As Hla Aye put it, "The authorities were acting under the belief that there are no political prisoners. Everyone is a criminal. That's the simplest form of torture in prison."[6] Political prisoners experienced the humiliations of being chained and having to squat in positions of subservience during daily inspections. Until the early 2000s, they were not allowed to write, read newspapers or journals, or listen to the news. They were also often sent to prisons far from their homes in order to decrease the frequency of contact with their families. Monks who were arrested were disrobed and forced to wear the common prisoner garb, although fellow prisoners continued to show respect to them.

In addition, the prison officials provided poor quality food in insufficient quantities, resulting in malnutrition for those prisoners who could not obtain extra food from family members or friends. Political prisoners were generally denied sufficient water for bathing, leading to skin diseases and discomfort. Medical care in prison was deplorable, with little attention given to serious ailments and prisoners' families generally having to provide medicine themselves. In addition, prisoners who expressed defiance or demanded better treatment were beaten and often put in solitary confinement in dark, claustrophobic cells for lengthy periods. According to the Assistance Association for Political Prisoners, between 1988 and 2010 at least 139 political prisoners died while in prison as a result of the effects of torture, poor conditions, and lack of access to adequate health care.[7] The tremendous mental stress of living in such challenging conditions and guilt over the problems they had caused their families also took a toll on many political prisoners, and some deteriorated mentally.[8]

Although release from prison was what political prisoners lived for, when they were actually released, they faced another set of challenges. Many could not enjoy their freedom, knowing that other colleagues were still behind bars. It was not uncommon for some of their relatives, neighbors, and former friends to shun them, worrying that association with a former political prisoner could bring suspicion upon themselves. In addition, employers did not want to hire them, and they were often barred from continuing formal education, leaving them few opportunities to assist their families financially or reintegrate into society. Some found solace, while in prison and once released, in meditation and prayer, some felt compelled to resume underground political activities despite the risk, and some left the country, either to be able to find employment or to continue political organizing.

Militarization and Civilian Suffering in the Ethnic States

In the ethnic states of northern and eastern Myanmar, militarization has taken a terrible toll on the civilian population. Many hundreds of thousands of people have been subject to a range of human rights abuses, impoverishment, and the breakup of families and communities.[9] This is particularly true in areas where people have been displaced. Satellite imagery has confirmed local human rights groups' reports that between 1996 and 2010, over 3,700 civilian settlements in eastern Myanmar were destroyed by the tatmadaw or abandoned by villagers prior to an attack.[10]

Although large-scale battles occasionally took place, the tatmadaw generally sought to debilitate the ethnic nationalist armies through counterinsurgency tactics. This included the "four cuts" policy of cutting off enemy armies' access to information, supplies, recruits, and weapons to undermine their ability to fight.[11] The tatmadaw did this by depopulating areas and restricting movements of the civilian population under their control. Tatmadaw soldiers often looted homes, destroyed food stocks, and burned whole villages. Large areas were declared free-fire zones, making it impossible for villagers to return. Villagers often moved multiple times, rebuilding small houses when they could and living in hiding in the jungle when they could not. As of 2011, an estimated 450,000 villagers were internally displaced in southeastern Myanmar.[12]

As Lang (2002) has pointed out, in the conflict areas, the boundary between combatants and noncombatants became blurred, as tatmadaw soldiers viewed the villagers themselves as the enemy.[13] This was in part because they did not know who was supporting the ethnic nationalist armies and also because of their anger and desire to take revenge when their comrades were injured or killed by ethnic nationalist troops.[14]

Most dangerous were the areas where troops from both the tatmadaw and an ethnic nationalist army operated. Villagers were compelled to assist and pay taxes to both armies, resulting in impoverishment and insecurity. Village headmen came under particular suspicion, because they had to implement the demands of both sides. In several Karen areas, villagers regularly rotated the headman position or selected female village heads in an effort to reduce the amount of violence they might be subject to. They thought that the army officers might show more sympathy toward female village heads. However, as the Karen Women's Organization report *Walking amongst Sharp Knives* (2010) documents, a number of female village heads were raped, tortured, and in some cases, brutally killed by tatmadaw soldiers.[15]

Indeed, girls and women of all ages in conflict areas were vulnerable to rape and gang rape in any type of encounter with tatmadaw soldiers. This included during attacks, when tatmadaw soldiers crossed their paths outside the village, when tatmadaw soldiers were based in or near their village, while carrying out forced labor at army posts, and while portering for the army.[16] Tatmadaw soldiers carried out rape with impunity, and even in more stable areas, when families called for justice, they were almost always ordered to stay silent. In situations when tatmadaw soldiers believed men in a village had assisted the enemy army, wives could be held hostage until their husbands returned, and family members were sometimes tortured and killed in front of their children.[17]

After the regime's introduction of market-oriented economic reforms in the early 1990s, militarization of the ethnic states also increased to secure areas for resource extraction and large-scale infrastructure development projects.[18] However, from the late 1990s on, tatmadaw troops were not provided with adequate supplies or financial support, and military camps had to produce or procure their own food. Lack of rations and insufficient salaries drove soldiers to demand or steal food from villagers, to extort money, and to confiscate villagers' fields and plantations for the army's use.[19] Villagers were then compelled to work the land that had been taken from them.

In general, wherever tatmadaw camps were located, human rights abuses were common occurrences. Tatmadaw soldiers routinely demanded that villagers perform a variety of tasks, such as building and maintaining army posts, cooking for the troops, working on military-run farms and businesses, and portering supplies for the military. Porters were forced to carry very heavy loads, not provided sufficient food, and often left to die or killed if they collapsed along the way.

Because the ethnic nationalist armies attempted to block the movement of tatmadaw soldiers into their areas by planting land mines along jungle paths and around their camps, villagers were sometimes ordered to walk in front of tatmadaw patrols. If there were land mines along the way, the villagers, not the soldiers, would step on them. The tatmadaw also laid mines, and internally displaced villagers who foraged in the forest for food were in particular danger of stepping on a land mine. Villagers often do not know all the places where the various armies have laid mines, resulting in many injuries and deaths.[20]

Soldiers in the ethnic armed groups also committed human rights abuses and took harsh measures against people believed to be traitors.[21] While the ethnic armies tended to have closer connections to local populations and were more reliant on their support, they too demanded food and porters.

Loss of fields, food stocks, money, and time to work for themselves, along with frequent displacement, increased the chances that families in conflict areas could not feed themselves adequately. According to a report by the Back Pack Health Worker Team, there were "vitamin, protein, and iron deficiencies, malnutrition, and greater vulnerability to disease."[22] The same report noted that an average of 221 out of every 1,000 children in the conflict areas of eastern Burma died before reaching the age of 5,[23] and the lifetime risk of dying while giving birth in these areas is one in twelve.[24] The extent of suffering of people in the conflict areas is hard to fathom. Villagers lived in states of chronic insecurity, witnessed and experienced terrible violence, and lost homes, property, and loved ones. However, both Heppner (2005) and South (2007) have argued that it is important to stress the agency of internally displaced persons in Burma and to highlight their capacities rather than see them as passive victims.[25] Indeed, civilians in militarized areas strategized about how to handle their situation and responded in a variety of ways, including hiding temporarily or moving away (to a more secure area, deeper into the jungle, or to a neighboring country), trying to conceal and protect their food supplies, or joining an armed group. To a certain extent, this helped villagers maintain a sense of control over their lives. Nevertheless, the highly unequal power balance between armed soldiers and unarmed civilians meant that villagers could only seek to minimize, survive, or escape from abuses rather than prevent their occurrence altogether.

Economic Policies and the Difficulty of Making Ends Meet

In rural areas under government control and in less violent conflict areas, the government made some efforts to modernize the country's infrastructure. Local officials and army units extended roads, railroads, and irrigation channels, but in many cases they used civilian forced labor to do the work manually. For Burman and ethnic minority families alike, this meant having to send one member to work on such projects, often for two or three weeks at a time. Workers had to bring their own tools and food, and there was no medicine for those who got sick or were injured. Because parents needed to continue their own work to support their families, they often had to send teenaged children and even younger children in their place. While carrying out the work, soldiers in particular sometimes treated the laborers harshly, and the only way villagers could get out of the work was to pay someone to go in their place. In the early 2000s, the International Labor Organization's efforts to persuade the government to stop the use of forced labor resulted in improvements in some parts of the country but fewer in the ethnic states.

Inflation was a problem during much of the period from 1995 to 2011, and soldiers, local officials, and civil servants were not paid salaries sufficient to cover their living expenses. As a result, they resorted to various forms of extortion and taxation, and civilians did not dare to openly refuse or to protest, although in some cases people were able to reduce or avoid such payments. At the same time, nonagricultural jobs were scarce, and restrictions on the size of state bank loans and the sale of agricultural produce kept the agricultural sector weak. Increasingly, young single people and even young parents sought to migrate abroad to find money for themselves and their families. Because of its proximity and strong economy, Thailand drew the largest number of Burmese migrant workers, who then remitted money to their families through informal banking channels.

Thai Policies toward Burmese Activists

In comparison to Myanmar, Thailand provides a largely peaceful environment, a vast number of job opportunities (albeit in jobs Thais no longer want to do), and far greater provision of public and private services. Nevertheless, in the past, most Burmese in Thailand did not have official documents granting them permission to reside in the country, so they lived with insecurity, often faced exploitation, and could not always access the services they needed. The development of Thai government policies regarding activists in towns, refugees in camps, and migrant workers will be discussed in turn.

Between 1962 and 2010, thousands of activists who participated in demonstrations or were members of underground organizations in Myanmar fled to areas controlled by ethnic nationalist armies or to neighboring countries to escape arrest and continue their activities. Of the approximately 10,000 student activists who arrived in the border areas or crossed into neighboring countries after the 1988 demonstrations, several thousand joined armed groups, underwent military training, and engaged in battles against the tatmadaw and allied militias. Living in camps inside ethnic nationalist–controlled territories of Myanmar, they had more independence than refugees. Members of armed prodemocracy and ethnic nation-alist organizations who became sick or were wounded could unofficially access Thai hospitals, if their organizations could transport them there. However, the trauma of war, of killing, and of seeing friends killed, and the doubts some felt about whether they had made the right decision in joining the armed struggle deeply affected many. In addition, suspicions within and between members of the armed organizations regarding the infiltration of spies occasionally led to incidents in which individuals were detained, tortured, and in some instances, killed.

Other activists who came from inside Myanmar, including former po-litical prisoners, sought to continue nonviolent organizing, advocacy, and support activities from border towns and cities in Thailand. Over time, po-litical parties, women's organizations, relief organizations, human rights organizations (including the Assistance Association for Political Prison-ers), and media organizations representing various ethnic groups from Myanmar established themselves in Thailand. Some educational and social welfare organizations were also established by Burmese activists in exile. With funding from foreign donors and donations from friends abroad, they set up offices, often where they lived, with little separation between their work and their personal lives. The Thai government's official policy was to not allow such offices and to not grant asylum to political activists; in practice, however, there was generally tolerance as long as the groups kept a low profile.

Particularly from the 1990s on, the Thai government was caught be-tween a desire to maintain cordial relations with the Burmese military gov-ernment for national security and economic purposes and a desire to see a more legitimate and reasonable government in power in the country. Some people in the Thai government hoped that the activities of the Burmese organizations could contribute to bringing about political reform in Myan-mar, while certain Thai academics, nongovernmental organization leaders, and politicians expressed solidarity with Burmese who were struggling for the kinds of rights that they also valued and had worked for.

Nevertheless, members of the Thai business community and some fig-ures in the Thai military pressured successive Thai governments to culti-vate more friendly relations with the Burmese military government to enable trade and investment. As a result, Burmese activists' offices were sometimes raided before high-level Burmese government visits to Thailand, and Bur-mese activists were often arrested by the police when they went out, be-cause they did not have any legal identification. (Thais who are 15 years and older must carry national identity cards at all times.) Although they would always find ways to carry on, Burmese activists lived in a constant state of uncertainty, never knowing when Thai policy might change and whether they would be able to continue their activities or remain in the country.

Activists struggled to maintain their sense of well-being given their lack of stability in Thailand, the lack of improvements in Myanmar, and the fact that most had little personal money and few opportunities to get out of their offices and relax. In addition, many activists were still bothered by the violence they had witnessed or experienced in Burma and the guilt they felt, both for having avoided prison when other colleagues hadn't and for having left their families to fend for themselves. Even students felt this guilt, as older siblings are expected to provide financial contributions to younger siblings' educations and to provide support for their parents as they age.

Those who were integrated into organizations often held themselves together because of peer pressure to get on with life. Everyone else in the organization had gone through similar experiences (whether in Myanmar or in Thailand or both) and was managing, so it was expected that no one should fall apart because of it. In some cases, by keeping themselves fully engaged and feeling good about the work they were doing, they were able to maintain their morale. Nevertheless, many men in such organizations drank excessive amounts of alcohol as a method for coping, generally together with their colleagues. In some cases, this led to fights, accidents from driving while drunk, and cirrhosis of the liver. Female activists generally drank far less, if at all, and were sometimes able to relieve their stress through talking openly with friends or family about their feelings, although they did not always feel comfortable doing so, particularly regarding domestic violence and sexual abuse. Some gained self-esteem from the work they were able to do in women's and other types of organizations, but they also faced challenges from family members who were not always supportive of daughters and wives engaging in such work.

Thai Policies toward Refugees from Myanmar

The Thai government allowed refugees from Myanmar to establish refugee camps along the Thai-Myanmar border starting in 1984. Since the mid-1970s, the Thai government had been hosting several hundred thousand refugees from Cambodia, Laos, and Vietnam in large camps along its eastern border. Unlike those camps, the Karen, Karenni, and Mon camps along the Thai-Myanmar border were originally quite informal and were run by local relief organizations with support from international organizations. They functioned more like villages, and in many areas, refugees were able to cross back into Myanmar to farm plots near the border during the day. However, in the late 1990s, the Democratic Karen Buddhist Army, an army formed with the encouragement of the tatmadaw to counter the Karen National Liberation Army, began demanding that camp residents return to Myanmar and carried out nighttime attacks on the camps. In one instance, they burned a large camp a few kilometers from the town of Mae Sot to the ground. The Thai government decided to amalgamate the many small camps into a few large camps, put them under much tighter control, and restrict movement in and out of the camps. At that time, the total population of all the camps was approximately 140,000.

Like the governments in other countries that border Myanmar, the Thai government has not signed the United Nations Convention Relating to the Status of Refugees and its 1967 Protocol. The convention requires signatories to recognize as refugees those individuals who have a well-founded fear of being persecuted by their own government and to provide them with protection. The convention was originally written with the expectation that only small numbers of people would require such assistance at any given time. However, Thailand's neighbors have gone through long periods of turmoil and repression, creating a situation where potentially millions of people could have a justification for seeking refuge in Thailand.

Over time, Thai authorities decided that they had to set limits to minimize the flow of refugees. Civilians fleeing conflict areas in Myanmar were granted the right to stay only temporarily, not to become permanent residents, and from 1997 on, only those fleeing *active* fighting were officially allowed to reside in the camps. They also refused to allow Shan people, who are ethnically related to Thais, to establish refugee camps in Thailand after a massive tatmadaw campaign to depopulate central Shan State. Nevertheless, as many as 150,000 Shan who were driven out of their villages reportedly entered Thailand between 1996 and 2003, with most having to survive as migrant workers.[26]

While the refugee camps generally offered greater security than the conflict areas did, and all children had access to free schooling through high school, the refugees had no autonomy over their lives, very few economic opportunities, and no guarantee that they would ever be able to return home. As the years dragged on, morale declined. Teenagers felt frustrated that despite a high school education, they could not leave the camps to pursue jobs or further education. This was because of official restrictions on movement out of the camps as well as the fact that their camp curricula were primarily taught in their own languages, and they were not fluent in

Thai. Some joined the ethnic nationalist armies or worked for international organizations or schools in the camps, while others maintained tiny garden plots, sold food or basic items, or engaged in day labor outside the camps when possible. Problems with alcohol and drug use among young people emerged in the Karen camps.

Men had to deal with feelings of inadequacy, since they could not be the economic providers for their families but were largely dependent on handouts. In addition, they faced confinement, boredom, and tremendous worries about their family's futures. As a Karen documentary film, *The Violence that Is Everyone's Secret* (2006), makes clear, this stress was too often taken out on their wives and children.[27]

According to the International Rescue Committee psychosocial programme officer for the Karenni refugee camps in 2007, the number of mental health patients was increasing in those camps, because of dismal living conditions and the fact that many had been living there for almost two decades with no hopes for the future (author's interview in 2007). The programme officer also said that alcoholism and gender-based violence had become bigger problems. Rapes also happened in the camps, and women who were raped often suffered in silence or were blamed by their families, leading to depression.

Nevertheless, other aspects of camp life helped bolster resilience. People from the same villages tended to resettle together in the same camps, giving some comfort and sense of community. In addition, churches, temples, and mosques organized religious services and social activities that brought people together and to a certain extent established a sense of normalcy. Religious leaders sought to keep people's spirits up and help them cope with their suffering. School teachers and student groups held sports events and other types of competitions to keep young people happy and busy. Still, it was not easy to maintain a sense of well-being.

At times, the Thai government put pressure on the ethnic nationalist armies to negotiate with the Burmese government. The Thai authorities understandably wanted the refugees to be repatriated as soon as possible, but such talk always alarmed the refugees. As much as they wanted to return to their homelands, they worried that they could be forcibly sent back before it was safe to do so, given the presence of numerous armed forces in the ethnic states and the widespread planting of land mines. Western governments tried to ease the burden on Thailand, and between 2009 and 2011, more than 50,000 refugees from Myanmar were resettled in the United States alone, but new people continued to move into the camps as the conflict continued.

Thai Policies toward Migrant Workers

As Thailand's economy continued to grow throughout the 1990s and into the 2000s, labor shortages emerged in agriculture, commercial fishing, construction, light industry, and other low-wage, labor-intensive jobs such as housemaids and restaurant workers. Large numbers of migrant workers from Myanmar, as well as smaller numbers from Cambodia and Laos, flowed into Thailand to take these jobs, as well as jobs in stores, markets, and brothels, some of which served migrant communities. The number of Burmese migrant workers continued to rise throughout the first decade of the 2000s, with almost 1 million registered workers as of 2011, and as many or more unregistered workers.[28]

While it was possible for migrants to legally cross into Thailand at official checkpoints with day passes, they needed to be transported illegally to reach jobs in other parts of the country. Agents hid the migrants, led them over jungle trails, or paid off security personnel at check points to move them beyond the border areas. Agents also placed migrant workers in jobs, but often took advantage of them as well, including by taking their first few months' wages and leaving them with employers they never would have chosen on their own.[29] The most unfortunate young men found themselves working as unpaid captives on commercial fishing ships, while the most unfortunate young women were sold into locked brothels against their will. Migrant workers did better if they had friends or acquaintances who could introduce them to employers whom they knew.

Until 2009, Burmese migrant workers who crossed into Thailand were seen by the Burmese authorities as engaging in an illegal activity because they did not pay taxes to the Burmese government. They were also illegal in Thailand unless they could obtain a migrant worker card with the assistance of an employer. Processes for legally allowing migrants to work in certain sectors started in 1996, and the Thai government initiated an open registration procedure for one-year migrant worker permits in 2004. Beginning in 2007, Burmese migrant workers already in Thailand also had to have their nationality verified by the Burmese government. A few years later, they were able to apply from Myanmar and come on temporary passports.

Although holding a migrant worker card gave migrant workers legal status, the expense and difficulties of registering ensured that large numbers of migrant workers never obtained them. Those who didn't register had to fear arrest and deportation, particularly after annual registrations were over and roundups of undocumented migrant workers were carried out. Even having a migrant worker card didn't necessarily guarantee security, as some employers confiscated the cards so that migrant workers could not leave to find a better job.

In theory, documented migrant workers have most of the same rights as Thai workers (except the right to form unions), but in practice, they are treated quite differently. Migrant workers in Thailand, as elsewhere, are often underpaid or, in some cases, not paid at all and routinely compelled to work extremely long hours, frequently in unsafe or difficult conditions. Many have few or no days off and are forced to live in cramped quarters where they work. It can be very hard for migrant workers to access health services, because many do not have transportation, are not allowed to take time off work, or cannot communicate in Thai.

Migrant workers also face abuses at the hands of the Thai police and other security personnel, including beatings, theft, and extortion if they are caught without a migrant worker card or passport or if the authorities insist that their documents are not genuine and take them away.[30] No matter what abuse they have suffered, as Human Rights Watch has noted, "migrants suffer silently and rarely complain because they fear retribution, are not proficient enough in the Thai language to protest, or lack faith in Thai institutions that too often turn a blind eye to their plight."[31]

Female migrant workers are in particular danger of sexual abuse by employers and by Thai security personnel, but they rarely dare to report such incidents. Migrant workers in many areas live in temporary mixed-sex camps, sharing outdoor bathing areas and latrines, which can also make women vulnerable to verbal and sexual abuse. Moreover, domestic violence is common among migrant worker couples and families, and even though neighbors know what is going on, they seldom intervene, seeing it as a private matter.

Another problem that migrant parents faced until late 2009 was the inability to register the births of their children, as the parents had to have a Thai citizenship card or a passport to do so. This policy has changed. Beginning in the mid-2000s, Burmese children in Thailand were also legally allowed to attend Thai schools, although some school officials refused to accept the children, and parents were afraid to challenge them.

Thais generally look down on Burmese. This is in large part because they are portrayed negatively in both the Thai media and in Thai textbooks, which construct the Burmese as longtime enemies to foster a sense of Thai unity and national identity. Although many Thais responded with sympathy and generous donations after Cyclone Nargis devastated parts of lower Myanmar in 2008, and a number of Thais also greatly admire Aung San Suu Kyi, most Burmese in Thailand are acutely aware of the fact that they are not seen as equals.

Restoring Well-Being for Individuals, Communities, and the Country

Burmese in Thailand are often coping with a number of stresses and, in some cases, severe depression. As Pollock and Somwong put it, "Inherent in the situation of refugees or forced migrants is the experience of loss. Loss of loved ones, loss of home, loss of community, loss of work and material possessions. There are also psychological losses, such as loss of status, loss of belief in oneself, loss of trust in others, loss of future hopes, loss of personal invulnerability, and loss of power."[32]

No one knows how many Burmese are struggling with mental illness or trauma, in large part because those who are suffering generally do not seek formal assistance. In both Myanmar and in Thailand, the use of mental health services is stigmatized, and even if desired, such services are not readily available to those in rural areas. There are very few trained psychologists or psychiatrists; instead, monks, pastors, and priests frequently take on the role of counselors and healers. Burmese also frequently rely on meditation or prayer to help them cope with their feelings or to return themselves to a state of equanimity. In other cases, people turn to astrologers, spirit mediums, and other types of spiritual healers, who may use rituals or require the person to carry out certain activities, such as releasing fish and birds, to restore themselves. Burmese in crisis also look to family members, friends, and trusted elders for moral support, although such people may in some cases tell them to stop feeling sorry for themselves or even blame them. This is particularly true for women who are raped and who are, in some cases, even forced to marry the rapist. It is also generally true for women who are victims of domestic violence. As noted above, less positive ways that people deal with their stress and trauma include excessive drinking, particularly among men, using violence against others, and turning inward and becoming increasingly alienated from others.

Along the Myanmar border, communities and organizations have sought to develop services to assist people suffering from depression or trauma; these are detailed in the chapters that follow. Examining both community responses and the new services that have been developed is valuable in formulating methods for helping all those who have suffered inside Myanmar as well as those who remain in Thailand. Yet it is important to recognize that it is not only individuals who have been damaged, but also communities and society as a whole.

If permanent peace is established in the ethnic states, and if greater political openness in Myanmar means people can truly speak and act freely, then a broader process of healing may be able to begin. Those who have stayed in the country, along with those who return, will be looking for a guarantee of physical security, a more representative government that can be counted on to respond to citizens' pressing needs, and a reduction in the use of all forms of aggression. This will not be easy, as the country is awash in guns, as it was just after independence, and the practice of using violence to resolve problems has become embedded.

Large numbers of soldiers from all sides will need to be demobilized and reintegrated into civilian society. Those soldiers and members of other security forces who remain in uniform will need to be told that they will no longer be able to commit abuses against civilians with impunity, and this must be enforced. Civilians returning to ethnic minority areas will have to be able to rebuild their homes and communities in safe locations, free of land mines. They must feel that not only will they live in security, but also they will not be discriminated against.

Having been treated as dispensable for so many years, the people of Myanmar need to be able to restore their dignity as human beings, as members of communities, and as citizens. New relationships of trust and accountability must be established between the government and society and between peoples of all ethnicities and religions. If this can be achieved, then Burmese citizens throughout the country will finally be able to experience a sense of wholeness, tranquility, and well-being.

Notes

1 The terms "Bamar" and "Myanmar" have been used interchangeably in Burmese. However, the English terms became politicized after the military government changed the country's official name from Burma to Myanmar in 1989 without any consultation process. There is also disagreement regarding which term, if either, is more inclusive of all the ethnic nationalities in the country. Although most citizens now use "Myanmar," some prodemocracy activists and ethnic nationalists continue to use Burma. In this chapter, I use Burma when referring specifically to the pre-1989 period and Myanmar in all other instances. I use "Burmese" to mean all citizens of Burma; however, it should be noted that some members of ethnic nationalities do not like to be called Burmese, because they feel that "Burmese" and "Burman," the term for the majority group, have become indistinguishable in most people's minds.

2 See Christina Fink, *Living Silence in Burma: Surviving Military Rule* (London: Zed Books, 2009), for a lengthier description of the social and political context in Burma before military rule began, as well as for a more detailed picture of life under military rule.

3 Assistance Association for Political Prisoners (Burma), *Spirit for Survival* (Mae Sot, Thailand: Assistance Association for Political Prisoners, 2001); Moe Aye, *Ten Years On: The Life and Views of a Burmese Student Political Prisoner* (Bangkok, Thailand: Louise Southalan, 1999); Amnesty International, *Unsung Heroines: The Women of Myanmar* (London: Amnesty International, 2000b); Amnesty International, *Myanmar: The Institution of Torture* (London: Amnesty International, 2000a); Amnesty International, *Myanmar's Political Prisoners: A Growing Legacy of Injustice* (London: Amnesty International, 2005).

4 Assistance Association for Political Prisoners (Burma), *Spirit for Survival*, 19.

5 Ibid., 20.

6 Fink, *Living Silence in Burma*, 175.

7 Assistance Association for Political Prisoners (Burma), *Burma Prisons and Labor Camps: Silent Killing Fields* (Mae Sot, Thailand: Assistance Association for Political Prisoners, 2009), 3.

8 Assistance Association for Political Prisoners (Burma), *Spirit for Survival*, 39–42.

9 Amnesty International, *Myanmar: Lack of Security in Counter-Insurgency Areas* (London: Amnesty International, 2002); Amnesty International, *Crimes against Humanity in Eastern Myanmar* (London: Amnesty International, 2008).

10 Thailand Burma Border Consortium, *Internal Displacement and Protection in Eastern Burma* (Thailand Burma Border Consortium, 2011), 16.

11 Martin Smith, *Burma: Insurgency and the Politics of Ethnicity* (London: Zed Books, 1999), 258–262.

12 Thailand Burma Border Consortium, *Internal Displacement and Protection in Eastern Burma*, 11.

13 Hazel J Lang, *Fear and Sanctuary: Burmese Refugees in Thailand* (Ithaca, NY: Southeast Asia Program Publications, Cornell University, 2002), 57.

14 Christina Fink, "Militarization in Burma's Ethnic States: Causes and Consequences," *Contemporary Politics* 14, no. 4 (2010): 450, doi:10.1080/13569770802519367.

15 Karen Women's Organization, *Walking amongst Sharp Knives* (Thailand: Karen Women's Organization, 2010).

16 Women's League of Burma, *System of Impunity* (Thailand: Women's League of Burma, 2004); Karen Women's Organization, *Shattering Silences* (Thailand: Karen Women's Organization, 2004); Karen Women's Organization, *State of Terror* (Thailand: Karen Women's Organization, 2007); Shan Human Rights Foundation and Shan Women's Action Network, *License to Rape* (Thailand: Shan Human Rights Foundation, 2002).

17 Karen Human Rights Group, *Dignity in the Shadow of Oppression* (Thailand: Karen Human Rights Group, 2006), 43–44.

18 Smith, *Burma*, 42–44; Ashley South, "Conflict and Displacement in Burma/
   Myanmar," in *Myanmar: The State, Community, and the Environment*, ed.
   Monique Skidmore and Trevor Wilson (Canberra: Asia Pacific Press, 2007), 67–69,
   http://epress.anu.edu.au/wp-content/uploads/2011/03/ch0436.pdf.

19 Amnesty International, *Myanmar: Lack of Security in Counter-Insurgency Areas*.

20 Landmine Monitor, *Burma/Myanmar: Landmine Monitor Report 2007*, 2007,
   http://www.icbl.org/lm/2007/burma.html.

21 Amnesty International, *Myanmar: Lack of Security in Counter-Insurgency Areas*,
   30–31.

22 Back Pack Health Worker Team, *Chronic Emergency: Health and Human Rights in
   Eastern Burma* (Thailand: Back Pack Health Worker Team, 2006), 38.

23 Ibid., 32–33.

24 Ibid., 41.

25 Kevin Heppner, *Sovereignty, Survival and Resistance: Contending Perspectives on
   Karen Internal Displacement in Burma* (Thailand: Karen Human Rights Group,
   2005), 30–31; South, "Conflict and Displacement in Burma/Myanmar," 55.

26 Shan Human Rights Foundation, *Charting the Exodus from Shan State* (Thailand:
   Shan Human Rights Foundation, 2003), 6.

27 Kaw Lah Lah Films and Karen Women's Organization, *The Violence that Is
   Everyone's Secret*, Documentary Film, 2006.

28 Mahidol Migration Center, "Thailand's Low Skilled Migration Policy: Progress
   and Challenges," in *Submission to the UN Committee on Migrant Workers,
   September 11, 2011*, 2011, 1,
   http://www2.ohchr.org/english/bodies/cmw/docs/DGD/MMC_19092011.pdf.

29 Physicians for Human Rights, *Looking for a Hidden Population: Trafficking of
   Migrant Laborers in San Diego County* (Boston: Physicians for Human Rights,
   2004), 33–38.

30 Human Rights Watch, *From the Tiger to the Crocodile: Abuse of Migrant Workers
   in Thailand* (New York: Human Rights Watch, 2010), 39–44.

31 Ibid., 2.

32 Jackie Pollock and Pranom Somwong, *Seeking Safety, Meeting Violence: Migrant
   and Refugee Women's Journey from Burma* (Chiang Mai, Thailand: Migrant Action
   Program/CARAM Asia, 2001), 3.

Bibliography

Amnesty International. *Crimes against Humanity in Eastern Myanmar*. London:
   Amnesty International, 2008.

———. *Myanmar: The Institution of Torture*. London: Amnesty International, 2000a.

———. *Myanmar: Lack of Security in Counter-Insurgency Areas*. London: Amnesty
   International, 2002.

———. *Myanmar's Political Prisoners: A Growing Legacy of Injustice*. London: Amnesty International, 2005.

———. *Unsung Heroines: The Women of Myanmar*. London: Amnesty International, 2000b.

Assistance Association for Political Prisoners (Burma). *Burma Prisons and Labor Camps: Silent Killing Fields*. Mae Sot, Thailand: Assistance Association for Political Prisoners, 2009.

———. *Spirit for Survival*. Mae Sot, Thailand: Assistance Association for Political Prisoners, 2001.

Aye, Moe. *Ten Years On: The Life and Views of a Burmese Student Political Prisoner*. Bangkok, Thailand: Louise Southalan, 1999.

Back Pack Health Worker Team. *Chronic Emergency: Health and Human Rights in Eastern Burma*. Mae Sot, Thailand: Back Pack Health Worker Team, 2006.

Corporal, Lynette Lee. "Psychological Woes Haunt Burmese Refugees." *Inter Press Service*, June 27, 2007.

Fink, Christina. *Living Silence in Burma: Surviving Military Rule*. London: Zed Books, 2009.

———. "Militarization in Burma's Ethnic States: Causes and Consequences." *Contemporary Politics* 14, no. 4 (2010): 447–462. doi:10.1080/13569770802519367.

Heppner, Kevin. *Sovereignty, Survival and Resistance: Contending Perspectives on Karen Internal Displacement in Burma*. Thailand: Karen Human Rights Group, 2005.

Human Rights Watch. *From the Tiger to the Crocodile: Abuse of Migrant Workers in Thailand*. New York: Human Rights Watch, 2010.

Karen Human Rights Group. *Development by Decree: The Politics of Poverty and Control in Karen State*. Thailand: Karen Human Rights Group, 2007.

———. *Dignity in the Shadow of Oppression*. Thailand: Karen Human Rights Group, 2006.

Karen Women's Organization. *Shattering Silences*. Thailand: Karen Women's Organization, 2004.

———. *State of Terror*. Thailand: Karen Women's Organization, 2007.

———. *Walking amongst Sharp Knives*. Thailand: Karen Women's Organization, 2010.

Kaw Lah Lah Films and Karen Women's Organization. *The Violence that Is Everyone's Secret*. Documentary Film, 2006.

Landmine Monitor. *Burma/Myanmar: Landmine Monitor Report 2007*, 2007. http://www.icbl.org/lm/2007/burma.html.

Lang, Hazel J. *Fear and Sanctuary: Burmese Refugees in Thailand*. Ithaca, NY: Southeast Asia Program Publications, Cornell University, 2002.

Mahidol Migration Center. "Thailand's Low Skilled Migration Policy: Progress and Challenges." In *Submission to the UN Committee on Migrant Workers, September 11, 2011*, 2011. http://www2.ohchr.org/english/bodies/cmw/docs/DGD/MMC_19092011.pdf.

Physicians for Human Rights. *Looking for a Hidden Population: Trafficking of Migrant Laborers in San Diego County.* Boston: Physicians for Human Rights, 2004.

Pollock, Jackie, and Pranom Somwong. *Seeking Safety, Meeting Violence: Migrant and Refugee Women's Journey from Burma.* Chiang Mai, Thailand: Migrant Action Program/CARAM Asia, 2001.

Shan Human Rights Foundation. *Charting the Exodus from Shan State.* Chiang Mai, Thailand: Shan Human Rights Foundation, 2003.

Shan Human Rights Foundation and Shan Women's Action Network. *License to Rape.* Chiang Mai, Thailand: Shan Human Rights Foundation, 2002.

Smith, Martin. *Burma: Insurgency and the Politics of Ethnicity.* London: Zed Books, 1999.

South, Ashley. "Conflict and Displacement in Burma/Myanmar." In *Myanmar: The State, Community, and the Environment,* edited by Monique Skidmore and Trevor Wilson, 54–81. Canberra: Asia Pacific Press, 2007. http://epress.anu.edu.au/wp-content/uploads/2011/03/ch0436.pdf.

Thailand Burma Border Consortium. *Internal Displacement and Protection in Eastern Burma.* Bangkok, Thailand Burma Border Consortium, 2011.

Women's League of Burma. *System of Impunity.* Thailand: Women's League of Burma, 2004.

Part II.

Assessment, Intervention, and Programs

Chapter 3

Assessments and Interventions

Strengths-Based Approaches in

Contexts of Displacement

Nancy Murakami and Thandar Shwe

Naw Wah[1] is a 20-year-old ethnically Karen female referred to a migrant community mental health counseling center by an outpatient medical department following multiple visits for headaches and abdominal pains. At her most recent medical visit, she reported waking at night in a sweat and being unable to go back to sleep. Naw Wah's mother told the medic that Naw Wah sometimes screams in her sleep.

During her initial visit with the mental health counselor, Naw Wah reported the following: When she was 15, the military attacked her village in Burma. She remembers how she and her family hurriedly gathered what belongings they could carry when they heard that soldiers had arrived, and they ran from their home. When they entered the fields at the edge of her village she looked behind and saw homes burning, and she can vividly remember the screams from other families also trying to flee amid sounds of gunfire. Her brother and sisters were crying, and she comforted the youngest, who clung to her as hard as she could while they ran. After days of walking with others from their village, they crossed a river and finally arrived at a refugee camp in Thailand.

When she was 18, her family left the camp, where life was exceedingly difficult for all of them, and moved to a small house near the Burma border where many other Burmese families from her village had relocated. Barely able to make ends meet, she remembers how her parents often argued about finances and the difficulties of life in Thailand. Her younger brother was now beginning to disrespect her and her parents.

When Naw Wah started working at a migrant school one month ago, she began to reexperience terrifying memories of her family's flight from their village and had to quit after working only two weeks. The family is facing eviction from their home because they can no longer afford the rent. When asked about her sleep, she reported that she has dreams of her home burning and of her youngest sister dying in her arms, even though she is still alive. When she wakes she is too scared to go back to sleep. She has told no one other than the medic and the counselor about these dreams.

As Naw Wah continued talking about her family's difficulties, she became increasingly angry and began to speak harshly to the counselor. Naw Wah said she never wanted to come to the counseling center because she is not crazy and she only wants medication to help her sleep better. At this point, she stood and said that she did not want to say anything more and would like to leave. Her mother encouraged her to sit and talk more with the counselor, but Naw Wah walked outside.

What might you do if you were the counselor? What internal and environmental strengths can you already identify in Naw Wah? How might Naw Wah's current experiences be related to her past? What would you want to assess further? What might be ways to engage Naw Wah in services at the center? Who might make up Naw Wah's coordinated care team?

The story of Naw Wah demonstrates a range of experiences that displaced refugees face and also reveals an array of engagement opportunities for psychosocial and mental health workers providing services in humanitarian emergencies. This chapter includes questions to consider when assessing and addressing psychosocial and mental health issues in conflict and displacement settings.

Frameworks

In the humanitarian emergency of a refugee's forced displacement, the needs and struggles of the individual, the family, and the community are broad and complex. Separation from friends and neighbors, disconnection from land, loss of home (both physical and cultural), death of loved ones, physical and psychological trauma, and disorientation in a foreign environment are just a few of the prima facie challenges faced by the estimated 42 million forcibly displaced people around the world.[2] For many of these individuals and families, these challenges are embedded in a web of extreme poverty—caught in a desperate struggle for basic survival, consumed by the lack of reliable access to basic goods, continually living in extreme stress under constant threat of disease. Despite this seemingly hopeless reality, refugees are surviving and healing, and through this are demonstrating the resiliency and strength that humans possess and are capable of developing, fostering, and drawing on in these times of indescribable hardship and devastation.

In the vast refugee settings around the world, basic assessments of and services for physical health, safety, sanitation, housing, and family reunification have become more commonplace, but recently there is growing recognition that psychosocial and mental health are areas of critical need that require similar attention. It is crucial to acknowledge and address the psychological struggle to begin to understand the complexity of refugee displacement. These processes are difficult to engage in, for the survivors as well as those who provide services in these settings, because of commonly limited language to describe psychological experiences and the universal stigma associated with mental health issues. Normalizing some of the survival experiences and highlighting an individual or community's inherent skills and abilities to cope with past and current challenges, namely the inherent survival frame, can often serve as a launching point to engage people in mental health services while lessening stigma associated with the psychological, physical, or social manifestations of surviving displacement.

Jack Saul, psychologist and director of the International Trauma Studies Program in New York City, highlights the normalcy of trauma reactions and their relationship to community, saying, "an inevitable consequence of natural and human-caused disaster is what we refer to as 'collective trauma,' the shared injuries to a population's social, cultural and physical ecologies."[3] The Sphere Project's *Humanitarian Charter and Minimum Standards in Disaster Response* recognizes a community's valuable role in its own healing through its approach to "offer our services in the belief that the affected population is at the centre of humanitarian action, and recognize that their active participation is essential to providing assistance in ways that best meet their needs, including those of vulnerable and socially excluded people."[4] Survivors in refugee settings have histories of persecution, often violent, with blatant disregard for human rights, and inherent in their traumatizing events are the destruction of their interpersonal connections, agency, and empowerment. Therefore, psychosocial and mental health assessment and services are best developed, trained, and implemented within both a trauma and a human rights framework. Viewing mental health and psychosocial experiences through a trauma lens enables the conceptualization of behaviors, problems, and symptoms in relation to a person's traumatic history, and it also helps us recognize once-adaptive responses that have become maladaptive over time, rather than viewing them as simply pathological. In these human-centered models, trauma reactions are normalized, the multilevel impacts of trauma are recognized, the self-efficacy and expertise of survivors are valued and fostered, and the involvement of community members in the development and implementation of services is essential.

Framework questions to consider when working in these settings:

1. What is the history of displacement/conflict/trauma in the region?
2. What types of terms are used to describe struggles within the community, how are individual and collective difficulties conceptualized, and how is the community involved in any services to address struggles?

Psychosocial Health and Mental Health

Psychological and psychiatric struggles are recognized in communities all around the world and are understood to be the result of a variety of causes, including spirit possession, the will of God, chemical imbalance, a normal reaction to an abnormal event, a disruption of harmony in one's earlier life, angry ancestors, or a curse.[5] In the global mental health field, an equally broad array of terms is used to describe these struggles and the services developed to address them. Theresa Betancourt and Timothy Williams have described two primary intervention paradigms in the field as "psychosocial" and "clinical/psychiatric" approaches.[6] The Inter-Agency Standing Committee (IASC) uses the phrase "mental health and psychosocial support," identifying "psychosocial" as the continual interconnection of psychological and social processes to describe any support that "aims to protect or promote psychosocial well-being and/or prevent or treat mental disorder."[7] The World Health Organization defines health as "a state of complete physical, mental and social well-being and not merely the absence of disease or infirmity," and it differentiates between social interventions and psychological interventions by the intended primary effects of the intervention, although acknowledges secondary psychological and social effects, respectively.[8] In this chapter, "psychosocial and mental health" will be used to describe conditions and approaches grounded in the intersection of a person's psychological functioning or state and environmental and interpersonal experience (psychosocial) and his or her psychiatric health (mental health).

Stressors associated with conflict and disaster are known to increase risk for psychological, interpersonal, and behavioral issues in affected populations.[9] According to recent estimates, in low- and middle-income countries, only about one in five people needing psychological, neurological, or substance abuse treatment actually receives it.[10] In conflict and disaster settings, it is not unreasonable to assume that the needs for psychosocial and mental health are greater, as are the limitations on resources, skewing this ratio even further. As more psychosocial and mental health services are developed and offered in these complex humanitarian emergencies, our first programmatic aim should be to create contextually appropriate and ethical psychosocial and mental health services that use the inherent strengths, resiliencies, and resources of those they are intended to support. Recognizing the interplay of these needs and services is also important, as Betancourt and Williams point out that "provision [of psychosocial care] may lead to improvements in general symptoms among persons both with and without specific disorders. This first line of response may be enough to reduce symptoms below a threshold of clinical significance for large proportions of the population."[11]

Psychosocial and mental health questions to consider when working in these settings:

1. How are psychosocial and mental health issues described and understood by the community and by agencies? What are the literal translations as well as the descriptive meaning of psychosocial and mental health terms in the local language?
2. What psychosocial and mental health services exist in the community?

Strengths-Based Approaches

A strengths-based approach to assessment and services is fundamental in the field of social work[12] and is gaining traction in other professional fields as a valuable framework for psychosocial and mental health work. Unlike disease-, deficit-, or problem-based models, a strengths approach explores and emphasizes the resources and capabilities that individuals and communities have (both historical and current) to cope with struggles and suffering. A strengths-based model places value on people's inherent and acquired protective factors and on the resiliency in their surviving and healing, and it also recognizes the benefits of incorporating these into any services they receive (from assessment through discharge). In a strengths model, the service provider helps clients identify and use strengths they already possess or possessed in the past and supports clients to foster their internal and environmental strengths.[13] The Sphere Project's core standard of a people-centered humanitarian response emphasizes the importance of these capacities, recognizing that "[d]isaster-affected people possess and acquire skills, knowledge and capacities to cope with, respond to and recover from disasters."[14] When people identify these skills, knowledge, and capacities as having value and as resources to draw on for their current coping and heal-ing, symptoms can feel less overwhelming, challenges can seem less daunt-ing, and the sense of self-efficacy can be greater.

Strengths-based questions to consider when working in these settings:

1. What are some identified individual and community strengths?
2. Are programs and services operating from a strengths-based perspective?

Assessment

An assessment is the gathering of pertinent information that informs design or implementation of programming and services. The target of an assessment may be an individual, a family, a community, or an agency. In psychosocial and mental health work, the assessment is fundamental in guiding the service provider and the client to identify the client's current and historical experiences and functioning, strengths and resources, pri-mary needs and goals, and risks and vulnerabilities. Thorough assessments also reveal potential barriers to engagement by identifying sociohistorical, economic, political, cultural, and other factors that could affect services, including prior efforts to address psychosocial and mental health issues in the community. Strong assessments recognize the role of culture in the presentation and understanding of symptoms, the symptom pathology, and client-service provider interactions. Segal and Mayadas note additional assessment components that are important for refugee families and can be applied to other displaced populations: guiding the client to discriminate between realistic and unrealistic expectations, evaluating problem-solving abilities, identifying the transferability of skills to a new context, and gaug-ing learning capabilities and motivation for adaptation.[15]

An assessment may begin even before initial direct engagement with a client (e.g., during information gathering from the client referral source) and continues throughout the work with the client. Assessments may be conducted formally (e.g., structured questionnaire, intake interview) or in-formally, such as a casual conversation during an unexpected encounter with a client. Assessments help prioritize needs while identifying the avail-ability of both internal and external resources, which is particularly impor-tant when resources such as medications, specialized knowledge and skills, or clinical facilities are limited.[16] Assessments identify members of the sup-port system, determine the broadness of the treatment team, and define and enhance the quality and effectiveness of services to be provided. As-sessments also inform the design, implementation, and ongoing evaluation of interventions, with the wider aim of ensuring the appropriateness and sustainability of a service or program.

A thorough assessment for displaced individuals must include an exploration of experiences and functioning from pre-flight through post-flight, with an emphasis on transformation, adaptation, and decompensation. Pre-flight experiences may include early childhood trauma that may shape responses to later traumatic experiences, as well as the presence of strong attachment or support systems that may be drawn on as resiliency factors to cope with stressors. Similarly, pre-flight experiences such as lack of access to basic needs or preexisting mental illness may shed light on developmental issues that continue to affect the client's functioning. Flight experiences may include witnessing the deaths of others, loss of family and community, disrupted education and health care, and chronic fear for safety. Post-flight experiences may include loss of status and role in the family or community, discrimination, unstable housing, limited access to culturally familiar resources, unemployment, and linguistic barriers. Assessing experiences and functioning across these time periods is helpful for more immediate clinical processes such as differential diagnosis or performing a mental status exam, but more broadly for client engagement, a more holistic understanding of the client, and a comprehensive treatment plan.

Knowledge of cultural norms regarding how issues are handled, both individually and by the greater community, will guide the service provider toward more accurate assessments that in turn shape appropriate services. For example, in Burmese communities, as in many communities around the world, family and community members play a broad and vital role in the care of an individual, and their participation in the initial assessment can be invaluable. Involvement of a person's support system (e.g., family, agency) in psychosocial and mental health care can positively affect the time it takes clients to initiate services, their continued engagement in services and adherence to treatment, and, ultimately, much-needed healing.

Assessment questions to consider when working in these settings:

1. What structures are already in place for conducting individual or community-level assessments?
2. What have prior needs assessments in the community focused on and revealed?

Systems and the Environment

We know that individuals can affect their environment and, reciprocally, can be affected by their environment, but this knowledge is not always put to best use in assessments and interventions for psychosocial and mental health support. Systems theories (e.g., Bronfenbrenner's ecological systems theory)[17] recognize the dynamic interplay of the "parts" of a system and the value of understanding and working at each of the system levels as well as at their intersections. For example, James Karls's Person-In-Environment perspective highlights that individuals cannot be holistically understood without taking into account their environment[18]—social, political, familial, cultural, spiritual, economic, and physical. This construct is often viewed as an alternative to the more common medical model of understanding and caring for patients, and is intended to be applied at assessment, intervention, and evaluation levels.[19] From the ecological-systems perspective, an individual's struggles arise from the environment rather than from the pathology of the individual; thus, focusing on one's environmental stressors and their intersections instead of focusing only on the individual's functioning will lead to broader intervention opportunities.[20] These perspectives, which espouse the idea that the environment—cultural, social, political, geographical—is in continual flux, are particularly relevant in humanitarian emergency and displacement contexts and can guide the nature of psychosocial and mental health services. For example, when lack of immigration documentation hinders freedom of movement, when active fighting in the area prevents people from safely leaving their homes, and when armed police officers stand outside the front gate of a health clinic, it is clear that environmental factors must be considered when establishing services.

Systems and environment questions to consider when working in these settings:

1. What are some environmental factors that may affect people's current functioning and their engagement in psychosocial and mental health services?
2. How can these environmental factors inform assessment approaches?

Interventions

Many people who experience stressful or terrifying events, even in conflict and disaster, are capable of self-managing their reactions by employing a repertoire of coping skills developed throughout their lifetimes, and they can recover without ever needing specialized services. For some, however, their naturally developed coping mechanisms may be overwhelmed, resulting in the development of chronic reactions that require additional support and treatment.[21] Furthermore, factors such as developmental age, health status, prior trauma history, sense of agency, and presence of a support system also affect a person's ability to cope with stressors and trauma.

The diversity of psychosocial and mental health interventions that have evolved around the world for displaced people—interventions that work in a particular sociocultural context—is a reflection of the remarkable creativity and determination that communities and programs possess in the universal effort to alleviate psychological suffering. Common psychosocial and mental health services include a broad range of activities, from prayer circles, activity-based groups (e.g., crafts, gardening), workshops, yoga, case management, and women's groups to mental health interventions such as supportive counseling, pharmacotherapy, individual/family/group therapy, self-help groups, and peer support. Services that develop organically from existing supportive practices and those established collaboratively with communities are more likely to be culturally syntonic and to complement services already offered in the community. The purpose of the interventions may be prevention (e.g., awareness-raising for indicators of suicide risk and what to do when someone is showing signs of suicide), health promotion (e.g., men's and women's groups to discuss safe relationships), symptom reduction (e.g., affect-regulation skills), or curing/treating (e.g., medication). The duration of the intervention can range from a single contact to years of engagement, and the setting of the intervention may be a medical clinic, a client's home, a community leader's compound, a school classroom, a safe house, or a community sports field.

Mental health services are commonly viewed through the cultural lens of the Western world, often taking the form of individual psychotherapy from a clinical social worker or psychologist or medication management from a psychiatrist. It is important to recognize, however, that psychosocial and mental health care occur universally through traditional means as part of our basic human tenet to want to reduce suffering and provide support. This often takes the form of consulting with religious leaders and elders or seeking treatment from traditional healers. Even if these traditional forms of care are not immediately identified as psychosocial and mental health services, global mental health workers must recognize the effect of traditional practices on the mind and interpersonal wellness, and they ought to be conceptualized as part of psychosocial and mental health care. All forms of psychosocial and mental health support need to be explored to inform the development and implementation of new or complementary services. Simply introducing interventions that have been successful in other contexts may prove to be ineffective, unsustainable, or even inappropriate and harmful without proper assessment and understanding in the new setting.

Intervention questions to consider when working in these settings:

1. How can you determine what psychosocial support and mental health services already exist within the community?
2. What are the current types of services, who is accessing them, and who is providing them?

Service Setting

The setting in which assessments and interventions are conducted informs and is informed by the services delivered. For example, in the acute phase of a disaster, the aim and quality of mental health work is markedly different than that offered to sequestered refugees who have survived chronic displacement for decades. Psychosocial and mental health services are often delivered under the umbrella of other services, such as inpatient care or reproductive health care in a clinic setting, but they can also be the primary service of an agency or program, such as at a counseling center or a women's safe house, or they can be offered in parallel with other services, such as at a mental health center located in a hospital that has a range of health departments. Whether the psychosocial and mental health services are identified as an agency's "primary service" may determine the level of expertise given to delivering such services, the prioritization of resources, and ultimately the way in which services are used and valued. The varied settings in which the services are offered can also drastically affect perceptions and expectations of the care that is provided (e.g., when a building has both mental health counseling services and HIV services), as well as access to the services (e.g., school-based programs offered during the school year only to youth attending that school), and the quality of the service delivery (e.g., activities in spaces where privacy cannot be maintained).

Service setting questions to consider when working in these settings:

1. What are the settings in which current psychosocial and mental health services are offered?
2. How might these settings be affecting services and service delivery?

Coordination and Integration of Services

The needs of an individual or a community affected by conflict or displacement can take on great breadth. The services available to the individual or the community would ideally be integrated across all systems of engagement, but more often services are provided in uncoordinated ways, risking redundancy or contradictory interventions. To avoid these pitfalls, there are serious efforts to adopt interdisciplinary, multisectoral approaches with the inclusion of the affected community in both receiving and providing support and healing.[22] In many settings, there is also effort to integrate psychosocial and mental health services into programs and systems already trusted and used by the community. Initial assessments can determine where services can most effectively be offered, who should be part of the coordinated care team, and what communication is authorized across the system. Coordinated services may involve regular communication of all stakeholders to identify and discuss needs and goals, to delineate roles of service providers, to plan the order of service provision, to discuss changes in the clients or service providers, to report environmental changes that may affect the clients or providers, and to remain familiar with community, agency, and governmental policies and practices that may affect stakeholders. Having a psychosocial and mental health voice as part of the interdisciplinary care team offers the added benefit of providing psychoeducation to other disciplines about these specialized needs and their effect on many aspects of a person's daily functioning—from the ability to get children ready for school each day to attending mandatory meetings before resettlement.

Coordination of services questions to consider when working in these settings:

1. Are psychosocial and mental health services in the community coordinated?
2. What multisectoral strategies and approaches are currently in place?

Service Providers

Providers of psychosocial and mental health support for those displaced by disaster and conflict often come from varied educational backgrounds, experiences, and training. Most often the facilitators of services are community members or leaders, paraprofessionals, teachers, or religious leaders, and they may be members of the community, individuals from the diaspora of the community, or foreigners. While some community members providing mental health care may not have background or training in these fields, they often possess greater cultural and personal connection to clients' experiences compared with those from outside the community. They may have firsthand knowledge of the traumatic experiences and can relate to the environments in which the clients are currently surviving. Other prominent advantages that community members may have are cultural and linguistic expertise, understanding of stigmas and barriers that may affect engagement in services, respected status within the community, awareness of current and past health services in the community, knowledge of community priorities, and a sense of belonging to the community, to name but a few. Individuals from outside the community (e.g., foreign mental health professionals) may also be providing direct services to clients or may be supporting and training those who are. The degree of service provision provided directly by people from outside the community is often influenced by the level of knowledge and skills of local service providers, access to mental health interpreters, and the culture of the agency or program regarding the roles of foreigners.

In both assessment and intervention, the role of the service provider is active and collaborative with the client and with the systems with which the client interacts. Just as there is a range in the mental health knowledge of these services providers, there is also variability in service delivery skills, and so ensuring that practices such as maintaining client confidentiality and having therapeutic boundaries are understood and respected is critical.[23] Given the difficulty and intensity of this work, all service providers, regardless of their level of training and experience, need support to lessen the likelihood of vicarious trauma, compassion fatigue, and burnout. When conducting assessments and providing interventions, providers are often told detailed histories of loss, suffering, and despair in addition to the client's current hopelessness and struggles, causing many providers to hold on to both the client's distress and the client's hope until the client can tolerate the former and maintain the latter. These memories and feelings can overwhelm even the most seasoned clinician if care for the provider is not available, destigmatized, and accepted.

Service provider questions to consider when working in these settings:

1. Who are the service providers and what are their strengths and skills?
2. What systems are in place to support service providers?

Ethics and Patient Rights

Most clinical disciplines have codes of ethics, practice guidelines, or moral oaths that guide practitioners to maintain the highest standards of ethical practice and humanistic work. Similarly, the first protection principle of the Sphere Project's *Humanitarian Charter and Minimum Standards in Disaster Response* ("Avoid exposing people to further harm as a result of your actions") outlines a framework of ethics for people of any discipline participating in humanitarian response work:

The form of humanitarian assistance and the environment in which it is provided do not further expose people to physical hazards, violence or other rights abuse. Assistance and protection efforts do not undermine the affected population's capacity for self-protection. Humanitarian agencies manage sensitive information in a way that does not jeopardise the security of the informants or those who may be identifiable from the information.[24]

This principle recognizes that services that are intended to be helpful have the potential to be harmful and thus, for individuals and communities that have already been traumatized, disempowered, and abused, adhering to these standards is of utmost importance. This principle also acknowledges a population's "capacity for self-protection" and service providers' responsibility to value and protect this strength. This principle notes the necessity of protection of information gathered during the work, which is both fundamental in health work and imperative for clinical and security reasons, particularly for those who have been or may continue to be subjected to violation of trust, ongoing conflict, trauma, and exploitation. It is important that all service providers respect the policies and procedures related to ethics and client rights of their agencies or programs, as well as codes of ethics of their individual disciplines or licenses.

Confidentiality and consent to treatment are additional rights that need to be protected. As Kathleen Allden et al. discuss, in crisis and conflict settings, there are unique challenges to informed consenting that must not be ignored, including enhanced power differentials and histories of human rights abuses, such as forced signatures on unexplained documents,[25] so implementation of privacy practices must be done thoughtfully. Patient health information is protected in the United States under the Standards for Privacy of Individually Identifiable Health Information, and many nations have comparable standards of privacy in health care.[26] Refugee camps that adhere to standards such as those of the Sphere Project have guidelines for protecting the rights of service recipients,[27] but in many humanitarian emergency contexts, privacy standards have not been established. It is important to talk with clients about their rights when they initially engage in services and throughout their care.

Ethics and patient rights questions to consider when working in these settings:

1. What ethical standards are in place, what is their adherence level, and how are they monitored?
2. How might ethics and patient rights be affecting delivery of services?

The Thai-Burma Border

Application of the above approaches is demonstrated in this section through descriptions of psychosocial and mental health programs currently operating along the Burma border in Thailand. The authors extend special thanks to current and past staff of Première Urgence-Aide Médicale Internationale (PU-AMI) who contributed to this section by providing written material[28] and discussions about the humanitarian emergency situation of refugee camp–based Burmese living along the Thai-Burma border.

Paw Htoo is an ethnically Karen, 22-year-old Christian female from Rangoon, Burma, who completed the equivalent of a third-grade education. Her three brothers, mother, and stepfather reside in Burma. Her family has always struggled financially, and her stepfather, who drinks alcohol excessively, regularly quarrels with her mother and often beats her. Paw Htoo and her siblings have also been beaten by their stepfather.

When Paw Htoo was 11 years old, a man from her community offered to reunite Paw Htoo with her father in Bangkok, Thailand, but instead he trafficked her to a border town in Thailand. Paw Htoo worked as an indentured servant until, at age 13, she fled and reunited with her father following attempts to locate him by distributing a photograph into the community. Her father cared for her and sent her to school, but after a short time she quit school, left her father, and began working on a farm. After being denied earnings despite multiple attempts to receive her pay, Paw Htoo attempted suicide by taking an overdose of medicine from the market. She was hospitalized for one month in a Thai hospital then discharged to an organization where she stayed for months before leaving without informing the organization. Paw Htoo attempted suicide twice more following incidents of interpersonal conflict, and each time was reconnected with the organization to which she had been discharged following her first hospitalization. Paw Htoo reported feeling overwhelming shame, sadness, frustration, and disappointment following these events and thinking that she would no longer seek connection with anyone. The organization referred Paw Htoo to mental health counseling following the third suicide attempt.

Paw Htoo authorized her counselor to communicate with the referral organization. The organization provided information about Paw Htoo's previous services and history of psycho-pharmaceutical treatment; details about her suicide attempts and indicators of increased suicide risk; and her mental status presentation over time, her interpersonal strengths, and her history of early withdrawal from treatments and services.

The counselor assessed that Paw Htoo's suicide risk was high and needed to be addressed immediately; that the patient continued to be affected by her history of early separation from family and the deceit and exploitation during her trafficking; that Paw Htoo has difficulty trusting people and getting close to others, that she has a history of non-adherence and early withdrawal from treatment that should be discussed and monitored, that she exhibits resilience that should be further explored and fostered, and that more time is needed to determine whether the patient meets criteria for any mental health diagnoses.

In response to the patient's suicide history, the patient and counselor collaboratively developed a suicide safety plan in the initial session. To develop the individualized plan, the counselor assessed the following: Paw Htoo's warning signs (thoughts, feelings, behaviors) that a crisis may be developing, things Paw Htoo likes to do to take her mind off problems, her healthy coping skills, and who can provide her support within twenty-four hours.

The counselor and patient identified the following strategies to cope with distressing feelings and thoughts that could lead to risky behavior such as suicide: tell someone; rest; find someone to talk to; write down or draw positive memories, experiences, or qualities about herself; be around other people; sing, take a walk, or do something she enjoys; do not drink alcohol; avoid going where she might harm herself; contact the counselor or the organization if she thinks about suicide.

The counselor taught the patient basic muscle relaxation techniques, which Paw Htoo enjoyed and found effective, noting that she was significantly more relaxed after practicing the skill. The counselor implemented basic counseling with the patient, which included techniques for managing thoughts associated with suicide risk, and began to teach the patient about connections between thoughts, feelings, and behaviors. Paw Htoo was assigned practice tasks for home.

Paw Htoo and her counselor began developing a treatment plan together. The patient was selective about what information the counselor was authorized to share with partner programs, and the counselor honored this. The patient and counselor agreed that services would be coordinated with the organization where the patient lives, to enhance sustainability of the patient's safety, the skills learned in treatment, and the patient's follow-through in care. The patient agreed to return in three days for a follow-up session during which they would discuss services the patient would engage in.

The counselor was optimistic that the patient would return for her follow-up appointment; however, she did not. One month following the initial session, a partner program informed the counselor that the Thai police had brought Paw Htoo to them. The program arranged for the counselor to meet the patient in their setting, hoping this would better facilitate engagement; however, Paw Htoo left the program before the counselor arrived. Months later, the patient visited the counselor and agreed to return to the organization where she had received services; however, that organization was unable to accept her because of her lack of adherence to program rules in the past. The patient left upon learning this news, and her current location is unknown.

COUNSELOR'S REFLECTION

The information provided by the partner organization and by Paw Htoo created a fuller picture of the patient's functioning, her history, suicide risk factors, protective factors, and history of engagement in service; however, Paw Htoo's primary presenting problem was never clear. The counselor wishes she had better helped the patient identify and prioritize her needs, identify how the counselor could be most helpful to her, and understand the role and collaborative approach of counseling services. The counselor helped Paw Htoo begin to identify her internal and environmental resources and stressors, but there are several bio-psychosocial factors the counselor would like to assess further, including the patient's support system in Thailand, the patient's psychiatric treatment experience in the Thai hospital, the patient's journey to Thailand and her trafficking experience, and the patient's familial relationships and history, including her childhood abuse. One of the greatest challenges was Paw Htoo's unstable environment and social support system, so the counselor wishes she had provided assistance with concrete and social needs, such as housing; had identified a support group or other women's groups that the patient could join; and had explored the possibility of including the patient's father in her treatment. The counselor respected Paw Htoo's decisions regarding authorization to share information with other organizations and adjusted her approach based on the patient's history and engagement with other programs. The counselor is hopeful that Paw Htoo will again reach out to the counselor or the organization when she is in need of support.

Approximately 2.5 million Burmese migrant workers are estimated to be living in Thailand, an additional estimated 129,000 refugees are living inside the official refugee camps along the Burma border in Thailand,[29] and an estimated 200,000 refugees are living outside the camps.[30] Another 400,000 people are estimated to be living in the southeastern region of Burma as internally displaced persons (IDP).[31] These numbers represent people affected by decades of war, economic struggle, family separation, violence, torture, and flight. There are no reliable data to confirm the prevalence of psychosocial and mental suffering of these people. However, anecdotal reports suggest that psychological distress is rampant and that it affects individuals, families, and entire communities; that it is associated with domestic violence, substance abuse, and suicide; and that individuals and programs working in these communities want to better understand and address it.

Along the border of Burma and Thailand, psychosocial and mental health awareness and services within the Burmese community have been gradually increasing. Few studies have been conducted to assess mental health in or outside the camps along the border. Nevertheless, community-based and nonprofit organizations, international nongovernmental organizations, and university research teams have initiated services in both settings. The heightened awareness and the growth of services have prompted development of assessment tools, protocols, interventions, and programs to facilitate better understanding of psychosocial and mental health needs and to promote stability and holistic health of individuals, families, and communities.

Access to eastern regions of Burma remains restricted for foreigners and sometimes dangerous and difficult for Burmese; therefore, psychosocial and mental health services have become more comprehensive, specialized, and accessible to the Burmese community in western Thailand, where foreign and Burmese individuals are providing training, consultation, and services. Knowledge and skills are reaching farther into Burma, however, as more community members and health care workers receive training in Thailand then return to Burma. For example, organizations like Karen Department of Health and Welfare and the Back Pack Health Worker Team, whose medics are trained in Thailand, are beginning to incorporate psychosocial health awareness and supportive services into the care they provide to communities in the regions of eastern Burma. Medics and health workers who are trained at Mae Tao Clinic and then return to Burma to live or work are also spreading knowledge of psychological health and treatment at family, community, and organizational levels and integrating it with traditional approaches to addressing suffering in these communities.

Mae Tao Clinic Mental Health Counseling Center

The Mae Tao Clinic (MTC),[32] commonly called "Dr. Cynthia's Clinic" after cofounder Dr. Cynthia Maung, is a health care facility and training center established to provide accessible quality health care, regardless of ability to pay, to displaced people of Burma along the Thai-Burma border. Dr. Cynthia Maung, a Burmese medical doctor and displaced activist from the 1988 prodemocracy movement, established these health care services for students, villagers, and thousands of others forced to flee Burma during years of widespread human rights abuses and violent and oppressive military rule. Starting as a single building in 1989, MTC has expanded to include around a dozen outpatient and inpatient departments, where approximately 150,000 visits and over 3,000 live births occurred in 2012 alone.[33] In addition to the current extensive medical services, MTC promotes general health through partnerships with many community-based organizations.

As the displaced Burmese population grew, Dr. Cynthia and other community leaders recognized the need to expand the clinic's services to include psychosocial and mental health support. In response to Dr. Cynthia's appeal for a fuller understanding of mental health needs and for establishment of services, the nonprofit organization Burma Border Projects (BBP)[34] established a long-lasting partnership with MTC. In 2006, following years of community- and clinic-based needs assessments, the MTC Mental Health Counseling Center was constructed and today provides psychosocial and mental health services, trainings, community awareness, and consultation for MTC and the broader community. The Mental Health Counseling Center's clinical services include an amputee support group in a centrally located space that is wheelchair and crutches accessible; a support group in the "patient house," where patients stay when receiving multiday outpatient services; and sessions in patients' homes when they are unable to travel to MTC or when community-based services are indicated. With training and support from BBP, counselors also visit other departments at MTC to meet bed-bound patients on the inpatient units, to meet with psychiatric patients who live at MTC, and to provide coordinated care for patients receiving services from the full range of outpatient and inpatient departments.

PATIENTS

Patients of the Mental Health Counseling Center include individuals and families affected by psychological trauma, loss, land mine accidents, domestic violence, substance abuse and dependence, gender-based violence, economic struggles, imprisonment, HIV/AIDS, mental illness, and daily struggles of life inside Burma and along the border. Many patients present with symptoms of depression, posttraumatic stress disorder (PTSD), and anxiety. Some present with symptoms of schizophrenia, substance abuse, bipolar disorder, and other mental illnesses. Most initial encounters are unscheduled and range from minutes to hours. Most patients attend sessions accompanied by a support person—a relative, neighbor, friend, or religious figure—who is actively engaged in their care. Patients often appear confused and apprehensive when they first arrive at the Mental Health Counseling Center, but they often leave smiling and expressing gratitude to the treating counselor and other staff. Sessions are conducted on mats on the floor and have a semi-structured format. Patients' children may sit with patients during a session or, when more strict privacy is needed, are cared for by staff during the meeting. Staff offer patients water or tea to drink; at times patients join the staff for lunch.

SERVICES

The atmosphere of the Mental Health Counseling Center is relaxed and welcoming, which is a notable difference from other MTC departments, which are usually busy, crowded, and loud. Patients are referred to the Mental Health Counseling Center by other clinic departments, community members, other Mental Health Counseling Center patients, and community-based organizations around Mae Sot. When people arrive inquiring about services or expressing need for services, they are greeted by staff, then an available counselor who speaks the patient's preferred language immediately begins the engagement process.

During a patient's initial encounter, the counselor begins to implement fundamental counseling skills through facilitating the development of trust, expressing empathy, being nonjudgmental, exhibiting nonverbal cues that are consistent with verbal messages, active listening, and maintaining confidentiality. Early in the initial encounter, the counselor explains what to expect during the session and throughout care. Many first-time patients are unfamiliar with the concept of mental illness and psychosocial suffering and thus have little or no framework for understanding the services or sometimes even why they were referred. For others, psychosocial and mental health services are laden with stigma. Some patients are only familiar with individuals who are suffering from severe mental illness, and they believe that the Mental Health Counseling Center is only for such individuals. Because the Mental Health Counseling Center was initially located above the Voluntary Counseling and Testing Department, which provides services to HIV-affected patients, some people believed that the Mental Health Counseling Center was for only HIV-positive patients. Some patients believe that because the Mental Health Counseling Center is based in a medical clinic, if they do not receive medication for treatment (e.g., if they receive solely counseling services), then they have received no treatment at all. These are some of the misconceptions addressed early in service provision through psycho-education and by allowing the patient space and time to share thoughts, feelings, and concerns. The counselors ask patients whether they want anyone present during the initial assessment and seek permission to document what the patients report for clinic records.

ASSESSMENT

Assessment of patients' presenting problems and bio-psychosocial history begins when they enter the clinic or are referred and will continue throughout engagement in services. MTC counselors recognize the potential impact of sociocultural factors on the counseling relationship and in particular during the assessment phase. Decades of war in Burma have affected people's trust of other individuals, ethnic groups, and systems and agencies. Therefore, both cultural differences and cultural similarities between the patient and the counselor can significantly affect patient assessment, as the patient selects what to share and what to withhold. Counselors also understand the critical role of language. Since many people of Burma speak multiple languages, a patient may communicate initially in the preferred language of the counselor; however, it is the counselor's responsibility to assess the patient's preferred language and communicate in that language directly or through an interpreter who is proficient in mental health terms in both languages. Counselors address additional potential barriers, including deference to health care providers, involvement of foreigners in their treatment, and mental illness stigma. In many mental health settings, a collaborative relationship between patient and health care provider is a goal and is understood to be best practice; however, in the Burma border context, as in many settings, the hierarchy in health care systems is customary; therefore, a collaborative approach is thoughtfully framed and discussed with patients in order to maintain engagement in treatment.

At the Mental Health Counseling Center, the assessment is viewed as developing the theory of the causes of a patient's presenting problems based on history and current functioning. It sets the initial road map for the patient's treatment. The assessment determines whether treatment is indicated, what the appropriate treatment should be, and whether that treatment can best be provided exclusively by the Mental Health Counseling Center, exclusively by another individual or organization, or through collaborative care with another organization. The assessment is holistic and individualized, taking into account such things as the patient's culture, religion, support system, and bio-psychosocial-spiritual identity. Counselors understand that the priority of needs held by the patient, as well as others involved (e.g., caregivers and counselors) may differ and that each should be explored. Counselors understand that their own biases and judgments can affect the work they do and so they must remain aware of the "self" in their work and seek support from colleagues when it is interfering with the patient's care.

During the initial assessment, the counselor explains confidentiality and its limits. At the Mental Health Counseling Center, everything a patient shares is confidential unless the patient gives her or his consent to share information. The only exceptions are when someone is in serious danger; there are allegations of abuse against a nongovernmental organization, United Nations staff, or Thai military; or the patient is under the age of 15. Following the initial assessment, counselors collaborate with the patient and any caregivers to develop an individualized treatment plan. The counselor helps the patient identify obstacles to following the plan and the possibility of treatment non-adherence, and they attempt to problem-solve these. The counselor and patient also agree to modify the plan as the patient's needs change or services at the Mental Health Counseling Center or in the community change.

INTERVENTIONS

The Mental Health Counseling Center's services have included supportive counseling, psycho-education, and relaxation; affect-regulation training, intensive case management, and medication management; an amputee/injury support and physical therapy group, a patient-house support group, and patient advocacy. Because discordance between patients' expectations and standard medical or mental health practice is common, patients are provided extensive psycho-education about any recommended services. For example, the practice of gradually increasing medication dosage to determine the optimal dose may be perceived by the patient as an indicator of being "sicker," so patients are informed of these practices before initiating medication, and they are reminded of them every time a dosage change is indicated.

Special attention at the Mental Health Counseling Center is directed to patients at risk for suicide, domestic violence, or substance abuse, and to aggressively psychotic patients. All reports of suicidal thought are taken seriously and explored by the counselor in a nonjudgmental fashion. Patients who report a suicide plan must meet with a supervisor and be further assessed before leaving the Mental Health Counseling Center. In the case of high suicide risk, patients will remain in the medical inpatient department for monitoring or counselors will take shifts in monitoring the patient in the outpatient Mental Health Counseling Center, even sometimes staying overnight with the patient. If the patient's needs cannot be met at Mae Tao Clinic, the patient will be transferred to a Thai hospital for inpatient psychiatric services. When domestic violence is reported to a counselor, the patients (e.g., husband and wife) will often be seen individually until the counselor assesses that it is safe for the patients to have joint or family sessions. Counselors validate the right for people to live without violence and inform patients of community resources available to domestic violence victims. When domestic violence is present, counselors also assess whether medical services are needed and whether the violence needs to be reported to authorities. For any patient reporting drug or alcohol use, the physical, psychological, and social risks of substance abuse and dependence are discussed. Family members often express the greatest concern about substance use and, with patients' consent, will be actively engaged in substance abuse services, which include harm-reduction approaches of psycho-education, counseling, and medication. Medic counselors closely monitor substance-dependent patients who are treated with medication to manage withdrawal. Psychotic patients exhibiting aggression are one of the greatest challenges to the counselors and the mental health systems of MTC. There are several patients with severe mental illness residing on the grounds of MTC, often requiring intensive medical, social, and psychiatric care that exhausts both inpatient and outpatient teams. This is one patient population whose needs have not yet been fully captured, and further development of a comprehensive care system for these patients is needed.

SERVICE PROVIDERS

Mental Health Counseling Center counselors are identified within the Burmese community as individuals who exhibit leadership skills, compassion, and an interest in the field of mental health and social services. Counselors represent multiple ethnic groups of Burma, and their diversity in language proficiency often enables services to be offered in patients' preferred languages. They have a variety of training and professional backgrounds ranging from midwifery to botany, but at MTC, all receive training on psychological trauma, mental illness, risk assessment and management, substance dependence, engagement and counseling skills, and safety planning. Counselors who also have medic training are the prescribers of psychotropic medication at the Mental Health Counseling Center and are the monitors of medication management.

Training and education at the Mental Health Counseling Center is provided by social workers, psychologists, and psychiatrists, as well as by locally trained counselors, medics, and paraprofessionals. BBP, which has partnered with MTC for fifteen years to provide psychosocial and mental health support, has taken a lead role in the training and capacity building of counselors, with BBP staff based at the Mental Health Counseling Center and also brought in for consultation and projects. All counselors receive on-the-job training in job responsibilities and many receive a multiday didactic and practical training soon after joining the team. All new counselors are provided training materials to develop their psychosocial and mental health knowledge. They shadow experienced counselors in their daily work and have regular consultation with other counselors and partner organization professionals to learn the required skills. Counselors receive continuing education through training in the Mental Health Counseling Center and in the community, individual or group supervision, and a multi-day annual training in the Mental Health Counseling Center. All counselors are encouraged to identify their own learning needs and the learning needs of their colleagues and to seek additional training and support when needed. Additional trainings are developed as needed in order to ensure high-quality service provision; for example when several suicides occurred in the community a few years ago, a specialized suicide and safety-planning training was developed and implemented.

One staffing challenge experienced at the Mental Health Counseling Center, as well as at other community agencies, is the high personnel turnover caused by resettling in third countries, returning to Burma, returning to refugee camps, or seeking higher-paying employment elsewhere. MTC invests heavily in its staff by providing extensive training and support, and new counselors are eager learners and passionate care providers; however, environmental and psychosocial factors hinder the development of a robust experienced team of counselors and necessitate frequent hiring and training of new team members.

RECENT CHALLENGES

With indicators of increasing safety and stability inside Burma in recent years, there is growing need to anticipate and address the psychosocial challenges of people of Burma returning home, either by individual choice or by political mandate, after months or decades of displacement. While there have been talks about mass repatriation, no definitive time lines have been announced and little preparation planning has been seen, leading to increased anxiety for many in the community. For some, repatriation means returning to land and people they once thought they would never see again, reestablishing stability in their homeland, and returning to documented status; but for many it also means leaving well-established communities and support systems, being exposed to trauma reminders from the time of fleeing, returning to areas that have changed, facing questions or fears of ongoing volatility in Burma, and, for children born in Thailand, returning to a homeland where they have never actually lived. Some people mistrust that peace will remain in their regions and that human rights will be respected, while others—from regions where land mine explosions,[35] interethnic fighting, and forced child labor continue[36]—wonder whether peace and security will ever return. Counselors and patients alike face uncertainties about remaining in Thailand, returning to Burma, or resettling in a third country.

Première Urgence-Aide Médicale Internationale Refugee Mental Health Program[37]

Since 1984, large numbers of ethnic minorities of Burma have fled from their communities to the nine official refugee camps along the Thai-Burma border, called temporary shelters.[38] The refugee situation in Thailand is one of the most protracted in the world, with many refugees having lived in the camps for close to twenty-nine years. Because Thailand is not party to the 1951 Refugee Convention, it does not recognize the official status of refugees in the country, and so refugees are not granted rights to movement or employment and must remain in the camps or face possible deportation to Burma. This long-term confinement has major implications for physical and psychological health and livelihoods. Nongovernmental organizations are primarily responsible for provision of health services in the camps, and Human Rights Watch recently released a report on the effects of camp living on refugee livelihoods: "As long as Thailand maintains its closed camp policy and forbids refugees from working legally outside the camps, the cutbacks in direct humanitarian assistance and reprogramming of aid toward promoting livelihoods are not likely to result in greater self sufficiency, but rather to more destitution and increased reliance on risky, illegal employment outside the camps to make ends meet."[39] Food security is another growing problem in the camps, with inability to earn income and food ration reductions cited as the first and third most pressing problems faced in the camps in a 2012 study.[40] This, coupled with restriction in livelihood and income-generating activities, adds to the stress of living as a refugee and compounds psychological trauma from fleeing home communities.

Première Urgence-Aide Médicale Internationale, previously called Aide Médicale Internationale (AMI), is an international nongovernmental organization (NGO) whose mandate is a comprehensive response to the essential needs of populations suffering from humanitarian crises in emergencies until autonomy and dignity can be obtained. PU-AMI's Thailand program began its humanitarian work inside Burma in Kayah State in the 1980s, following military-ethnic conflict in the region. Shortly thereafter, AMI projects expanded into the Karen and Mon states, providing basic curative and preventive care in areas controlled by insurgent groups and conducting activities that promoted the training of native community health workers.

In 1995, the Karen National Union, a political organization representing the ethnic Karen people of Burma, lost the battle for their headquarters in the city of Manerplaw to the Burmese military, resulting in mass fleeing of populations to the Thai-Burma border to seek refuge. As the population fled the region, AMI followed to provide medical assistance to the displaced population in Thailand. Initial operations were located in Mae Ra Ma Luang from 1995 to 2002, and expanded to Nupo in 1997, Umpiem in 2001, and Mae La in 2005, all in Tak Province, Thailand, where it continues to operate today. The organization continues to provide health services, free of charge, to populations in need thirty years later.

A COMPREHENSIVE APPROACH TO HEALTH

PU-AMI's Thailand mission promotes a comprehensive definition of health. Its programs integrate activities that aim to provide treatment for physical ailments with awareness-raising to promote mental well-being and social cohesion for communities it serves. PU-AMI Thailand offers health promotion and disease prevention in Mae La camp and offers a range of services in all three Tak Province camps, including clinical services; disease surveillance/control; "vertical programs" focusing on specific entities such as HIV/AIDS, tuberculosis, and mental health; and activities in malaria control. Training is a key focus of PU-AMI activities, to equip refugee staff with tools to conduct program activities and to reinforce partner capacities to collaboratively address health issues.

PU-AMI's Mental Health Program reinforces coping mechanisms of refugees through culturally appropriate individual and group counseling services and therapies while addressing the larger social well-being of the community by promoting increased awareness of mental health disorders, decreased stigma and social exclusion, and increased self-reliance. Furthermore, PU-AMI works to empower communities by training local staff and building partnerships with local community-based organizations (CBOs) and NGOs to improve the protection of refugees through increased multisectoral coordinated efforts.

With the possibility of refugees voluntarily returning to Burma in the near future, in addition to providing essential health services for the refugee population, PU-AMI also focuses on preparing them for return and for other durable solutions, such as resettlement or integration into hosting communities.

ASSESSMENT OF NEEDS

Communities respond to stressors in unique ways, so a needs assessment is an important first step in understanding issues in a community, defining and developing a program or service plan, and evaluating services. PU-AMI has conducted two in-depth assessment studies along the Thai-Burma border to better understand the prevalence of psychological distress and effective strategies for healing. In 2006, PU-AMI conducted a mental health assessment in Mae La and Umpiem camps in response to what appeared to be high rates of psychosomatic symptoms at the camp health facilities.[41] Following the results of the study, PU-AMI's Mental Health Program was developed and first implemented in 2007 in the three Tak Province camps. As more data became available, Mental Health Program activities were modified to better meet the community's needs. In 2013, a second mental health study was conducted in two Tak Province camps. This "Rapid Ethnographic Assessment" documented basic positive and negative coping behaviors, documented perception and usage of existing mental health facilities, and better defined population needs and motivations to inform future program development.[42] Results of these studies are discussed below.

Before 2007, PU-AMI focused primarily on physical health; however, its health facilities had considerable numbers of patients presenting with psychosomatic complaints. PU-AMI's initial mental health needs assessment revealed a high prevalence of nonpsychotic mental disorders, with 36–38 percent of the respondent population demonstrating signs of depression, 13–15 percent manifesting anxiety, 3–17 percent experiencing PTSD, and upward of 66 percent of the total respondents reporting sleep disorders.[43] Reinforcing these findings of high rates of depression and anxiety among refugee camp populations, a study conducted by Barbara Lopes Cardozo et al. in Mae Hong Son, a northern Thai province, showed upward of 40 percent of the interviewed population experiencing depression and about the same proportion experiencing anxiety, related to factors such as the micronutrient content of the food ration and the policy to forbid movement, employment, and cultivation of land outside the camps.[44]

Mental health data collected by PU-AMI in Tak Province camps during 2012 showed that 56 percent of new patients seen by PU-AMI psychosocial workers suffered from nonpsychotic mental disorders such as anxiety and depression, 8 percent suffered from acute or severe psychosis that required medical intervention, and the majority of follow-up patients suffered from severe mental health disorders. Since the beginning of the mental health program, PU-AMI has seen a steady increase of new patients referred to mental health services, resulting in a doubling of the new-patient load from 2007 to 2011.

PU-AMI's 2013 study looked at the community's understanding of psychosocial and mental health issues, approaches to healing, and barriers to accessing care. Participants reported a range of stressors in the community, including familial and interpersonal challenges, environmental difficulties, and internal emotional issues. Some participants discussed traditional practices to address mental health issues, such as tying string around one's wrist to help with spirit possession; however, many lamented the loss of traditional healing approaches, possibly caused by loss of or separation from family and elders who pass on knowledge and traditions. The study also identified lack of knowledge about mental health and limited vocabulary to discuss psychological issues as primary barriers to seeking and receiving psychosocial and mental health care. Participants discussed coping skills used to manage distress, including prayer and consulting religious leaders, community involvement, and being in nature, as well as alcohol and drug use and aggressive behavior. As one participant explained, "we live here with a lot of worry. Some relax the stress with religion, some relax with drugs."[45] Several service recommendations were developed out of this study, including increased community-based interventions, changes in mental health nomenclature and treatment structure to align more with familiar methods of support and healing, increased support of religious leaders who reported limited efficacy when addressing individuals with mental health issues, and normalization of mental health issues and support.

ACTIVITIES TO PROMOTE MENTAL HEALTH

The assessments described above demonstrate the critical need for psychosocial and mental health support to strengthen coping mechanisms and foster resiliency in the refugee population living in protracted and restrictive displacement. The complicated and uncertain living situation of refugees can further compound underlying mental health disorders, resulting in actions that may disrupt the community as a whole, so interventions must be multilevel. Similarly, both internalized and community stigmatizations of mental illness need to be addressed to reinforce healing. Pre-flight, flight, and post-flight factors affect the mental health of refugees, so it is critical to explore diverse and enduring stressors across these experiences.[46] Because psychosocial struggles have broad impact, it is also essential to have a comprehensive multisectoral service approach in which a collaborative network of agencies and disciplines work together to provide services and to identify service gaps.

Focusing on a strategy of empowering communities to take initiative in promoting well-being, PU-AMI trains refugees to serve as psychosocial workers (PSWs) for their local communities. Currently, a team of eighteen PSWs in the three Tak Province camps conduct a range of activities based on World Health Organization guidelines, from counseling to community awareness-raising for mental health. Taking into account the cultural specificities of the local communities, PU-AMI recruits PSWs from all ethnic groups represented in the three camps. As the mental health team itself is small and the target population is large (78,000 beneficiaries in the three camps), a training-of-trainers approach was adopted to maximize the reach of the message and the provision of the following core services of the PU-AMI Mental Health Program.

Individual and Group Counseling

Supportive counseling, focused on providing emotional support and development of cognitive behavioral understanding, is offered to individuals and small groups. The counseling does not aim primarily to cure, but rather to support and improve coping mechanisms. It aims to help people improve self-control through education and social skills and boost resilience through mobilization of self-support and self-reliance.

Expression and Relaxation Therapies

PSWs conduct expression and relaxation therapies to promote mental well-being. Art and music are powerful tools to express feelings and have proven to be beneficial to the patients' state of mind. Relaxation therapies, such as yoga, simple massage, breathing exercises, and meditation are recommended tools to deal with stress and sleeping disorders.

Awareness-Raising and Community Education

Existing literature on mental health in conflict and postconflict settings highlights the communal effects of psychosocial dysfunction,[47] so the social component of the Mental Health Program addresses psychosocial problems at a community level. PU-AMI conducts awareness-raising activities with CBO leaders to gain support and alliance with local leaders while also disseminating information through PSWs and partner organizations. In response to its 2013 assessment, PU-AMI will enhance its community education on prevailing psychosocial problems to increase community-wide self-awareness and self-help. Community education also assists in reducing stigma and increasing awareness about available services.

Follow-Up and Home Visits

Home visits facilitate understanding of problems through observation of living conditions. They facilitate connection with the patients' social environments and opportunities to provide information to family and friends to improve social support networks.

Medical Treatment for Severe Cases

In severe cases, medical treatment is provided to patients by PU-AMI medics and certified clinical doctors with counseling support provided by the PU-AMI mental health officer, mental health supervisor, and camp-based PSWs. Sessions on recognizing mental health disorders have been incorporated into the annual medic trainings, and all medics are taught skills to recognize the signs of severe mental disorders that may require treatment. Clinical doctors in close collaboration with the mental health officer or supervisor develop treatment programs based on the Sphere Project standards and the World Health Organization and Mental Health Gap Action Programme intervention guide for severe cases of psychosis and other disorders.[48] In some cases, PU-AMI refers patients to Thai hospitals for psychiatric assessment and treatment. PSWs and medics also follow up with home visits to ensure medication adherence and provide education and support to patients' caregivers.

RECENT CHALLENGES

Camp residents experience high rates of anxiety and depression related to a range of experiences including camp confinement and resettlement-related family separation but, more recently, believed also to be related to uncertainty surrounding refugee repatriation following peace talks in Burma. The lack of control of their situation leads to additional stress affecting both individuals and communities. Some people turn to substance use to combat this stress, further exacerbating issues of anxiety, depression, sleep disorders, and interpersonal conflict. A social approach to mitigating this stress is necessary to promote healthy behaviors and mental well-being and to increase community agency at a time when this may feel very limited.

The Mae Tao Clinic Mental Health Counseling Center and the PU-AMI Refugee Mental Health Program are just two models of psychosocial and mental health services for the displaced people of Burma. Like others, these programs recognize the complexity of the environment, the historical context, and mental health issues, and they also recognize the necessity of identifying the strengths within both individuals and communities as the starting point for psychosocial and mental health care.

Conclusion

The stories of Naw Wah and Paw Htoo demonstrate the effect of decades of oppression, violence, and lack of needed health infrastructure in Burma, as well as community and agency responses to psychosocial and mental health needs. Promoting mental health is no longer only a critical component for achieving health and well-being in these refugee communities—it is now a necessity for a nation that is rebuilding. The growing recognition that psychological needs cannot be ignored and in fact should be prioritized is leading to more holistic and coordinated approaches to addressing the struggles of displaced populations around the world. The approaches to developing and implementing the services highlighted at the beginning of this chapter can guide psychosocial and mental health services in any context of humanitarian emergencies. By standing up to address psychosocial issues, communities are taking on one of the greatest global health challenges of our time.

Notes

1   Client stories are composites of narratives told along the Thai-Burma border.
2   United Nations Secretary General, "Message for World Refugee Day," http://www.un.org/News/Press/docs/2012/sgsm14353.doc.htm.
3   Jack Saul, *Collective Trauma, Collective Healing: Promoting Community Resilience in the Aftermath of Disaster* (New York: Routledge, 2014), 1.
4   The Sphere Project, *Humanitarian Charter and Minimum Standards in Disaster Response* (Geneva: The Sphere Project, 2011), 23.
5   Première Urgence-Aide Médicale Internationale (PU-AMI), Rainy Dawn Warf, "Mental Health Seeking Behavior: A Rapid Ethnography of Two Burmese Refugee

Camps," 2013 *PU-AMI Mental Health Study* (Thailand: Première Urgence-Aide Médicale Internationale, 2013), 15; Sylvester Ntomchukwu Madu, "Traditional Healing Systems and (Western) Psychotherapy in Africa," in *African Traditional Healing: Psychotherapeutic Investigation; World Council for Psychotherapy,* ed. Sylvester Ntomchukwu Madu, Peter Kakubeire Baguma, and Alfred Pritz (Vienna: World Council for Psychotherapy, 1997), 30.

6 Theresa S Betancourt and Timothy Williams, "Building an Evidence Base on Mental Health Interventions for Children Affected by Armed Conflict," *Intervention* 6, no. 1 (2008): 39.

7 Inter-Agency Standing Committee, "Mental Health and Psychosocial Support in Humanitarian Emergencies: What Should Humanitarian Health Actors Know?," *Global Protection Cluster Group and IASC Reference Group for Mental Health and Psychosocial Support in Emergency Settings* (Geneva, 2010), 1, http://www.who.int/mental_health/emergencies/what_humanitarian_health_actors_should_know.pdf.

8 "WHO Definition of Health," World Health Organization, http://www.who.int/about/definition/en/print.html; WHO, *Mental Health in Emergencies* (Geneva: WHO Department of Mental Health and Substance Dependence, 2003), 2.

9 Sphere Project, *Humanitarian Charter,* 333.

10 World Health Organization and Mental Health Gap Action Programme, *mhGAP Intervention Guide for Mental, Neurological and Substance Use Disorders in Non-specialized Health Settings* (Geneva: World Health Organization, 2010), 1.

11 Betancourt and Williams, "Building an Evidence," 41.

12 Rosalie J. Russo, "Applying a Strengths-Based Practice Approach in Working with People with Developmental Disabilities and their Families," *Families in Society* 80, no. 1 (January/February 1999): 25.

13 Charles D. Cowger, "Assessing Client Strengths: Clinical Assessment for Client Empowerment," *Social Work* 39, no. 3 (1994).

14 Sphere Project, *Humanitarian Charter,* 56.

15 Uma A. Segal and Nazneen S. Mayadas, "Assessment of Issues Facing Immigrant and Refugee Families," *Child Welfare* 84, no. 5 (September/October 2005): 577.

16 WHO, *A WHO Educational Package: Mental Disorders in Primary Care* (Geneva: World Health Organization, 1998).

17 Urie Bronfenbrenner, "Ecological models of human Development," *International Encyclopedia of Education* 3, 2nd ed. (Oxford: Elsevier, 1994), reprinted in *Readings on the Development of Children,* 2nd ed., ed. Mary Gauvain and Michael Cole, 37–43 (New York: Freeman, 1993), http://www.psy.cmu.edu/~siegler/35bronfebrenner94.pdf.

18 "NASW Social Work Pioneers,"
http://www.naswfoundation.org/pioneers/k/karls.html.

19 Ibid.

20 René D Drumm, Sharon W Pittman, and Shelly Perry, "Social Work Interventions in Refugee Camps: An Ecosystems Approach," *Journal of Social Service Research* 30, no. 2 (2003): 70.

21 Judith Herman, *Trauma and Recovery: The Aftermath of Violence—From Domestic Abuse to Political Terror* (New York: Basic Books, 1997), 33.

22 Inter-Agency Standing Committee, *IASC Guidelines on Mental Health and Psychosocial Support in Emergency Settings* (Geneva: Inter-Agency Standing Committee, 2007).

23 American Psychological Association, *Resilience and Recovery after War: Refugee Children and Families in the United States* (Washington, DC: American Psychological Association, 2010), http://www.apa.org/pubs/info/reports/refugees.aspx.

24 Sphere Project, *Humanitarian Charter*, 33.

25 Kathleen Allden et al., "Mental Health and Psychosocial Support in Crisis and Conflict: Report of the Mental Health Working Group," *Prehospital and Disaster Medicine* 24, suppl. S2 (July/August 2009): s225. http://pdm.medicine.wisc.edu.

26 "Summary of the HIPAA Privacy Rule," *OCR Privacy Rule Summary,* US Department of Health and Human Services, last revised May 2003, http://www.hhs.gov/ocr/privacy/hipaa/understanding/summary/index.html.

27 Sphere Project, *Humanitarian Charter*, 25–43.

28 This section includes written material from an unpublished Première Urgence-Aide Médicale Internationale (PU-AMI) document titled "2013 BBP MH Chapter Draft," which was drafted by multiple staff of PU-AMI for the purpose of this book and then incorporated into this chapter.

29 The Border Consortium, *Programme Report January–June 2013* (Thailand: The Border Consortium, 2013), 8, http://theborderconsortium.org/resources/resources.htm#reports.

30 The Border Consortium, *Programme Report January–June 2012* (Thailand: The Border Consortium, 2012), viii, http://theborderconsortium.org/resources/resources.htm#reports.

31 The Border Consortium, *Programme Report January–June 2013*, 20.

32 Mae Tao Clinic, http://www.maetaoclinic.org.

33 Mae Tao Clinic. *Annual Report 2012* (Mae Sot, Thailand: Mae Tao Clinic, 2012), 5, 10, http://maetaoclinic.org/wp-content/uploads/2013/04/mtc-annual-report-2012.pdf.

34 Burma Border Projects, http://www.burmaborderprojects.org.

35 "Politically Explosive," *Economist*, July 13, 2013,
http://www.economist.com/news/asia/21581775-failure-clear-landmines-casts
-doubt-myanmars-peace-processes-politically-explosive.

36 "Child Soldiers Forced to Fight in Burma's Kachin Conflict," *Irrawaddy*,
http://www.irrawaddy.org/archives/25026; "Ethnic Rifts Strain Myanmar as It
Moves toward Democracy," *New York Times*, April 4, 2013,
http://www.nytimes.com/2013/04/05/world/asia/ethnic-rifts-strain-myanmar-as-it
-moves-toward-democracy.html?pagewanted=all&_r=0.

37 This program description was adapted from an unpublished PU-AMI document
titled "2013 BBP MH Chapter Draft," which was drafted by PU-AMI staff for the
purpose of this book and then incorporated into this chapter. Note that the
original document used the country name Myanmar; however, the chapter authors
have changed the country name to Burma.

38 *Protracted Displacement and Militarisation in Eastern Burma* (Thailand: Thailand
Burma Border Consortium, November 2009),
http://theborderconsortium.org/resources/resources.htm.

39 Human Rights Watch, *Ad Hoc and Inadequate: Thailand's Treatment of Refugees
and Asylum Seekers* (Human Rights Watch, September 2012).

40 ET Jackson and Associates Ltd (evaluator), *Adaptation, Resilience and Transition:
Report of the Formative Evaluation of Camp Management in the Burmese Refugee
Camps in Thailand. Long Report* (Canadian International Development Agency,
Australian Agency for International Development, Act for Peace, September 2012).

41 Première Urgence-Aide Médicale Internationale (PU-AMI), L Clouin, *Major
Psychological Needs among Population Living in Thai-Burmese Border Temporary
Shelters—Tak Province, Maela and Umpium*, unpublished, November 2006.

42 Première Urgence-Aide Médicale Internationale, "Mental Health Seeking Behavior."

43 Première Urgence-Aide Médicale Internationale, *Major Psychological Needs*.

44 Barbara Lopes Cardozo et al., "Karenni Refugees Living in Thai-Burmese Border
Camps: Traumatic Experiences, Mental Health Outcomes, and Social
Functioning," *Social Science & Medicine (1982)* 58, no. 12 (June 2004): 2640.
doi:10.1016/j.socscimed.2003.09.024.

45 Première Urgence-Aide Médicale Internationale, "Mental Health Seeking
Behavior," 20.

46 Matthew Porter and Nick Haslam, "Predisplacement and Postdisplacement
Factors Associated with Mental Health of Refugees and Internally Displaced
Persons: A Meta-analysis," *JAMA* 294, no. 5 (reprinted) (August 3, 2005): 603.

47 Barbara Lopes Cardozo et al., "Karenni Refugees"; Richard F Mollica,
"Communities of Confinement: An International Plan for Relieving the Mental
Health Crisis in the Thai-Khmer Border Camps," *Southeast Asian Journal of Social*

Science 18, no. 1 (1990); Florence Baingana, "Mental Health and Conflict," *Social Development Note: Conflict Prevention and Reconstruction* 13 (October 2003), http://worldbank.org/conflict.

48   World Health Organization and Mental Health Gap Action Programme, *mhGAP Intervention Guide*, 2010.

Bibliography

Allden, Kathleen, L Jones, I Weissbecker, M Wessells, P Bolton, TS Betancourt, Z Hijazi, A Galappatti, R Yamout, P Patel, and A Sumathipala. "Mental Health and Psychosocial Support in Crisis and Conflict: Report of the Mental Health Working Group." *Prehospital and Disaster Medicine* 24, suppl. S2 (July/August 2009): s217–s227. http://pdm.medicine.wisc.edu.

American Psychological Association. *Resilience and Recovery after War: Refugee Children and Families in the United States.* Washington, DC: American Psychological Association, 2010. http://www.apa.org/pubs/info/reports/refugees.aspx.

Baingana, Florence. "Mental Health and Conflict." *Social Development Note: Conflict Prevention and Reconstruction* 13 (October 2003). http://worldbank.org/conflict.

Betancourt, Theresa S, and Timothy Williams. "Building an Evidence Base on Mental Health Interventions for Children Affected by Armed Conflict." *Intervention* 6, no. 1 (2008): 39–56.

The Border Consortium. *Programme Report January– June 2012.* Thailand: The Border Consortium, 2012. http://theborderconsortium.org/resources/resources.htm#reports.

———. *Programme Report January– June 2013.* Thailand: The Border Consortium, 2013. http://theborderconsortium.org/resources/resources.htm#reports.

———. *Protracted Displacement and Militarisation in Eastern Burma.* Thailand: Thailand Burma Border Consortium, November 2009. http://theborderconsortium.org/resources/resources.htm.

Bronfenbrenner, Urie. "Ecological models of Human Development." *International Encyclopedia of Education* 3, 2nd ed. Oxford: Elsevier, 1994. Reprinted in *Readings on the Development of Children*, 2nd ed., edited by Mary Gauvain and Michael Cole, 37–43. New York: Freeman, 1993. http://www.psy.cmu.edu/~siegler/35bronfebrenner94.pdf.

Burma Border Projects. http://www.burmaborderprojects.org.

Cowger, Charles D. "Assessing Client Strengths: Clinical Assessment for Client Empowerment." *Social Work* 39, no. 3 (1994): 262–268.

Drumm, René D, Sharon W Pittman, and Shelly Perry. "Social Work Interventions in Refugee Camps: An Ecosystems Approach." *Journal of Social Service Research* 30, no. 2 (2003): 67–92.

Herman, Judith. *Trauma and Recovery: The Aftermath of Violence—From Domestic Abuse to Political Terror.* New York: Basic Books, 1997.

Human Rights Watch. *Ad Hoc and Inadequate: Thailand's Treatment of Refugees and Asylum Seekers.* Thailand: Human Rights Watch, September 2012.

Inter-Agency Standing Committee. *IASC Guidelines on Mental Health and Psychosocial Support in Emergency Settings.* Geneva: Inter-Agency Standing Committee (IASC), 2007.

————. "Mental Health and Psychosocial Support in Humanitarian Emergencies: What Should Humanitarian Health Actors Know?" In *Global Protection Cluster Group and IASC Reference Group for Mental Health and Psychosocial Support in Emergency Settings.* Geneva: Inter-Agency Standing Committee, 2010. http://www.who.int/mental_health/emergencies/what_humanitarian_health_actors _should_know.pdf.

Irrawady. "Child Soldiers Forced to Fight in Burma's Kachin Conflict." http://www.irrawaddy.org/archives/25026.

Jackson, ET, and Associates Ltd (evaluator). *Adaptation, Resilience and Transition: Report of the Formative Evaluation of Camp Management in the Burmese Refugee Camps in Thailand. Long Report.* Canadian International Development Agency, Australian Agency for International Development, Act for Peace, September 2012.

Lopes Cardozo, Barbara, Leisel Talley, Ann Burton, and Carol Crawford. "Karenni Refugees Living in Thai-Burmese Border Camps: Traumatic Experiences, Mental Health Outcomes, and Social Functioning." *Social Science & Medicine (1982)* 58, no. 12 (June 2004): 2637–2644. doi:10.1016/j.socscimed.2003.09.024.

Madu, Sylvester Ntomchukwu. "Traditional Healing Systems and (Western) Psychotherapy in Africa." In *African Traditional Healing: Psychotherapeutic Investigation; World Council for Psychotherapy*, edited by Sylvester Ntomchukwu Madu, Peter Kakubeire Baguma, and Alfred Pritz, 27–40. Vienna: World Council for Psychotherapy, 1997.

Mae Tao Clinic. http://www.maetaoclinic.org.

————. *Annual Report 2012.* Mae Sot, Thailand: Mae Tao Clinic, 2012. http://maetaoclinic.org/wp-content/uploads/2013/04/mtc-annual-report-2012.pdf.

Mollica, Richard F. "Communities of Confinement: An International Plan for Relieving the Mental Health Crisis in the Thai-Khmer Border Camps." *Southeast Asian Journal of Social Science* 18, no. 1 (1990): 132–152.

NASW Foundation. "NASW Social Work Pioneers." http://www.naswfoundation.org/pioneers/k/karls.html.

New York Times. "Ethnic Rifts Strain Myanmar as it Moves toward Democracy." April 4, 2013. http://www.nytimes.com/2013/04/05/world/asia/ethnic-rifts-strain-myanmar-as-it -moves-toward-democracy.html?pagewanted=all&_r=0.

"Politically Explosive." *Economist*, July 13, 2013.
   http://www.economist.com/news/asia/21581775-failure-clear-landmines-casts
   -doubt-myanmars-peace-processes-politically-explosive.

Porter, Matthew, and Nick Haslam. "Predisplacement and Postdisplacement Factors
   Associated with Mental Health of Refugees and Internally Displaced Persons: A
   Meta-Analysis." *JAMA* 294, no. 5 (reprinted) (August 3, 2005): 602–612.

Première Urgence-Aide Médicale Internationale (PU-AMI). Clouin, L. "Major
   Psychological Needs among Population Living in Thai-Burmese Border Temporary
   Shelters—Tak Province, Maela and Umpium." Thailand: Unpublished, November 2006.

———. Warf, Rainy Dawn. "Mental Health Seeking Behavior: A Rapid Ethnography of
   Two Burmese Refugee Camps." *2013 PU-AMI Mental Health Study*. Thailand:
   Première Urgence-Aide Médicale Internationale, 2013.

Russo, Rosalie J. "Applying a Strengths-Based Practice Approach in Working with
   People with Developmental Disabilities and their Families." *Families in Society* 80,
   no. 1 (January/February 1999): 25–33.

Saul, Jack. *Collective Trauma, Collective Healing: Promoting Community Resilience in
   the Aftermath of Disaster*. New York: Routledge, 2014.

Segal, Uma A, and Nazneen S Mayadas. "Assessment of Issues Facing Immigrant and
   Refugee Families." *Child Welfare* 84, no. 5 (September/October 2005): 563–583.

The Sphere Project. *Humanitarian Charter and Minimum Standards in Disaster
   Response*. Geneva: The Sphere Project, 2011.

United Nations High Commissioner for Refugees. "2013 UNHCR Country Operations
   Profile—Thailand."
   http://www.unhcr.org/pages/49e489646.html.

United Nations Secretary General. "Message for World Refugee Day."
   http://www.un.org/News/Press/docs/2012/sgsm14353.doc.htm.

US Department of Health and Human Services. "Summary of the HIPAA Privacy
   Rule." *OCR Privacy Rule Summary*. Last Revised May 2003.
   http://www.hhs.gov/ocr/privacy/hipaa/understanding/summary/index.html.

World Health Organization (WHO). *Mental Health in Emergencies*. Geneva: World
   Health Organization Department of Mental Health and Substance Dependence,
   2003.

———. "WHO Definition of Health."
   http://www.who.int/about/definition/en/print.html.

———. *A WHO Educational Package: Mental Disorders in Primary Care*. Geneva:
   World Health Organization, 1998.

World Health Organization and Mental Health Gap Action Programme. *mhGAP
   Intervention Guide for Mental, Neurological and Substance Use Disorders in
   Non-specialized Health Settings*. Geneva: World Health Organization, 2010.

Chapter 4

Community-Based Mental Health
and Psychosocial Assistance

Whitney Haruf, Jessica Bowes, Naw Dah Pachara Sura,

and Kathleen Allden

Theoretical Underpinnings

According to the UN Office for the Coordination of Humanitarian Affairs
(OCHA) definition, a complex emergency is characterized by extensive violence and loss of life, massive displacement of people, widespread damage to
societies and economies, and the need for large-scale, multifaceted humanitarian assistance, as well as obstructions to such assistance by political and
military constraints including security risks for the relief workers themselves.[1] From this definition and perspective, one can understand that a multisector coordinated approach to providing mental health and psychosocial
support is essential. To promote such an approach, the UN established, with
General Assembly Resolution 48/57, the Inter-Agency Standing Committee
(IASC). The committee consists of the heads of UN agencies such as OCHA,
United Nations Population Fund, UN High Commissioner for Refugees,
World Food Program, World Health Organization, and United Nations
Children's Fund, working along with the World Bank, the International
Committee for the Red Cross, the International Federation for the Red Cross,
and three large nongovernmental organization (NGO) consortia covering
hundreds of international NGOs. Between 2004 and 2007, the IASC orga-
nized a task force on "Mental Health and Psychosocial Support in Emergency
Settings." The resulting guidelines were published in September 2007.[2]

Providing mental health and psychosocial support for societies in developing countries affected by war, natural disaster, and political instability
presents a constellation of interrelated problems that require solutions tailored to each context and input from multiple disciplines, ranging from
medicine, nursing, psychology, social work, and public health to anthropology, social sciences, and political activism. The primary goal of the
IASC guidelines is to encourage humanitarian actors and affected communities to plan, establish, and coordinate a set of basic minimum responses using a multisector approach, with the aim of protecting and
improving people's mental health and psychosocial well-being in the midst

of a complex emergency. The guidelines outline a hierarchy of risk and describe corresponding levels of psychosocial and mental health interventions using a schematic known as the intervention pyramid.[3] The guidelines also flag potentially harmful interventions, such as "single incident debriefing," which has now been shown to be potentially damaging and therefore should not be used in these populations.[4]

The principles of the IASC guidelines and the intervention pyramid were discussed in chapter 1. Programs described in this chapter are Burmese community-based organizations that illustrate the levels of intervention presented in the guidelines.

Examples of Psychosocial and Mental Health Programs at or near the Burma Border

CONTEXTUAL BACKGROUND OF THE PARTNERSHIPS

The importance of building partnerships with local actors, organizations, and affected individuals cannot be stressed enough. The only way to build on available resources and capacities is to work closely with local partners to draw on their experiences, resilience, and strength. Working from a strengths-based perspective with a commitment to empowerment through knowledge-sharing and collaboration draws on principles of indigenization and requires the outsider to engage in self-reflection. "Indigenization" is the process of adapting knowledge or ideas imported from one culture to fit the needs of a local culture, and the development of indigenous research agendas, theories, frameworks, and solutions created by indigenous actors so that the end product is most relevant to their society.[5] One must examine and draw on the inherent strengths and resilience of the local community, as well as adapt techniques and theories so as not to place them on top of another culture's unique situation and characteristics. To do this, one must assume that the power differentials in place in societies globally and locally are at work in one's relationships, whether overtly or subtly. There is no formula for understanding how one's social positionality will interact with both the culture that one is an outsider to and the unique experiences and living histories that each party brings to the relationship. However, there will undoubtedly be moments when these ingrained systems of oppression play out.

Authors Jessica Bowes and Naw Dah are currently working together in the Mae Sot region of the Thai-Burma border. Jessica works for Burma Border Projects (BBP) as the adult mental health and psychosocial services director. Naw Dah works for the Karen Department of Health and Welfare (KDHW) as the mental health coordinator. Jessica and Naw Dah are currently working closely together on developing a mental health program for KDHW. Jessica is a white, educated, middle-class woman from the west coast of America with heritage stemming from Eastern European Jewish and Irish and German Catholic roots. Naw Dah is an ethnically Karen woman raised in Karen State until her early teenage years, when she moved to the Thai side of the Thai-Burma border to attend school. She has lived in Thailand since her move twelve years ago, while her parents and other family members reside in her native village. These two authors stress the point that where a person comes from helps create who she or he is, and this unquestionably enters into every relationship. Because of Jessica's background, she must be aware of stepping into a role of "expert" or a position of power and must shy away from asserting herself, slipping into "othering" her Karen colleagues, or speaking more than she listens. Naw Dah should be wary of "othering" Jessica, discrediting Karen cultural knowledge and wisdom gained from life experiences, or deferring to Jessica in the face of Western and Karen cultural contradictions. The ways their identities intersect are complex, but keeping one eye on these issues at all times, working slowly, and listening deeply will serve them, their working relationships, and the resultant outcomes well.

KAREN DEPARTMENT OF HEALTH AND WELFARE

Saw D is a 34-year-old health worker from Karen State who attended a three-day mental health training as part of his annual program training with the KDHW. Trainers discussed how fear, anger, and sadness generated by trauma can grow, spread, and cause long-term reactions in the body and mind. Saw D spoke up. He said that he had never before considered how all these things are connected. Three years ago his 4-year-old daughter died from lack of access to health care. After her death he found himself thinking too much and not wanting to talk with others, leading to a long period of isolation. He started worrying that other people would think he was crazy because they said that he should just have another baby and everything would be fine, but he could not make himself forget the loss of his child. The group used Saw D's story to highlight how and why trauma symptoms persist, how a community's response to one's emotions affects one's mental health, and then began to talk about coping skills and cultural norms for healing from trauma. One participant stated, "There are many people I've seen in villages in Karen State who had trauma, and we all just thought they were crazy because of how they behaved. People were scared of them, didn't know what to do to help or what was wrong . . . now I think I understand better."

KDHW was established over twenty years ago to provide free primary health care and disease-specific health care programs to the thousands of displaced people in all seven districts of Karen State in Burma. Karen make up the third-largest ethnic group in Burma. Karen State, also known as Kayin State in Myanmar, is a region highly affected by war, violence, political oppression, forced relocation, and many forms of human rights abuse.

KDHW trains indigenous staff as community health workers and medics to deliver services through their thirty-seven mobile health clinics (MHCs), each of which employs an average of ten local staff and serves a population of 3,500 to 5,000 individuals. From these MHCs, health workers address problems such as malaria, vitamin deficiency, intestinal parasites, and trauma injuries from land mines through treatment and prevention via community education and health promotion activities.

The efficacy of MHCs' mobility is twofold. First, they are prepared to pack up and move at any moment in the event of a security threat and, second, about half of the clinic staff regularly travels within their designated coverage area to provide education, host awareness-raising events, and provide disease screenings. These "backpack" medics and health workers receive their initial six months of training at KDHW's central office, located in Thailand. Medics and health workers return annually or semiannually to the central office for further trainings.

Given the stresses they face in their work, KDHW health workers are particularly at risk of developing a number of mental health problems such as anxiety, depression, and posttraumatic stress disorder (PTSD). They must endure perilous security situations because clinics and mobile medic teams have often been the targets of human rights violations by the Burmese military.[6] Furthermore, as professionals who repeatedly listen to narratives of fear, pain, and suffering from their patients, KDHW health workers may be susceptible to developing vicarious trauma, compassion fatigue, and ensuing burnout.[7] Under these demanding circumstances, normal coping mechanisms may prove ineffective, and health workers may develop persistent psychological symptoms, greatly increasing their risk for drug and alcohol dependence and abuse. Additionally, such mental health issues may adversely affect health workers' performance, leading to compromised efficacy in treating their target populations. The medics and community health workers have shown marked resilience in the face of trauma. However, KDHW leaders recognize that further support for health workers is needed to maintain their mental well-being and are trying to address this need.

Community-Based Interventions (Outreach, Support Groups, Training, and Education)

The second-largest layer of the intervention pyramid, community-based interventions, involves psychosocial support and mental illness prevention. These programs can take a range of forms depending on the target community's needs. KDHW, in partnership with BBP, has been developing a mental health program with a focus on psycho-education, promotion of healthy coping, and improvement of KDHW health workers' own well-being. This is meant to be a first but important step toward the inclusion of mental health services in all its work by demonstrating the importance and benefits of mental health workshops at an experiential level with health workers themselves. Because mental health issues are considered taboo and few people are willing to admit or often even recognize mental illness as a health issue, KDHW and BBP aim to utilize the health workers as a gateway to the community. A starting point must therefore be to help health workers articulate mental health as an important issue to themselves and to patients in the field. To do this, one must meet the health workers where they are and with a curriculum that is accessible to them.

The primary goal of this project is to develop the first culturally competent Karen mental health and counseling program, with two main objectives: first, to reduce health workers' risk of developing negative mental health effects by enhancing self-care and encouraging culturally appropriate ways of coping; and second, to train health workers about basic mental health concepts and culturally relevant counseling skills to better serve their patients. This will contribute to the sustainability of KDHW's work as a whole, and, ultimately, will improve the quality and stability of community-based health care in Karen State.

KDHW and BBP are working on a customized curriculum for mental health training of KDHW health workers that draws together traditional Karen training methods, Karen cultural ways of knowing, and Western social work–based mental health and counseling principles. The curricula and educational materials for workshops are developed based on what is most relevant to the learning needs of the health workers. The training topics include an exploration of stigma and discrimination of mental illness in the community; understanding principles of mental health and its contributing factors; self-care and coping skills; understanding stress and trauma; counseling techniques; and positive communication skills. For longer trainings, more information on substance abuse/dependence and mental illness basics is provided.

The process of curriculum development is conducted in a trainer-of-trainers (TOT) model, with the aim of building the capacity of the KDHW mental health team to have an in-depth knowledge of the content and a familiarity and confidence in the training methods and materials. The TOT model has been used in the health sector to transfer knowledge from more highly trained professionals to others working in the field with strong community ties who have not had the same level of education.[8] "In resource-poor countries with few mental health professionals, the training of community-level workers builds capacity to deliver psychosocial care to large populations of survivors" and ensures that the programs are appropriate and sensitive to the culture and language of the program participants.[9] The model prescribes that the mental health professional is responsible for planning and implementing the trainings, preparing lectures and experiential activities, and developing materials for both the trainees and those who will use the services. The trainees then develop the skills to train more community members, allowing a larger number of services to be offered where mental health professionals are scarce.

KDHW and BBP are employing the TOT model with the aim of phasing out the presence of a BBP trainer altogether as the KDHW staff gain more confidence in the material and in their skills as trainers. After the initial project phase, the KDHW mental health workers will be able to conduct trainings with help from BBP consultants, and after the second phase, they will be able to conduct trainings independently, with BBP supervision if so desired.

Despite the TOT model's high success rates and far-reaching design, it is not free from drawbacks. Because the goal is to eventually phase out the presence of trained professionals, the material could become watered down as successive groups of trainers provide trainings. In a field as varied, dynamic, and nuanced as mental health, certain concepts are bound to be lost through misunderstanding or the chosen focus of a particular trainer, and when that trainer has not been exposed to a full education in mental health, some key ideas or approaches may go missing. Furthermore, community psychosocial workers are often tasked with addressing and providing training on challenging, specialized, and high-needs cases. For this reason, it becomes important that a mental health professional be available for ongoing supervision or technical advising as needed, to uphold both the quality of care offered in the community and to support the well-being of the community-level workers.

As curricula are developed, KHDW and BBP are conducting trainings to pilot training materials and exercises. Trainings take place in various areas along the Thai-Burma border and are provided either at the beginning or end of the health workers' semiannual or annual refresher trainings. BBP and KDHW trainers interview the program coordinator of the group scheduled to receive the training to gain a sense of the health workers' levels of experience, exposure to past mental health trainings, and interest in various topics. Based on participation, pre- and post-feedback, and evaluations, BBP and KDHW trainers adjust the materials and exercises accordingly for future trainings. In this way, the training program evaluation process during the pilot stage is both qualitative and quantitative. It is crucial to the success of the project that the health workers (beneficiaries) are included in all phases and activities.

Curative Interventions (Individualized Treatment and Referral for Those with Mental Illness)

The very top of the intervention pyramid, covering the smallest area, is dedicated to specialized, individualized mental health interventions for people struggling with more severe conditions, whether triggered by an organic or biological cause, extreme experiences, or some combination of factors. These services can take the form of inpatient or outpatient care, talking or medication therapies, outreach, rehabilitation, or medical, legal, or social assistance. A number of factors are causing more community-based organizations in the border region, including KDHW, to recognize the great need for more extensive mental health and psychosocial services, and also to actively advocate for the creation and inclusion of such programs within their existing structures.

Recognizing the need for mental health services in Karen State, KDHW is in the planning stages of including mental health services at each of its MHCS. Because the medics and health workers in the community are well respected, trusted, and looked to for answers regarding illnesses, they are often approached by community members for assistance with mental health problems for family, friends, or neighbors. Furthermore, because there are no state-run health clinics or mental health institutions in Karen State, patients struggling with severe symptoms are brought to the MHCS for services. Each of the KDHW staff members specializes in one medical field, such as malaria, tuberculosis, or immunization, and thus they have little to no knowledge of or access to resources about mental health and mental illness issues. They are often faced with trying to help affected community members to the best of their ability despite a lack of training and a duty to fulfill their other job requirements.

KDHW is expanding its program to include a "mobile counselor" at each of its clinics. This counselor will be a community health worker who receives specialized training in mental health, mental illness, and chemical dependency issues, as well as culturally sensitive counseling techniques. He or she will be the focal point in the region for providing counseling, instituting principles of psychological first aid, facilitating community discussions about these topics with the aim of destigmatizing mental health challenges, and providing psycho-education and trainings at respective clinics. Hence, the mental health focal point will be a community health worker who provides both curative and preventive services. Because of the high level of basic need in Karen State, the lack of knowledge around mental health challenges, and the overwhelming stigma of mental illness, KDHW acknowledges the need to begin a larger conversation about these matters at a community level among both its health workers and villagers before employing backpack counselors.

FORTUNE: SHAN BURMESE PSYCHOSOCIAL ORGANIZATION

Dink is a 13-year-old Shan girl from Burma who is developmentally delayed from cerebral malaria in early childhood. After the family was forced to flee Burma, Dink suffered from anxiety and social phobia; her daily functioning became very limited. In Thailand, she had only her sister and brother to care for her, and because they had very few options for mental health support and limited understanding of her disabilities, they treated her poorly and kept her on the porch night and day under harsh conditions. The director of a local Burmese community organization called Fortune learned of Dink's situation and began doing regular home visits, giving material and emotional support to her and her siblings, but knew Dink needed services beyond his scope. He found an orphanage in a nearby city that accepted her into its facility and began to provide physical therapy and rehabilitation. Fortune's director stayed in touch with the girl and her siblings. He reported that her family was very grateful, not only because it eased their own burden but because they knew Dink was receiving care and support that they were unable to give her.

Shan Burmese are the largest ethnic minority group in Burma. Like the Karen, these villagers have experienced widespread and systematic persecution for decades, and the attacks have not abated despite recent steps by the Burmese government toward reform, such as easing media restrictions and releasing some political prisoners.[10] For example, in April 2013 over one thousand Shan from sixteen villages were forced to flee their homes because of new military operations by the Burmese army. Human rights violations include executions, beatings (including of children), forced labor, conscription as porters, use as "human shields" with resulting death and injuries from land mines recently laid in the villages, and looting and destruction of villagers' property.[11] At times the oppressive effect of the Burmese army is even more far-reaching; for instance, in March 2011 over 30,000 villagers were displaced by large-scale military offensives, including documented gang rapes of village women by the Burmese army.[12] The effect of this displacement forces some Shan to live in the jungle in unofficial IDP (internally displaced persons) camps inside Shan State, whereas others seek refuge in neighboring Thailand. An estimated 6 million Shan have been driven over the border into northern Thailand. However, unlike the Karen, the Shan have been denied official recognition as refugees and therefore are not afforded international assistance through registered refugee camps.[13] Many eke out a living working, often seven days a week, on Thai-owned farms, plantations, and factories across northern Thailand.

Fortune, a Shan Burmese community-based organization (CBO), was formed under the support, guidance, and training of a US-based organization called SalusWorld, in response to the mental health and psychosocial needs of the Shan migrant workers in thirteen outlying communities around Fang in northwest Thailand. SalusWorld staff, including coauthor Whitney Haruf, provided the technical expertise in mental health and organizational development for a small group of Shan schoolteachers and medics eager to step into the role of part-time peer counselors and educators. SalusWorld's capacity-building approach and partnership with Fortune progressed to the point where Fortune currently functions independently and has grown in its capacity well beyond the initial trainings provided to them, finding innovative ways to strengthen the migrant communities in which its members live. Fortune's programs consist of a variety of interventions that fulfill all three mental health–related categories of the intervention pyramid: support groups, outreach, training, and education on the community-based level; counseling, home visits, and coping strategies on the preventive level; and referral to specialists for those with mental illness on the curative level. Each level of the intervention pyramid and its corresponding interventions, as demonstrated by Fortune's activities in the Shan migrant communities, will be discussed in turn.

Community-Based Interventions (Outreach, Support Groups, Training, and Education)
Fortune has led a variety of activities and outreach services since its inception, responding and adapting through each phase of its existence and slowly growing into its identity over time. One of Fortune's key tenets has

always been direct outreach to the Shan migrant communities spread out over the areas surrounding Fang near the border of Shan State. While Fortune is associated with Tin Tad Clinic, a small medical clinic in Waing Wai village that provides Shan migrants with free medical care, it became clear at an early stage that having a counseling center based solely at the clinic would not provide the support the community needed. Migrant workers laboring on orange and onion farms and in brick-making factories often work seven days a week, which, unless someone is seriously ill and forced to visit the clinic, does not allow for visits during clinic operating hours. Many of the migrants have no legal standing and feel insecure traveling away from the farms where they reside.

Fortune's response was to visit the farms in the evening, after the migrants had finished laboring for the day. It created a space to meet with the workers out of makeshift quarters, laying down mats and setting up electric generators. To attract attention to this unknown subject of mental health and begin educating migrants on psychosocial issues, the staff presented puppet shows with homemade puppets to entertain the workers while educating them about such things as alcohol abuse, domestic violence, and HIV/AIDS. They also drew cartoons on large posters pertaining to the subject of stress, such as depicting a woman carrying two baskets on a pole in the traditional farmer fashion, one that was manageable and represented a healthy amount of stress, and another that was so heavy it was backbreaking and represented an unhealthy amount of stress. These cultural adaptations for understanding concepts of mental health proved useful to the migrants attending.

The psycho-educational outreach slowly grew to embody further education on a variety of subjects relevant to migrants' lives, using several kinds of media to attract interest. In its current metamorphosis, Fortune members and volunteer youth provide outreach to a different community each month to educate migrant workers about the foundations of mental health, in particular stress, as it is deemed most applicable to their daily lives. They also inform the community of other services specifically catering to Shan people, including Tin Tad Clinic and a program Fortune has developed and received outside funding for called the Migrant Worker Empowerment Program. This program staffs a Fortune member at the Fang District Office (a Thai government outpost) whose sole purpose is to offer administrative support and interpretation for Shan migrant workers who come to the district office to apply for a temporary work permit and other services. Fortune also shows an educational video it created, which portrays the story of a young man who becomes HIV-positive after sleeping with a prostitute (not an uncommon occurrence in Burmese migrant communities across Thailand) and his process of grappling with his HIV status. The video includes scenes portraying him visiting the Tin Tad Clinic for testing and receiving the diagnosis, breaking this news to his wife, struggling with feelings of denial and anger, starting medications, and then finally reconciling with his wife. This is often the first time Shan migrants have heard of the causes and treatment for HIV. Following the video showing, Fortune closes the outreach by distributing snacks and practical items such as laundry soap or kitchen utensils to the families.

Another key component of Fortune's programming involves identifying and connecting with natural leaders, helpers, and concerned citizens in the migrant communities—a few of whom hold the distinction of resident traditional healer—and bringing these individuals on board to serve as community networkers. The community networkers currently come from seven of the migrant communities, have been selected and trained by Fortune staff, and are given a transportation stipend by Fortune in return for being on-the-ground resources monitoring the well-being of the Shan migrants at the farm and offering on-site support and basic counseling services to those in need. The community networkers have a monthly meeting with Fortune to discuss the mental health and psychosocial problems their fellow workers are facing, share the counseling that was provided, and receive suggestions and guidance from Fortune members—in essence, this meeting acts as an informal case consultation. In cases of difficult peer/client situations, Fortune follows up with the clients directly and gives more focused assistance to the community networker. All these outreach activities in the migrant communities, in essence, promote healthy living and resiliency; they also provide mental health resources where needed.

Because the teachers and medics who make up Fortune are viewed as leaders in the community, easier trust-building and faith in the mental health and psychosocial activities Fortune offers is facilitated. As can be typical for many community-based organizations, Fortune's role does not stop here, however; the community faces a variety of shortages and only a select few have had the educational opportunities and experiences needed to meet these shortages, so Fortune fulfills other roles in the Shan community as well. The director of Fortune teaches Shan traditional dancing and drumming to Shan children and adolescents. Fortune holds performances in temples and event centers across the area, with the express desire of preserving Shan cultural traditions and bestowing them in the younger generations while in the midst of assimilation into Thai school systems and society. Fortune has also created a community center for children and youth to attend after school, where it provides extracurricular education in such areas as English-language exercises, arts and crafts, and computer skills. As part of the Migrant Worker Empowerment Program, a member of Fortune broadcasts a weekly program through the local Shan radio station, sharing information about the Thai legal system and migrant worker rights. Fortune, through its extensive community outreach, has become a fixture in the Fang area and now networks with leading Thai and international organizations working in the area. In addition, to better monitor its work, Fortune has created extensive tracking and reporting systems and is currently in the process of analyzing data collected from a comprehensive community-based survey it recently conducted.

Preventive Interventions (Counseling and Emotional Support, Coping Strategies)

Whereas community-based interventions are provided for a significant portion of an affected population, preventive interventions are used with a smaller segment of the population that has been severely affected by traumatic situations. Paralleling this smaller demographic, Fortune provides supportive services to Shan migrants experiencing the impact of traumatic events, but serves a smaller percentage of the population through these efforts. Differences in opinion are often voiced by cross-cultural mental health professionals on best practices for ethnic Burmese receiving counseling services and on whether group or individual counseling is most culturally relevant; Fortune has sidestepped the debate by providing both types.

While Fortune staff are available at various times at Tin Tad Clinic, the majority of the individual counseling services provided are through home visits in the migrant communities, recognizing that those most in need often are unable to avail themselves of these services at the clinic because of a variety of obstacles and limitations. Fortune members, either through their own contacts or through the community navigators' referrals, visit at-risk Shan migrants on a regular basis to listen to their problems and provide support. Occasional referrals also are made to Fortune by Shan traditional healers with whom Fortune has created a trusted relationship and who recognize both the value of Fortune's work and, at times, their own limited capacity to aid those with mental illness. As one Shan spirit medium stated, he is only able to help those with mental disturbance half the time, and can refer those who need additional assistance to Fortune.

Another component of Fortune's preventive interventions is a monthly support group. The support group is held in the local Buddhist temple (the vast majority of Shan are Buddhist), in the Fortune office, or in various migrant communities, and offered to specific populations, such as women or youth. The topics vary according to both the overall general findings from informal needs assessments Fortune has gathered and the immediate needs of each group. Topics frequently discussed in the support groups are family conflict, domestic violence, alcohol abuse, divorce, and stress and worry. Fortune members take turns leading the group, introducing the topic using their own life experience, and then giving space for everyone attending to voice their concerns and personal struggles. Out of this shared interaction, group members naturally support each other, offering suggestions and practical assistance. There is frequently the recognition that these struggles are shared struggles, as nearly everyone not only can identify with the effects of violence and displacement in their lives but also can acknowledge the ways they have shown resiliency in the face of such hardships.

Curative Interventions (Referrals to Specialists for Those with Mental Illness)

Mental disorders that present prior to an emergency are often exacerbated following the emergency; the emergency can also be a significant enough stressor to trigger the onset of a mental disorder. While the percentage of the population suffering from mental illness during the aftermath of a complex emergency is a small percentage of the whole population, they are the most vulnerable and show the greatest need. In such a low-resource setting as rural northwest Thailand, and with the added factor of Shan Burmese being undocumented in the country, few specialized psychiatric services are provided for those with mental illness.

Fortune has provided for those in its community with severe mental illness or in altered states of mind to the best of its ability; however, referral to trained professionals and facilities in outlying areas is necessary for this select population. Fortune members have gone to some length to find feasible resources for clients with psychiatric and developmental disabilities. For instance, staff members have taken clients to Chiang Mai, a city three hours away, to meet with psychiatrists and receive treatment in psychiatric hospitals. They have advocated for undocumented clients in local hospitals, explaining their clients' conditions and paying for psychiatric medications. Fortune has referred clients in psychiatric distress to Shan traditional healers, including spirit mediums, traditional medicine doctors, astrologers, and palmists. It has also expanded its reach from referral to psychiatric specialists and built relationships with staff at nearby facilities such as orphanages to place youth with severe disturbances in their care, as can be seen in the following case.

FOUNDATION FOR EDUCATION AND DEVELOPMENT:
BURMESE MIGRANT HUMAN RIGHTS ORGANIZATION
Palu died at age 34 from TB and HIV/AIDS far from his home and family. He was an ethnic Burman man from Rangoon who received end of life care for over three years at a temporary shelter for migrants in southern Thailand operated by a Burmese community organization called FED (Foundation for Education and Development). In his last days, Palu was incredibly thin with a greyish pallor to his skin and a vacancy in his eyes. He suffered a great deal through his illnesses and his death may have come as a relief. The health coordinator of FED and his coworkers cared for Palu until his death. They gave him reassurance and support, including sharing lessons from Buddhist teachings to help ameliorate Palu's fears and enable him to prepare for his impending death. Palu had been employed by a fishery; the fishing industry in Thailand is known for human rights abuses. Fishing boats typically dock at isolated ports where the only surrounding facilities are bars and brothels charging extortionist prices and pressuring the men to use the services, thereby exposing them to high risk of contracting HIV. When Palu died his funeral service was very simple and brief, with some construction worker friends and shelter staff in attendance.

Southern Thailand, with its paradisiacal beaches and turquoise waters, has a thriving tourist industry, attracting vacationers from all over the world. Burmese migrants, perhaps unremarked by foreign travelers, are the backbone of this service industry. Their proficient English-language skills enable them to hold jobs as wait staff, hotel clerks, and shop assistants. They also work in remote areas tourists do not often frequent, laboring on Thai-owned farms, plantations, and fisheries, and working construction. Because of their illegal status and vulnerability in the country, exploitation is rampant, and workers experience as normal, and even expected, situations such as no salary for months or unsafe work conditions. Many highly publicized reports have come out in recent years of Burmese migrants as victims of both sex and labor trafficking. One common report involves young men trafficked by Thai fishing industries. According to a report by the International Organization for Migration (IOM), the men are promised jobs and lured onto boats where they are kept indefinitely, working eighteen to twenty-two hours a day, often near starvation, and even killed by boat captains if too sick or weak to continue working.[14] It is so bleak that some risk suicide, throwing themselves overboard when far out to sea, to escape the servitude. The fishing industry is notorious for its human rights abuses, but other industries that feed on illegal labor are often not much more humane.

Burmese migrants face many difficulties and have little recourse for dealing with exploitation and deportation. For example, when coauthor Whitney Haruf was working in Khao Lak, a staff member with FED told her that 150 migrants in Tablamu, a fishing village they had visited a few days prior, had been arrested for not having proper work permits. Threats of deportation and other extreme kinds of stress can take a heavy toll on the migrants' psychological condition, not to mention traumatic experiences already endured under Burma's military regime before arriving in Thailand.

FED is a grassroots human rights organization based in southern Thailand in Khao Lak, Phang Nga Province. FED has been active in providing services to Burmese migrants since the 2004 Indian Ocean tsunami severely struck parts of southern Thailand, including Khao Lak. Many Burmese migrants of illegal status living in the area who survived the tsunami received limited aid from the Thai government; a Burmese human rights activist founded FED in response to the needs of the Burmese community. FED's purpose is to support Burmese migrant workers in the area, including fighting for labor rights and giving legal assistance, providing education for the migrant workers' children, offering shelter to the most vulnerable, and running a number of other health and educational programs. FED has expanded since its inception; its current facilities consist of an administrative and legal office, a learning center for Burmese migrant children, a small orphanage/children's home, a Women's Education and Development Association Center, a small health clinic, and a temporary shelter for patients and migrants in need. FED also has a branch office in Mae Sot, and there is consideration of developing a branch inside Burma in the near future, too.

Unlike Fortune and KDHW, FED is not providing services for a specific ethnic group; the ethnic makeup of the Burmese migrant population in the Khao Lak area is diverse because of its location and opportunities for employment. The ethnic groups include Dawei, Mon, Rakine, Karenni, Burman, Chin, and Myeik. While FED's primary focus is not mental health and psychosocial services, it has incorporated psychosocial support in a number of its programs. Concurrently, FED recognizes the need for more comprehensive psychological supportive services and in recent years has taken steps to enhance its programs, in particular its community health program, by partnering with international NGOs to provide technical expertise on culturally relevant mental health and psychosocial issues. One such partnership has been with SalusWorld, mentioned earlier. Looking to build the capacity of FED staff to address the current challenges they are facing in serving their communities, SalusWorld staff, including coauthor Whitney Haruf, have begun to provide technical assistance to FED's community health workers, teachers, women's association staff, and interns.

Community-Based Interventions (Outreach, Support Groups, Training, and Education)

Foundational to FED's community-based interventions are its outreach programs, which have proven to be highly effective in connecting with and providing services for an extensive number of marginalized migrants. At times, staff will drive for several hours to reach distant Burmese communities that otherwise would have no access to much-needed resources. One prime example of FED's innovative outreach is its community health worker (CHW) program. The CHW program trains Burmese who live in migrant communities, such as on farms and in fisheries, to treat basic medical problems, and efforts are being made to train increasing numbers of migrant workers. Recently, a program that began as seventeen CHWs employed by FED grew over a mere five weeks to eighty-nine CHWs, through a training-of-trainers model. With assistance from the health coordinator, each of the seventeen CHWs were responsible for training five new CHWs across twelve communities on basic health care. The program was so successful that FED has plans for advanced trainings. FED supplemented a health manual from the World Health Organization with psychosocial training material provided by coauthor Whitney Haruf that covers basic counseling skills and progressive relaxation practice, incorporating for the first time mental health interventions into the standard community health curricula. FED staff expressed a desire for further training regarding psycho-education, and specifically on the effectiveness and benefits of counseling, how it differs from taking medication, and how to provide short-term brief counseling in order to adapt to the demands and mobility of the migrant worker lifestyle.

Another thriving outreach program under the umbrella of FED is the Women's Education and Development Association (WEDA). WEDA staff run health and psycho-education groups several times a month in migrant communities across the area, catering largely to women but inviting men to participate too. They educate clients on reproductive health issues such as family planning, pre- and postnatal care, and immunizations. They have developed materials that work for an illiterate audience, drawing pictures depicting various reproductive health issues. Staff members also hold focus groups on women's rights and gender-based violence and provide vocational training to women. They give support to domestic violence survivors and meet with the survivors' husbands—recognizing that most Burmese women don't leave their husbands—to talk about making changes in the husband's behavior. In addition, WEDA does medical checkups in the community and provides health education for Burmese students and teachers every two weeks.

FED employs several other fruitful outreach projects to educate and inform migrant workers. FED's Health Department broadcasts a weekly radio program through collaboration with a local Thai station to educate migrants about health concerns and to publicize resources offered by FED and others in Khao Lak. FED also has a staff person working three days a week at a local Thai hospital providing free Burmese-Thai translation and supplying Burmese patients with information about FED's health services for further care after discharged. It also provides emergency transport and financial assistance to migrants who need medical care.

One of FED's strengths is in its collaboration with a variety of governmental and nongovernmental organizations. FED has invested in building positive relations with local Thai government officials and other authorities through facilitation of special events and workshops to build friendship and understanding between local Thais and Burmese migrants. The special events, according to FED's website, include "sports tournaments among different Thai and Burmese communities, jointly held religious ceremonies and other community-focused activities."[15] All these community peace-building activities make a difference in strengthening ties between local Thais and their Burmese neighbors, with the aim not only of improving relations but also of decreasing violence toward Burmese migrants by Thais in the Khao Lak area. In addition, relationships have been cultivated with international organizations in the area, as well as with other Burmese CBOs and community groups. For instance, FED has developed and deepened its partnership with Mae Tao Clinic; Dr. Cynthia Maung, its founder and director, visited FED's office in Khao Lak and invited FED staff to take part Mae Tao's supplemental health trainings. In addition, Mae Tao Clinic sent three staff to work in FED's community health worker program for one year.

FED's education programs have provided education for migrant workers' children when nothing else existed for them and have developed a number of thriving educational programs. In brief, it has created learning centers (unofficial schools); a nursery for children under five years; and educational support toward integration into Thai schools, including an outreach program for youth ages 12 and 13 who have completed their studies at the learning centers and who want to continue their education under FED's tutorship in order to qualify for the local Thai middle schools.

Preventive Interventions (Counseling and Emotional Support, Coping Strategies)

Training the CHWs in basic counseling skills is a significant step toward providing for the emotional well-being of the CHWs' patients. Concurrently, if coping strategies such as progressive relaxation are offered in the migrant communities to those the CHWs determine are destabilized and struggling because of stress and other factors, these efforts can lead to preventive interventions and hopefully help alleviate some of the mental and emotional disturbances in the migrants they treat. In addition, WEDA staff provide aspects of psychosocial support and counseling to the women they serve, such as domestic violence support groups and individual meetings with women who have reproductive health problems.

While incorporation of mental health and psychosocial counseling in the stricter sense may not be applied extensively at this time, an increasing number of the staff has incorporated basic counseling skills such as active listening and giving encouragement in a natural, organic fashion in their work with migrants. The head of FED's Health Program has implemented the most direct therapeutic interventions at FED. He mans the small medical clinic, providing not just first aid care for all Burmese migrants that drop in during the week but also offering counseling support while treating these patients. He provides ongoing counseling for patients residing at FED's temporary shelter, located adjacent to the medical clinic. The shelter is often at full capacity, housing approximately twenty people and supplying free food and lodging to those migrants who are most vulnerable or seriously ill, including rape and domestic violence survivors and patients with serious medical problems such as HIV, tuberculosis, or malaria.

FED's health coordinator stated that many of the patients suffer from depression, due in large part to being ill and lacking medical supplies to adequately treat their illnesses. They often express feelings of hopelessness and worry about a quickly approaching death. He gives encouragement and emotional support and attempts to lift their spirits out of their bleak situations through talking to them about Buddhist dharma, or teachings of the Buddha, as a way to cope with their suffering. For those who do pass away while in the shelter, he prepares the body of each patient, says prayers for the patient, and arranges the funeral rites and cremation. The fact that he looks after the patients from the time of sickness through the dying process shows the extent of his caring as a medic and counselor, and expands the general Western notion of therapy from attending to one's emotional well-being to an incorporation of support for one's spiritual well-being, too.

Curative Interventions (Individualized Treatments and Referrals for Those with Mental Illness)

For those in the migrant communities who suffer from severe and prolonged emotional disturbance and undiagnosed mental illness, the options for psychiatric support available to FED are very limited. Similar to Fortune, FED staff provide for those in extreme states as best they can through community structures and access to limited medications. However, whenever they are able, they refer these individuals to specialized psychiatric services, such as local Thai hospitals, and continue to offer supportive services to them through the length of their treatment.

Notes

1   United Nations Office for the Coordination of Humanitarian Affairs, *OCHA Orientation Handbook on Complex Emergencies* (Geneva: United Nations, 1999).

2   Ibid., ii–ix.

3   Inter-Agency Standing Committee, *IASC Guidelines on Mental Health and Psychosocial Support in Emergency Settings* (Geneva: Inter-Agency Standing Committee, 2007), 5–13.

4   Ibid., 1–5; Suzanna C Rose et al., "Psychological Debriefing for Preventing Post Traumatic Stress Disorder (PTSD)," in *Cochrane Database of Systematic Reviews*, ed. The Cochrane Collaboration and Suzanna C Rose (Chichester, UK: John Wiley & Sons, 2002),
    http://www.ncbi.nlm.nih.gov/pubmedhealth/PMH0010736/.

5   Jayashree Nimmagadda and Charles D Cowger, "Cross-Cultural Practice: Social Worker Ingenuity in the Indigenization of Practice Knowledge," *International Social Work* 42, no. 3 (July 1, 1999): 261–276, doi:10.1177/002087289904200302; Huang Yunong and Zhang Xiong, "A Reflection on the Indigenization Discourse in Social Work," *International Social Work* 51, no. 5 (September 1, 2008): 611–622, doi:10.1177/0020872808093340.

6   Karen Human Rights Group, *Enduring Hunger and Repression: Food Scarcity, Internal Displacement, and the Continued Use of Forced Labour in Toungoo District* (Thailand: Karen Human Rights Group, 2004); Karen Human Rights Group, *Attacks and Displacement in Nyaunglebin District* (Thailand: Karen Human Rights Group, 2010).

7   Kathleen M Palm, Melissa A Polusny, and Victoria M Follette, "Vicarious Traumatization: Potential Hazards and Interventions for Disaster and Trauma Workers," *Prehospital and Disaster Medicine* 19, no. 1 (March 2004): 73–78; I Lisa McCann and Laurie Anne Pearlman, "Vicarious Traumatization: A Framework for Understanding the Psychological Effects of Working with Victims," *Journal of Traumatic Stress* 3, no. 1 (January 1, 1990): 131–149, doi:10.1007/BF00975140; Ronnie Janoff-Bulman, *Shattered Assumptions: Towards a New Psychology of Trauma* (New York: Free Press, 1992); Ayala Pines and Christina Maslach, "Characteristics of Staff Burnout in Mental Health Settings," *Hospital & Community Psychiatry* 29, no. 4 (April 1978): 233–237.

8   Beverley Lloyd et al., "Building Capacity for Evidence-Based Practice in the Health Promotion Workforce: Evaluation of a Train-the-Trainer Initiative in NSW," *Health Promotion Journal of Australia: Official Journal of Australian Association of Health Promotion Professionals* 20, no. 2 (August 2009): 151–154.

9   Susan M Becker, "Psychosocial Care for Women Survivors of the Tsunami Disaster in India," *American Journal of Public Health* 99, no. 4 (April 2009): 654, doi:10.2105/AJPH.2008.146571.

10   Human Rights Watch, *World Report 2012: Burma* (Human Rights Watch, 2012), http://www.hrw.org/world-report-2012/world-report-2012-burma.

11   US Campaign for Burma, *Shan Human Rights Foundation: Urgent Update on the Human Rights Situation in Shan State, Burma*, April 5, 2013, http://www.uscampaignforburma.org/statements/3108-shrf-urgent-update-on-the -human-rights-situation-in-shan-state-burma.html.

12   Shan Human Rights Foundation and Shan Women's Action Network, *Rape Cases Documented During Burma Army Offensive in Northern Shan State Since 13 March 2011* (Shan Human Rights Foundation; Shan Women's Action Network, 2011), http://www.shanhumanrights.org/images/stories/Action_Update/Files/summary %20of%20rape%20cases%20during%20burma%20army%20offensive%20in%20n. shan%20state.pdf.

13   SalusWorld, "Thailand: Aiding Displaced Shan," http://salusworld.org/current/southeast-asia.php.

14   International Organization for Migration, *Trafficking of Fisherman in Thailand* (Thailand: International Organization for Migration, January 14, 2011), http://www.iiom.int/jahia/webdav/shared/shared/mainsite/activities/countries /doc/Thailand/Trafficking-of-Fisherman-Thailand.pdf.

15   Grassroots Human Rights Education and Development, "Public Relations and Community Peace Building," http://www.ghre.org/en/programs/migrant-development/336-public-relations-a -community-peace-building/.

Bibliography

Becker, Susan M. "Psychosocial Care for Women Survivors of the Tsunami Disaster in India." *American Journal of Public Health* 99, no. 4 (April 2009): 654–658. doi:10.2105/AJPH.2008.146571.

Grassroots Human Rights Education and Development. "Public Relations and Community Peace Building." http://www.ghre.org/en/programs/migrant-development/336-public-relations-a-community-peace-building/.

Human Rights Watch. *World Report 2012: Burma*. Human Rights Watch, 2012. http://www.hrw.org/world-report-2012/world-report-2012-burma.

Inter-Agency Standing Committee. *IASC Guidelines on Mental Health and Psychosocial Support in Emergency Settings*. Geneva: Inter-Agency Standing Committee, 2007.

International Organization for Migration. *Trafficking of Fishermen in Thailand*. Bangkok, Thailand: International Organization for Migration, January 14, 2011. http://www.iom.int/jahia/webdav/shared/shared/mainsite/activities/countries/docs/thailand/Trafficking-of-Fishermen-Thailand.pdf.

Janoff-Bulman, Ronnie. *Shattered Assumptions: Towards a New Psychology of Trauma*. New York: Free Press, 1992.

Karen Human Rights Group. *Attacks and Displacement in Nyaunglebin District*. Thailand: Karen Human Rights Group, 2010.

———. *Enduring Hunger and Repression: Food Scarcity, Internal Displacement, and the Continued Use of Forced Labour in Toungoo District*. Thailand: Karen Human Rights Group, 2004.

Lloyd, Beverley, Lucie Rychetnik, Michelle Maxwell, and Trish Nove. "Building Capacity for Evidence-Based Practice in the Health Promotion Workforce: Evaluation of a Train-the-Trainer Initiative in NSW." *Health Promotion Journal of Australia: Official Journal of Australian Association of Health Promotion Professionals* 20, no. 2 (August 2009): 151–154.

McCann, I Lisa, and Laurie Anne Pearlman. "Vicarious Traumatization: A Framework for Understanding the Psychological Effects of Working with Victims." *Journal of Traumatic Stress* 3, no. 1 (January 1, 1990): 131–149. doi:10.1007/BF00975140.

Nimmagadda, Jayashree, and Charles D Cowger. "Cross-Cultural Practice: Social Worker Ingenuity in the Indigenization of Practice Knowledge." *International Social Work* 42, no. 3 (July 1, 1999): 261–276. doi:10.1177/002087289904200302.

Palm, Kathleen M, Melissa A Polusny, and Victoria M Follette. "Vicarious Traumatization: Potential Hazards and Interventions for Disaster and Trauma Workers." *Prehospital and Disaster Medicine* 19, no. 1 (March 2004): 73–78.

Pines, Ayala, and Christina Maslach. "Characteristics of Staff Burnout in Mental Health Settings." *Hospital & Community Psychiatry* 29, no. 4 (April 1978): 233–237.

Rose, Suzanna C, Jonathan Bisson, Rachel Churchill, and Simon Wessely. "Psychological Debriefing for Preventing Post Traumatic Stress Disorder (PTSD)." In *Cochrane Database of Systematic Reviews*, edited by The Cochrane Collaboration and Suzanna C Rose. Chichester, UK: John Wiley & Sons, 2002. http://www.ncbi.nlm.nih.gov/pubmedhealth/PMH0010736/.

SalusWorld. "Thailand: Aiding Displaced Shan." http://salusworld.org/current/southeast-asia.php.

Shan Human Rights Foundation and Shan Women's Action Network. *Rape Cases Documented During Burma Army Offensive in Northern Shan State Since 13 March 2011*. Shan Human Rights Foundation; Shan Women's Action Network, 2011. http://www.shanhumanrights.org/images/stories/Action_Update/Files/summary%20of%20rape%20cases%20during%20burma%20army%20offensive%20in%20on.shan%20state.pdf.

Substance Abuse and Mental Health Services Administration. *Psychological First Aid for First Responders*. Substance Abuse and Mental Health Services Administration, 2005. http://store.samhsa.gov/shin/content//NMH05-0210/NMH05-0210.pdf.

United Nations Office for the Coordination of Humanitarian Affairs. *OCHA Orientation Handbook on Complex Emergencies*. Geneva: United Nations, 1999.

US Campaign for Burma. *Shan Human Rights Foundation: Urgent Update on the Human Rights Situation in Shan State, Burma*, April 5, 2013. http://www.uscampaignforburma.org/statements/3108-shrf-urgent-update-on-the-human-rights-situation-in-shan-state-burma.html.

Yunong, Huang, and Zhang Xiong. "A Reflection on the Indigenization Discourse in Social Work." *International Social Work* 51, no. 5 (September 1, 2008): 611–622. doi:10.1177/0020872808093340.

Part III.

Vulnerable Groups and Challenges

Chapter 5

Discovering Culturally Appropriate
Psychosocial Care for Children and Young People

Derina Johnson, Liberty Thawda, Sid Mone Thwe,

and Hay Mar San

An 11-year-old girl's mother abandoned her when she was young. She was ignored by the community and lived with a family who abused her physically, emotionally, and sexually. She never got the chance to attend school. During this time, her grandmother and her sister were living in Myawaddy [a Burmese town across the border from Mae Sot, Thailand], unaware that she was still alive. When they heard she was living in Mae Sot, they came to look for her. When they found her, she was in serious need of medical treatment, and they immediately brought her to Mae Tao Clinic. Every day while at the clinic, she went to Child Recreation Center to play. One day, there was an activity with color and the staff realized that she didn't even know her colors. Over the course of the two weeks she got healthier and was able to eat again. She seemed happier, always keen to play and laugh with other children.[1]

In many trauma-affected communities around the world, people addressing the well-being of children and young people face considerable challenges. In some places, concepts of psychosocial and mental health can be misunderstood or mistrusted; in others, well-intentioned interventions may be misapplied. At times, the inner worlds and needs of children remain elusive and unheard because of lack of knowledge of how to hear them or lack of confidence about how to help. In this chapter we outline efforts founded in and grown from community beliefs and approaches and argue for the importance of community-based collaboration, capacity building, and leadership.

International Best Practices

In enduring situations such as that on the Thai-Burma border, communities seek social services to mitigate the effects of ongoing forced displacement, chronic civil conflict, abuses in the home and in society, poverty, and discrimination. Providing these services is not an easy task, however.

Practitioners are challenged to find ways to overcome stigma and misunderstandings, link mental health to community beliefs, and ultimately integrate psychosocial development and well-being as part of a holistic community approach to the care of children.

When the international mental health community cannot agree on best practices or approaches, the question of where to begin can be overwhelming. In a survey of international experts on mental health and disaster management in middle- and low-income countries, Weiss, Saraceno, and their colleagues found that although there is a growing consensus about the need for social interventions, such as restoring social support networks and communities, much debate continues about clinical issues, priorities, and what model to follow.[2] More fundamentally, the applicability of Western trauma-related mental health concepts and psychiatric labels to children in non-Western settings generates heated discussions.[3] Also, differences of opinion about approaches suitable for the acute phase of an emergency versus contexts of chronic conflict create additional challenges.

Matters are further complicated in low-resource settings, where limitations of trained local actors, funding, and time often result in programs led by priorities and concerns of visiting foreign professionals rather than communities' needs. Clinical interventions require professional specialists not only to help commence programs but also to provide ongoing supervision and follow-up. In low-resource settings, long-term commitment by professionals is rarely possible or affordable. Unstable funding may result in well-intentioned but unsustainable initiatives. Good intentions and a short-term cascade of costly resources will not exact lasting change. Dipak Naker, writing on violence against children in Uganda, explains: "We have to resist appeasing our conscience in the short term, and think harder about what will work in the longer term."[4]

Patience and long-term commitment to repeating and reinforcing the same message are essential to attitude and behavior change and the integration of new ideas.[5] The introduction of a new idea is often a journey rather than a single action. According to Everett Rogers's innovation-decision process, this journey has five important stages: knowledge (and understanding), persuasion (change of attitude), decision (engagement in activities, leading to adoption or rejection of the innovation), implementation (use of innovation), and confirmation (reinforcement of the decision).[6] In addition, psychosocial programs that prioritize the acquisition of interest, understanding, and buy-in are more likely to end up creating a future of possibilities. Applying this type of framework may facilitate more cogent and reflective responses in critical situations, and thus be more likely to have the much-sought-after and needed effect.

The gradual process of change over time is a principal property of enduring psychological growth across many psychotherapy disciplines. Despite this, psychosocial projects in emergency or low-resource settings are frequently short term. Longer-term programs allow for more enduring process-enabling rather than project-based goals. Process-enabling programs with a long-term vision allow for gradual progress. These programs seek to meet community members where they are, resulting in more community-centered rather than practitioner-centered focus. Process-enabling methods support the integration of psychosocial practices and principles into adults' everyday interactions with children, thus aiding the generalization of well-being-promoting behaviors toward children within communities.

The nature of the approach to the community is also critical to an intervention's success; one author's interview captures this simply, "If the approach is not right and the community doesn't accept you, then even if you are considered a super counselor or a super doctor, you can do nothing."[7] Elisabeth Fries, writing about her time working with community health nurses in Democratic Republic of Congo, explained advice she received: "Go as a friend, share what you have and look for their resources."[8] Working with local partners and listening to local advice not only overcomes language issues but also makes programs more community relevant. This is especially important at the beginning, when laying the foundations of sustainable, accessible, appropriate mental health and psychosocial services. Silove, Steel, and Psychol warn against overrating outside expertise at the cost of community input. They emphasize that the best comfort can be found through fellow community members and thus effort should be made to ensure that programs seek out and use resources within communities.[9]

According to the World Health Organization, a community mental health approach facilitates care that is closely linked to the culture.[10] Successful community mental health models assure that the program has buy-in and ownership by community leaders and that it is implemented by those who are familiar, trusted, well-trained, and confident in dealing with the issues at hand.[11] Western models must be adapted and tested for suitability. Strengths and traditional practices should be integrated whenever appropriate. Sometimes international best practices and local customs can converge unexpectedly. One author witnessed an exchange between a Western psychiatrist and a well-respected local school director on the Thai-Burma border about the nature of disciplining children. The foreigner was recommending the use of time-out, expounding its benefits in the West. The director was reluctant and explained his own approach of meditation, which worked with his children—the child is instructed to sit and meditate for a certain number of minutes to calm his mind and allow a new perspective to form. Different cultures may have different ways of expressing the same ideas.

Without cultural sensitivity and relevance, psychosocial programming can risk creating a "carnival of interventions," a phrase used by Kolitha Wickramage to describe what he perceived as the "psychosocial playground" created in Sri Lanka after the 2004 tsunami.[12] According to Wickramage, foreign volunteers bringing unsolicited "toolboxes" for psychosocial and trauma recovery activities "added as much amusement as it did confusion."[13] In one instance, over one hundred families living in temporary accommodation were visited by a group of foreigners delivering "psychosocial therapy." Children were subjected to "healing" massage on their limbs and faces by the team members, who failed to explain what they were doing, mistakenly assuming the children had no English.[14] Similar experiences have been reported along the Thai-Burma border; one local psychosocial worker recalled such an event from her youth,

> We were told by the elders that we must go to see the performers as they had spent so much money to get here. We all stood around the performers; I could not see clearly, but I did get a glimpse of a man dressed in very different clothing jumping at the younger children. Many having expected a dance from the performers, walked away saying "but it was nothing!" They didn't understand what we were seeing or what they were trying to do. This group went to the school, the clinic, and all the boarding houses! Even a driver was made available to them at all times.[15]

Ananda Galappatti, while seeking to categorize the myriad of psychosocial interventions on Sri Lanka, discovered a 2001 directory of seventy-one discrete concurrent projects, the majority of which, according to Galappatti, came with poor or inadequate supporting principles, methodologies, tools, or processes.[16] Huge resources are at risk of being wasted to create and maintain such projects, as a psychosocial officer from the Thai-Burma border reflects: "If they want to do something psychosocial, they have to do something which will touch people's hearts. If it is too Western people will simply not understand, and it will be a waste."[17]

Interventions require comprehensive community needs assessments and sensitivity to the sociocultural context. The nature of children and childhood can present differences; for instance, activities cited as suitable for one group of children may not be understood or applicable in another context. There may also be universals. One community worker on the Thai-Burma border explained the core matter as he saw it: "Emotions are in the heart. If they don't have good care, whatever child, Burmese or English, if their parents don't love them, they feel sad. If a person makes a joke of them, they feel angry."[18]

Burma Border Context

In many parts of the world, children look to their parents and society for protection and care. The family has great potential to play a protective role in the lives of children and can act as an important buffer against adversity and trauma.[19] Despite recent rapid economic and political changes in Burma, children and families continue to face enduring hardships. The UN Children's Fund reports infant and under-5 mortality rates to be the highest among countries in the Association of Southeast Asian Nations (ASEAN).[20] Save the Children reveals that more than 90,000 Burmese children under age 5 die annually from preventable or treatable diseases.[21] Even with steady improvements in the last decade, one in three children under 5 years of age continues to be malnourished.[22] Conditions in remote and border regions of the country are even more critical, where lack of access to basic vaccinations and general health care lead to poor health and survival outcomes for children.[23] Although Burma's income continues to grow, health care and education remain low on the agenda. In "World Report 2013," Human Rights Watch reports that despite billions of US dollars acquired from natural gas sales to Thailand, the Myanmar government has yet to prioritize improvements in health care or education.[24] In accordance with its Millennium Development Goals, the Myanmar government has committed to "free and compulsory basic education of good quality" for all children by 2015.[25] Nevertheless, currently fewer than half of all children complete primary school, with even lower completion rates among poor rural communities.[26] The situation is worse for ethnic minority children. Prohibitions on using their ethnic language and on growing crops and poor access to education are some of the daily hardships faced by ethnic minority groups.[27] Human Rights Watch reports that the Myanmar government continues to deny humanitarian aid to northern areas of Burma, despite widespread military attacks on civilians, including killings, rape, torture, and forced labor.[28]

The situation in Mae Sot, Thailand, helps illustrate the difficult context confronting children at the Burma border. Mae Sot is one of three official immigration and export points along this border, and its strong manufacturing, construction, and agriculture sectors make it a chief destination for many coming across the border seeking employment and a new start. Mae Sot has an official population of 120,000; however, this does not include the large number of unregistered migrant workers and children living in the town. Figures from the Mae Sot–based Committee for the Promotion and Protection of Child Rights (CPPCR) suggest the migrant community is between 150,000 and 300,000 people, with children making up 10 percent.[29]

SAFETY AND SECURITY

According to the UN Special Representative for Children in Armed Conflict, who has pledged to end children's involvement in armed conflict by 2016, recent trends of terror tactics in chronic conflict situations, coupled with a lack of "clear front lines and identifiable opponents," make this an era of increased vulnerability for children worldwide.[30] The Burmese government signed a commitment in 2012 to prevent and end recruitment of children into the government armed forces, known as the Tatmadaw Kyi.[31] However, a 2013 report by Child Soldiers International cited evidence of ongoing recruitment of children into both state and rebel forces.[32]

Karen Human Rights Group (KHRG), a grassroots human rights organization in eastern Burma, cautions the world against complacency despite the region's tenuous cease-fire agreements. In a 2012 report, KHRG documented the unsystematic and incomplete clearing of land mines from around schools in villages, continuing to disrupt children's education as well as posing serious physical risks to children and villagers.[33] Forced labor, a common practice during military rule, is also ongoing in Karen State. Another KHRG report from March 2013 documented the forcing of villagers, including children, to work on the construction of a bridge in the state's Papun District. Villagers report having to work full time without pay or any indication of how many days, weeks, or months they will be further required to work.[34]

These ongoing civil conflict and human rights abuses in Burma have resulted in decades of flight for families and separated children into neighboring Thailand. The Back Pack Health Worker Team (BPHWT), which delivers primary health care to underserved and remote areas in eastern Burma, carried out a household survey of human rights violations in eastern Burma in 2006. The survey revealed that families forced to flee their homes were 2.4 times more likely to have a child under 5 die compared with those who had not suffered human rights violation.[35]

Crossing into Thailand illegally without documentation and the inability to register births within Thailand has given rise to a large number of children who are considered stateless. Statelessness can deny people their basic survival needs, including access to education and essential health care, leaving children at high risk for exploitation and abuse, fewer work options, fear of arrest, and uncertain future.[36] It is worth noting that there are at least three categories of children in this migrant context: children who have migrated with their parents to Thailand, children who are born to migrant parents in Thailand, and children who have traveled to Thailand without their parents. However, as their experiences often overlap, for the purposes of this chapter the term "migrant children" will be used to include all three categories.

All children in Thailand are covered by the 2003 Royal Thai Government Child Protection Act.[37] However, as with many other public services, lack of identification documentation, fear, and distrust of Thai authorities, as well as limited and unsystematic implementation of laws, often leave migrant children without the protection of the law.[38] A change in the Thai Civil Registration Act in 2008 meant that all children, regardless of their parents' legal status, could be issued a birth certificate by Thai government. Although this document does not equate to Thai citizenship, it does increase potential for future Thai residency and work permits.[39] Prior to this change, the responsibility of birth registration of migrant children had been undertaken by the CPPCR, a Burmese community-based organization in the border town of Mae Sot. In 2003, because of the lack of official processes available to undocumented Burmese migrants, CPPCR began issuing unofficial birth certificates, providing some proof of a child's identity while also helping migrant worker parents prove a child-parent relationship, thus protecting parents from accusations by Thai police of trafficking children.[40]

Children without legal documentation are at heightened risk for abuse, exploitation, and trafficking. Constant fears of arrest, fines, and deportation limit movement even around the community and result in families becoming effectively imprisoned in their homes. A Burmese community child protection worker in Mae Sot voiced concerns about the effect of this on children: "The children here, even the ones who have their parents, have some kind of feeling 'oh this is not our country' . . . they feel they will do something wrong, they worry."[41]

CHILD LABOR

Taking on "3D" jobs (dirty, dangerous, and demeaning), migrant workers continue to face social and economic hardships in Thailand. Unsafe working conditions, financial exploitation, and risk of trafficking continue to challenge their safety, freedom, and agency in the country where they sought refuge.[42] It is estimated there are 200,000 Burmese children living in Thailand and that children make up as much as 20 percent of the migrant workforce.[43] Thai labor law only permits the registration of children for employment from the age of 15 years.[44] A 2013 study by Chiang Rai Rajabhat University researcher Penpisut Jaisanit paints a grim picture of migrant child labor in northern Thailand. Jobs carried out by children are in three main categories: work in domestic service (the most common), karaoke bars and restaurants, and begging. The majority of these laborers were girls from Burma, many under the age of 15. Many reported working well over the four-hour-per-day legal work limit, and most reported physical and verbal abuse, as well as sexual harassment, especially those working in "entertainment centers." [45]

PARENTING

> *Parents are working so hard for their family's survival. . . . In the morning the parents go to work and only come home late in the evening. For many men their routine is then eating, drinking and sleep. . . . They say they do not have time, no time, no time.*[46]

These words from an experienced Mae Sot–based community worker are frequently echoed by community child protection workers. They provide insight into the reality of the demanding, relentless work and hardships of living in Thailand as experienced by migrant parents, limiting their ability to provide emotional sheltering for their children.[47] Overwhelmed with their own stresses and traumas, parents are unable to see beyond surviving one day to the next. They work long, hard hours and consequently struggle to have adequate time, energy, or patience with their children.

Parental support and monitoring has emerged globally as a consistent promotive factor of children's resilience across cultures and contexts, as well as a common protective factor against adversity.[48] This pattern has also been found along the Thai-Burma border migrant community, as revealed by the 2011 study by the International Rescue Committee investigating the community's concepts of child and family well-being.[49] The community identified parental instruction and guidance, positive role modeling, and supervision as key cornerstones to the well-being of children. However, the ongoing daily struggles faced by migrant parents and families can result in a very different reality for children and give rise to experiences of isolation in their own home.

HEALTH CARE

Under Thailand's Universal Health Care Coverage Scheme, 30 baht (approximately US$1) is the maximum a patient can be charged for a visit. This is a countrywide program to provide access to low-cost health care for the poor. According to a study in 2013 by Massachusetts Institute of Technology, this program has been credited with reducing infant mortality in Thailand by 30 percent in the ten years since its inception.[50] Those who are unregistered are outside this scheme. According to reports from the Thai government, in the northwestern province of Tak, adjacent to Karen State in Burma and home to hundreds of migrant communities, hospitals spent over 100 million baht (US$3 million) in 2012 treating those outside the scheme, such as unregistered migrant workers and members of ethnic hill communities.[51] Despite this, for many migrant workers and their families, health care in Thai facilities is simply not affordable. Seeking help is also coupled with fear of arrest, deportation, discrimination, and language and access difficulties. To some extent, the shortfall of free health care is taken up by Mae Tao Clinic (described elsewhere in this volume). Mae Tao Clinic provides a wide range of free primary and preventive health care to over 150,000 refugees, migrant workers, and others who cross the border from Burma.[52]

In 2009, the first-ever documented survey of the nutritional status of children in the migrant communities in Tak Province (Thailand) was carried out by the Shoklo Malaria Research Unit, a project that, since 1986, has tackled malaria along the Thai-Burma border. The researchers found that over 30 percent of migrant children suffered from malnutrition, with rates of stunting and underweight sometimes double those of children in other areas of northern Thailand. Levels of wasting or acute malnutrition, caused by a short-term deficiency in energy and nutritional intake, was three times higher for children in the migrant schools than for children living in the refugee camps.[53] The World Health Organization highlights how nutritional deficiencies can inhibit intellectual and physical potential, even resulting in lifelong disability. Combined with a lack of psychosocial care and stimulation, this can cause long-lasting consequences in all areas of children's development and mental health.[54]

EDUCATION

Family and education were among the top four reasons for leaving Burma, according to a 2008 International Rescue Committee survey of migrant communities along the Thai-Burma border.[55] Education is a universal human right and considered a key protective factor in helping children find solace and normality after conflict and adversity.[56] Despite the Thai government's extension of its Education for All program to include all children in Thailand regardless of their legal status, less than 20 percent of migrant children in Thailand are believed to attend school.[57] Documentation and fear of arrest continues to be a huge obstacle. The government policy allows a lot of flexibility in terms of what documentation is required to register a child in a Thai school; for instance, when a birth certificate or registration papers cannot be provided, a family biography can suffice. Nonetheless, implementation varies on a local level, and for parents who do not speak Thai, engaging with Thai school authorities can be daunting.[58] A 2013 report by Voluntary Services Overseas (vso), an international volunteer organization that has been working with the migrant community since 2005, revealed a number of additional factors contributing to this shortfall in migrant children accessing Thai schools. For many migrant workers living in remote agricultural areas, access and transportation can be serious obstacles. For others, the cost of materials and the related indirect costs have an effect on the family's potential earnings.[59] Lack of Thai language skills is a considerable barrier to many children, and some parents fear their child may lose their native language if sent to a Thai school.[60] Parents also worry about discrimination and bullying within Thai schools. vso revealed that many Thai teachers lack understanding of the community from which migrant children are coming and of how to manage a multicultural classroom.[61] Speaking at a conference on refugees, integration, and well-being in 2012, Mahidol Migration Center's Dr. Jerry Huguet cited unregistered workers' lack of job security as another reason for the low uptake of Thai education by the migrant community. Huguet suggested that an easier and less expensive registration process would result in greater job security and improved social status for migrant workers, who might, envisioning a more secure future in Thailand, be more likely to enroll their children in Thai schools.[62]

These factors have given rise to the establishment of numerous migrant learning centers, so called because they do not meet the Thai government criteria to be a school. Around Mae Sot, for instance, vso reports seventy-four migrant-run learning centers;[63] however some community workers estimate there are over one hundred. Although learning centers address many concerns of parents, a lack of comprehensive curricula and teacher training means many centers fall below accepted education standards.[64] Education at the migrant learning centers is unrecognized by both the Thai Ministry of Education and the Myanmar Department of Education, contributing to uncertain futures for graduates.

The combination of a lack of documentation and unrecognized educational qualifications can leave young people with limited future choices. To address this deficiency, a few small-scale initiatives around Mae Sot, to which academically strong students can apply, focus on intensive English education to put youth in a stronger position for employment with nongovernmental organizations (NGOs). For other students, intensive academic programs help them get into university either in Thailand or overseas. Vocational training options exist, such as the training and apprenticeship program run by the NGO Youth Connect Thailand, which aims to help bridge the gap between youth and prospective employers by equipping youth with Thai, practical math, life-skills training, and work experience.[65]

Unfortunately, many migrant children drop out of school at an early age. Understandably, parents may not see the benefit of an extended education in the face of poverty and hunger. Often the sense of obligation to support struggling parents leads many children to leave school themselves. In a focus group with adolescents facilitated by the author, a 12-year-old girl spoke of community pressures and expectations to leave school. Having learned to read and write, she felt it was regarded by her community that she had received sufficient education, and her responsibility was now to support her parents, despite her own hopes to continue her education.

For other children, accessing an education is the reason they are separated at a young age from their families, childhood home, and communities.[66] Haphazard school closures and unsafe conditions in Burma result in children being sent across the border to Thailand alone, to live with relatives or in "boardinghouses," the term given to accommodations linked to schools and often run by the teachers. The backgrounds of children at boardinghouses vary considerably, and there are often few material differences between boardinghouses, safe houses, and orphanages in the migrant community. Children in all three settings share common backgrounds of having been abused in the home, rescued from trafficking, orphaned, or abandoned, or of having parents in the late stage of HIV/AIDS or hepatitis. All three provide security and supervision, as well as consistent food, routines, and interactions with peers. For the purposes of this chapter we use the term "boardinghouse" to cover all three settings.

Parents' decisions to abandon children at boardinghouses occur for a host of social, economic, and practical reasons. Taking care of young babies prevents mothers from being able to work to provide for other children, and children with illnesses or disabilities can be particularly challenging in this setting. The desperate situation faced by some mothers is complex, as explained by a child protection worker:

> A mother delivers the baby then wonders—where will I stay, how will I feed this child? The husband is not here so she gives the child away or sells the child. A pregnant woman delivers a baby at Mae Tao Clinic, and then has to make the decision about what to do next—to go back to Burma, to work, where to live, how to eat. She cannot see the future, so she gives away the child or sells the child so she can travel back to Burma.[67]

Room to Grow Foundation is a small Canadian-based nonprofit organization focused primarily on supporting the basic needs of "unparented" migrant children around Mae Sot. Room to Grow's program coordinator described the traumatic experiences of many of these children, who have watched their parents or siblings die, or been abandoned or forced to work. She told of children whose lives have been so chaotic they do not know where they are; they are listless "sitting, doing nothing, looking out onto the road."[68]

The pressure on boardinghouses to provide for all the physical and developmental needs of children in their care is enormous. It is made more challenging by the children's heightened psychosocial needs, resulting from traumatic experiences, abandonment, and the social isolation brought about by their lack of documentation. Acting as teachers by day and boardinghouse care staff by night results in demanding schedules for staff. In some instances, as few as three staff can be responsible for as many as seventy children.

Psychosocial Initiatives for Children and Youth in the Migrant Community

Typically, over time, stability returns after emergencies, conflicts, and disasters. Unfortunately conditions have not stabilized in many parts of Burma, giving rise to a protracted emergency situation for hundreds of thousands of migrants and children along the border, for whom neither the Thai nor Myanmar government has assumed real responsibility. Such a chronic and enduring situation makes psychosocial programming more complex, as it involves simultaneously both acute (attacks and forced movement) and ongoing (conflict and poverty) problems.[69]

Since 2006, integrated psychosocial programs have been emerging in migrant communities' education and health sectors, bringing foreign technical expertise together with the inherent skills of the local community.

These programs sometimes bring very new concepts and ideas that challenge long-set ideas about child welfare and services, which at times require a considerable shift of perspective about the inner emotional worlds of children. A local child protection trainer considers this shift to be the most important element of her work, to guide the community toward understanding what can be harmful or hurtful to a child. Through being able to see the world from the perspective of a child, the trainer believes the community will be more capable and willing to respond sensitively to the emotional needs of children.[70]

The Inter-Agency Standing Committee's (IASC) guidelines on mental health and psychosocial support in emergency settings introduce clear principles for the development of psychosocial responses.[71] These principles are reviewed in chapter 1. On the Thai-Burma border, psychosocial programs are led by large and small international agencies and local organizations. Programs vary in terms of budget and personnel and as a result span a variety of needs and approaches. IASC's intervention pyramid provides a useful framework for the community programs provided to children and young people in migrant communities around Mae Sot.[72]

BASIC SERVICES AND SECURITY

At the bottom and widest layer of the IASC pyramid lies provision of basic services and security, which includes addressing people's physical needs, such as those for food, health, and shelter.[73] These responses can involve mobilizing community networks and social supports so that needs are met in culturally appropriate and participatory ways. In Mae Sot, the Burmese community instigated and continues to mobilize programs to address these basic services and security needs. For example, Mae Tao Clinic fills gaps in traditional government welfare services provision, acting as an umbrella network of social services in the community.[74] The clinic provides a broad spectrum of essential physical services, from nutrition and health care to education and a safe space to live, addressing the core facets of child protection, human rights, and, ultimately, the emotional well-being of migrant children.[75] The Child Protection Department at Mae Tao Clinic, initially an ad-hoc project to support needs as they arose, is now a comprehensive program with a holistic approach to child protection. The department takes responsibility for the support and monitoring of nutrition and hygiene programs at community migrant learning centers and boardinghouses, as well as leading programs for vitamin A supplementation, deworming, essential immunization, and supplemental feeding. The department also coordinates and oversees several boardinghouses in the community and was central in the creation of the comprehensive *Child Protection Policy and Procedures Guidebook* published in 2013 and designed for use by migrant learning centers, boardinghouses, and community-based organizations in the Mae Sot area.[76]

In 2009, community initiatives to respond to child abuse cases in Mae Sot gave rise to a community-based CPPCR-led child protection referral system (CPRS), with the goal of establishing a safe society for children. The migrant community took a leading position in the program, enabling solutions to be sought from an inherently culturally appropriate standpoint.

In 2010, the International Rescue Committee (IRC) joined this initiative and over the subsequent three years helped CPPCR and local partners develop a comprehensive and operational community-wide CPRS initiative. The initiative provides ongoing child protection and case management training to twenty child protection focal points, members of local child-related organizations responsible for the documentation, referral, and monitoring of child protection cases. Another facet of the IRC's involvement was to simultaneously increase confidence and cooperation between the migrant community and local Thai child protection officers in the regional Social Welfare Department and Ministry of Social Development.

COMMUNITY AND FAMILY SUPPORT

The IASC pyramid's second layer involves establishing community and family supports.[77] The Mae Sot migrant community is very familiar with fear and distrust resulting from disruption of their families and communities. Psychosocial programs focused on reestablishment of community supports and strengthening of the family unit make up a large number of the programs in Mae Sot.

Responding to the results of its 2011 study on migrant communities' concepts of child and family well-being, the IRC determined to implement a family-focused program designed to strengthen the protective capacity of families and reduce risk factors such as family separation and abuse.[78] The IRC selected and adapted Karol Kumpfer's Strengthening Families Program, a fourteen-week program targeting high-risk families, initially in the United States, which had been proven adaptable in over seventeen countries, including Thailand.[79] Focusing on concrete behavioral skills development, in-line with the results of IRC's study, the program included stress management, positive discipline, and anti-drug and anti-alcohol components. Cultural adaptations were made to examples, songs and games, and cultural and religious concepts. The program was also renamed the Happy Families Program or Chan Myae Pyaw Shwin Thaw Mi Thar Su

A Si A Sin in Burmese, to be more accessible and easily understood by the community.[80]

The program was run in partnership with Social Action for Women, a Burmese women's organization that provides shelter, health, and educational facilities for migrant women and children. The program targeted Burmese migrant and displaced families with at least one child between 8 and 12 years old. The program's objectives were to improve family functioning and cohesion and increase knowledge and use of positive parenting skills; improve children's behavior and build their social competence and resilience; and reduce or prevent parental alcohol and drug use. The program's technical staff, together with one community group leader, facilitated weekly two-hour sessions with the children and their parents. During the initial hour, parents and their children worked separately before coming back to participate together in the second hour. Initial results reported that 90 percent of parents liked the program and said they spent more time together as a family, needed to use less physical punishment, and were happier.[81]

One of the program's local trainers believed the strengths of the program lay in the core message to parents to spend time with children. He believed that by encouraging talking and sharing, family bonds would be improved and child protection bolstered, as children would feel more comfortable sharing time with their parents and may be more likely to disclose any abuse. The trainer explained how Burmese children are traditionally instructed to "pay respect to the monk, pay respect to the teacher, pay respect to the parent";[82] their individual voices, opinions, ideas and feelings are not sought or nurtured at home or in school. He believes the Happy Families Program helped change that norm, improving both the communication skills of children and the listening skills of their parents.

World Education has been working on the development of psychosocial understanding in migrant communities around Mae Sot since 2006. Led by Burmese staff with foreign technical support resources, World Education has supported psychosocial and child protection training for Burmese migrant community–based organization staff and school teachers. The training content focuses on psychosocial principles and on understanding the needs and development of a person, stress and trauma and their effects on children, and the general helping process in the classroom.

Seeking to establish a more comprehensive approach in schools for the psychosocial development of children, World Education brought together the Burmese mental health perspectives of Mae Tao Clinic's Counseling Center and international mental health professionals' perspectives from

Burma Border Projects (BBP) to produce the *Creating Opportunities for Psychosocial Enhancement COPE Teacher Training Manual*. This basic psychosocial training resource was translated into Karen and Burmese and covers topics from the psychosocial development of the person to the effect of stress and trauma on children to general classroom-based helping skills. The manual includes expressive activities for the classroom involving storytelling, drama, meditation, and writing, as well as self-care techniques.[83]

Migrant teachers have for the most part come directly from Burma and often have themselves survived many of the same traumas and hardships as their students. World Education soon discovered the self-care component to be a vital element in all teacher trainings. In response, training in that component was extended to students of post–high school programs. Training incorporated both didactic and experiential techniques to cover definitions, manifestations and symptoms of stress, coping skills, and a broad selection of relaxation techniques such as deep breathing, listening to your body, visualization, and muscle relaxation.

Comments by two teachers in Mae Sot who participated in the training provide insight into the experience of integrating daily psychosocial skills into personal and teaching practice. HT said, "I do yoga regularly and I have become more patient, better able to divide what to do, not do, what to do first, and what to do later. I can relate with others better and my stress level is reduced." CW applies muscle relaxation techniques when she feels overloaded with work and now shares it with her own students, "There are forty-four girls. Each morning when we wake up at 5:30 a.m., I lead the students in yoga, deep breathing, and muscle relaxation. The self-care training has been very useful for me."[84]

Another World Education community support measure consisted of a community mobilization project to complement the CPRS and increase awareness of child protection in the wider migrant community. World Education identified community mobilizers (adults regarded as dependable and influential persons within their communities) from twenty different local migrant communities around Mae Sot. These individuals were responsible for implementing child protection awareness and prevention activities to address issues directly related to their respective communities. Having a link back to the CPRS empowered local mobilizers to seek support for children and families in difficulty who may not trust or open up to someone outside their immediate community. A World Education program officer recollects one young boy in a village: "I noticed he had changed within a month. The child became quiet and had no confidence. I really wanted to talk with the mother but she was always avoiding me, she didn't want to talk to me."[85] She further explains, "I want to talk with people about how to look after their children. But they are travelling; they only listen for a little bit. I understand they are so busy; they are trying to survive, to have food to eat."[86] Directly placed within the community, the community mobilizers are able to gradually and more informally address issues and facilitate greater knowledge about abuse and protection needs of children. At the same time, they are best placed to instigate child protection referrals when necessary.

World Education, together with IRC, BBP, and CPPCR, supported the training of the community mobilizers and the development of activities when needed. Such community-based activities included practical safety awareness for children playing on the narrow busy roads or swimming in the swollen rivers during the rainy season. At other times, more complex and culturally sensitive matters needed to be addressed. In one instance, child to child sexual abuse cases arose in the community. Together BBP and World Education developed safe touch awareness building age-appropriate workshops. An information session was developed for the adults, to inform them of the content of the sessions and to raise awareness of the importance of protecting children from pornography and educating children about appropriate behavior. The workshops were delivered together with local partners in schools, community centers, and boardinghouses.

NONSPECIALIZED SUPPORTS

A community program reflecting the third layer of the IASC pyramid (focused, nonspecialized supports) is the Child Recreation Center (CRC) at Mae Tao Clinic. IASC describes nonspecialized supports as services for particular individuals, groups, or communities delivered by trained, supervised workers.[87] Established in 2011, the CRC is unique in the migrant community, providing a child-centered psychosocial play space for children while they attend the clinic, either as patients or while family members receive medical care. The center is run by psychosocial care workers from the local migrant community, who were trained and receive ongoing technical advice and support from BBP. The manager of the CRC also acts as the child protection focal point for Mae Tao Clinic, responsible for responding to child protection cases and connecting children with available legal and shelter services within the wider network of the community's child protection referral system.

The CRC serves as a friendly and welcoming space, an escape from the trauma and tension of illness and treatment. While the medical departments at Mae Tao Clinic treat symptoms, the CRC gives love and care to help children reconnect with peers, their community, and themselves as children.

Many CRC staff members have survived harsh experiences. During one training session, a participant recalled her own painful experiences as a child and for the first time linked what she was learning about child abuse to her own childhood. As distressing as it was for all to hear, BBP had the opportunity to model for the staff how to respond sensitively to possible future disclosures by children. Knowing how the Burmese culture values music and song, and in recognition of the ethnic diversity in the group, participants were invited to sing a song from their culture and ethnic language. In this way, the music provided a calming, comforting atmosphere in which the group was able to get to know each other through sharing the origins and meanings of their chosen songs.

Following the opening of the CRC in early 2011, ongoing weekly trainings incorporated an opportunity for staff to seek guidance on dealing with particular behaviors or issues pertaining to the children in their care. Self-care was also a key component of the weekly sessions.

According to the center manager, the children who come in to the CRC present with a broad range of psychosocial difficulties, including physical underdevelopment, fear of talking or playing with other children, aggression, or isolation. Many children who visit the CRC do not regularly attend school, and it is not unusual for children to lack basic knowledge, such as the names of colors. The CRC psychosocial care workers take a holistic approach in the care of these children. A regular daily routine provides structure—beginning each day with morning songs and washing hands—and, when necessary, haircuts and new clothes. A broad range of activities are provided, according to the needs of the children attending, including expressive art, music and dancing, learning and socialization games, and storytelling and relaxation. Each day ends with fruit and milk. The nature of the CRC allows for informal individual psychosocial supports for children, and ongoing supervision and training from BBP builds and reinforces the strengths of the community to care for their own children.

BBP's primary approach is to work within a community mental health framework, providing technical advice when needed and integrating mental health well-being into existing support services within the community. This approach minimizes extra demand on already stretched resources, and instead increases the mental health promoting capacity and effectiveness of programs already present and accepted by the community. With limited resources on the border, both in personnel and finances, it can make sense for smaller organizations to pool resources, building on their strengths to support each other's work. As a result, close community partnerships have formed between organizations working on the ground around Mae Sot.

Since 2011, two young women, one Karen and one Burmese and both with lived experience as young people in the refugee camps and border migrant community, have worked alongside the international mental health staff at BBP. As they became more familiar with the work of BBP and the ethos and language of mental health, they translated technical terms unfamiliar to the community. Instead of direct translations, they used more practical translations: for example, for "positive discipline" they use *tane mway swar sone ma chin*, which means giving discipline gently for the good of the child; and for "play therapy," *kasar nee phyit hnit theimt sway hnway ku nyi pay chin*, which means a way of comforting, discussing, and helping, using play.

Improving the skills and capacity of local staff allowed for more direct programs to be developed and delivered to children and facilitated the blending of cultural awareness with psychosocial goals and principles. BBP's Children's Psychosocial Development Program has established long-term partnerships with safe houses and boardinghouses, especially those serving vulnerable children referred after abuse, trafficking, or abandonment. Led by BBP's local Burmese staff, the program provides ongoing mental health training and support to staff, alongside separate psychosocial and life skills sessions to children and youth.

SPECIALIZED SERVICES

While there remains an unmet need on the border for more comprehensive specialized services for children acutely affected by traumatic experiences (the IASC's pyramid's fourth and final layer),[88] there are plans currently to address this. One small-scale response being delivered is a mentorship program, led by BBP in partnership with World Education, to support young people making risky decisions such as skipping school, running away, engaging in early sexual behavior, and creating disruptions in the community.

Mentoring involves a supportive relationship between an adult and a child or young person, including emotional care and advice and based on regular shared time, friendship, and fun.[89] Less formal than counseling, it involves many of the same supportive features. A meta-analysis by David DuBois and colleagues of seventy-three mentoring programs over ten years, primarily in the United States, found that mentoring programs have the capacity to serve as a promotive and preventive intervention, improving emotional, behavioral, social, and academic outcomes for young people.[90]

The BBP Youth Mentoring Program takes a strengths-based approach, focusing on developing and reinforcing a young person's positive decision-making skills and preventing problem behaviors. To begin, concrete long-term goals are identified in conjunction with the case management team. These goals often include increasing pro-social behavior, returning to school, or reducing incidences of running away. Next, together with the young person, the mentor identifies achievable short-term goals, which in the beginning can often simply involve committing to stay at the safe house or boardinghouse until the next session with the mentor. The mentor looks for the young person's strengths, and builds a trusting relationship through authentically engaging in an interest the young person enjoys, such as drawing or sewing, dancing or playing the guitar. Through developing and mastering these skills, opportunities arise for the mentor and young person to explore strategies to overcome challenges and to learn how positive change takes time. Central to the mentor's message is confidence that the young person is capable and filled with potential. The mentor works as an advocate of the young person, helping to bridge the strained relationships in their lives. Finally, the relationship is based in hope and belief in the young person's abilities rather than deficits, and in the capacity to make positive and safe decisions for the future. These steps reflect the six characteristics of a strengths-based approach as outlined by Charles Rapp and his colleagues. [91]

One case involved a 14-year-old boy who had changed schools and boardinghouses several times because of disruptive behavior and absenteeism. Child protection advocates managing his case were running out of options and patience as, despite the youth's assertions that he was happy in his present boardinghouse, his behavior continued to be disruptive and he was not attending school. A program officer with World Education volunteered to be a mentor for the young man under the guidance and support of BBP's director of child and youth services, who met with the mentor weekly to reflect on the growing relationship and process, as well as to discuss ongoing challenges. The mentor and young man also met weekly, the sessions initially focused simply on learning to play the guitar. The mentor was open with the young man about any information he heard about his behavior over the previous week, but did not dwell on the issue. Gradually the young man shared his frustrations, dreams, and goals, and the mentor explored strategies with him for overcoming challenges and managing his behavior. Over six months, the young man's behavior dramatically transformed. He began to take responsibility for his behavior, admit his wrongdoings, and contribute to his boardinghouse. In turn, the attitudes of those working with him changed. By the end of the six months, the youth had positive and supportive friendships, was well-liked, and was attending school.

Conclusion

The future of the children and youth living among migrant communities along the Burma border continues to be shrouded in uncertainty. Recent years have seen harsher restrictions in the migrant community and drastically reduced funding to the border regions. Concerns are intensified by whispers of repatriation and the closure of refugee camps. However, as highlighted by the 2012 documentary *Nothing about Us without Us*,[92] refugee and migrant communities continue to be left in the dark by those making decisions about their futures. When asked about the issue of repatriation during her visit to Mae Sot in June 2012, Nobel Laureate Aung San Suu Kyi replied, "I do not think you really need to 'return refugees back,' because if conditions were right, refugees would go back of their own free will."[93]

The recent reforms in Burma and preparations for the launch of the ASEAN Economic Community in 2015 have prompted beliefs that before long, abundant employment opportunities back home will entice many migrant workers to return. According to the former ASEAN secretary-general, Surin Pitsuwan, this mass exodus will leave Thailand with serious labor shortages.[94] A 2012 study by Malee Sunpuwan and Sakkarin Niyomsilpa suggests that the general feeling among Thai nationals toward the migrant community is not a positive one, revealing that the majority of respondents consider the migrant community and refugees to pose a threat to their personal safety.[95] Sunpuwan and Niyomsilpa found little support among Thais for granting permanent residence status to those who have lived long-term in either the refugee camps or in the migrant communities. There was equally little support found for granting permanent residency to stateless children of refugee or migrant worker parents, for which Sunpuwan and Niyomsilpa say Thailand is facing human rights challenges.[96]

There are many changes occurring on the border, as well as in Burma. It is not yet clear how the trauma, chronic transience, and separation have really affected children, their well-being, or their pathways toward future adulthood. There are still substantive gaps in programming, especially for smaller groups of the population. One underserved area is that of the psychological and social rehabilitation and reintegration of former child soldiers, which may be more timely now than ever as the Myanmar government has committed to end recruitment and release current child soldiers. There are many other areas in need of attention, such as that of girls and boys affected by sexual violence. There can be no denying that there is as great a need as ever now for psychosocial programming to help these children and young people retain a semblance of safety and security, as well as acquire strength, resilience, and hope for their futures.

This chapter has focused on examples of psychosocial practice from the Thai-Burma border that have prioritized the implementation of culturally sensitive and integrative interventions to promote the psychological well-being of children and youth in these trauma-affected communities. Although each protracted conflict or emergency situation around the world has unique characteristics, many aspects of these interventions can be globally relevant. Experiences and lessons such as those described in this chapter may serve as useful guides to policy makers and practitioners faced with similar challenges and opportunities. The central messages have been to meet a community where it is, put the community's needs above priorities and concerns of foreign professionals, and integrate the community in all aspects of the decision-making and delivery of services for their young people.

Notes

1   K, Child Recreation Center manager, in discussion with the author, October 18, 2012.

2   Mitchell G Weiss, Benedetto Saraceno, Shekhar Saxena, and Mark van Ommeren, "Mental Health in the Aftermath of Disasters: Consensus and Controversy," *Journal of Nervous and Mental Disease* 191, no. 9 (2003): 611, doi:10.1097/01.nmd.0000087188.96516.a3.

3   Sean Perrin, Patrick Smith, and William Yule, "Practitioner Review: The Assessment and Treatment of Post-Traumatic Stress Disorder in Children and Adolescents," *Journal of Child Psychology and Psychiatry* 41, no.3 (2000): 277, http://www.ingentaconnect.com/content/bpl/jcpp/2000/00000041/00000003/art00002.

4   Dipak Naker, "Creating Violence-Free Childhoods: What Will It Take?," *Bernard van Leer Foundation Early Childhood Matters* 116 (2011): 60, http://vps.earlychildhoodmagazine.org/wp-content/uploads/2011/06/ECM116_Creating-violence-free-childhoods_13.pdf.

5   Roger Clarke, "A Primer in Diffusion of Innovations Theory," unpublished paper, 1999, http://www.anu.edu.au/people/Roger.Clarke/SOS/InnDiff.html.

6   Everett M Rogers, *Diffusion of Innovations*, 5th ed. (New York: Free Press, 2003), 169.

7 S, a community project assistant with previous experience as a teacher, boardinghouse master, and trainer with families, in discussion with the author, August 15, 2012.

8 Elizabeth Fries, "Steps towards Empowerment for Community Healing," *Intervention* 1, no. 2 (2003): 42, http://www.interventionjournal.com/downloads/12pdf/1207%20Fries.pdf.

9 Derrick Silove, Zachary Steel, and M Psychol, "Understanding Community Psychosocial Needs after Disasters: Implications for Mental Health Services," *Journal of Postgrad Medicine* [serial online] 52 (2006), http://www.jpgmonline.com/text.asp?2006/52/2/121/25157.

10 WHO, "Community Mental Health Services Will Lessen Social Exclusion," World Health Organization (WHO), last modified June 1, 2007, http://www.who.int/mediacentre/news/notes/2007/np25/en.

11 Ibid.

12 Kolitha Wickramage, "Sri Lanka's Post-Tsunami Psychosocial Playground: Lessons for Future Psychosocial Programming and Interventions Following Disasters," *Intervention* 4, no. 2 (2006): 167, http://ourmediaourselves.com/archives/42pdf/WTF14.pdf.

13 Ibid., 167.

14 Ibid., 168.

15 H, a Karen psychosocial officer in Mae Sot, with experience of living in the UN-run refugee camps and the Mae Sot migrant community, in discussion with the author, September 10, 2013.

16 Ananda Galappatti, "What Is a Psychosocial Intervention? Mapping the Field in Sri Lanka," *Intervention* 1, no. 2 (2003): 5, http://www.interventionjournal.com/downloads/12pdf/1204%20Ananda%20 Galappatti.pdf.

17 H, in discussion with the author, September 10, 2013.

18 S, in discussion with the author, August 15, 2012.

19 United Nations, "Report of the Independent Expert for the United Nations Study on Violence against Children," Sixty-First Session, UN General Assembly, Item 62A, Promotion and Protection of the Rights of Children, August 29, 2006, 12, http://www.unicef.org/violencestudy/reports/SG_violencestudy_en.pdf.

20 UNICEF, *Situational Analysis of Children from Myanmar* (Myanmar: UNICEF, July 2012), 6, http://www.unicef.org/eapro/Myanmar_Situation_Analysis.pdf.

21 Save the Children, "Myanmar," last updated July 2012. http://www.savethechildren.org/site/c.8rKLIXMGIpI4E/b.6150543/.

22 UNICEF, *Situational Analysis*, 36.

23 Ibid., xvi.

24 Human Rights Watch, "World Report 2013: Burma (Events of 2012)," 7,
    http://www.hrw.org/world-report/2013/country-chapters/burma.

25 Government of the Republic of the Union of Myanmar Ministry of Education,
    "Education for All: Access to and Quality of Education in Myanmar" (Conference
    on Development Policy Options with Special Reference to Education and Health
    in Myanmar, Nay Pyi Taw, Myanmar, February 13–16, 2012), 2–3,
    http://yangon.sites.unicnetwork.org/files/2013/05/Final-UBW-presentation-12-2-12
    -UBW.pdf.

26 UNICEF, *Situational Analysis*, xvii.

27 Committee for Protection and Promotion of Children's Rights (Burma), *Feeling
    Small in Another Person's Country: The Situation of Burmese Migrant Children in
    Mae Sot Thailand* (Mae Sot, Thailand: CPPCR, 2009), 19.

28 Human Rights Watch, "World Report 2013," 1.

29 CPPCR, *Feeling Small*, 31.

30 Leila Zerrougui, "Special Representative for Children in Armed Conflict
    Statement to Security Council Working Group debate on Children and Armed
    Conflict" (June 17, 2013),
    http://childrenandarmedconflict.un.org/statements/open-debate-security-council
    -statement/.

31 Watchlist, "Children and Armed Conflict," Watchlist, April 2013,
    http://watchlist.org/wordpress/wp-content/uploads/Watchlist-CAC-Update-April
    -2013.pdf.

32 *Child Soldiers International*, "Chance for Change: Ending the Recruitment and
    Use of Child Soldiers in Myanmar," *Child Soldiers International* (January 2013): 2.

33 Karen Human Rights Group, "Abuses since the DKBA and KNLA Ceasefires:
    Forced Labour and Arbitrary Detention in Dooplaya," *Karen Human Rights
    Group Field Report* (May 7, 2012), http://www.khrg.org/khrg2012/khrg12f2.pdf.

34 "Papun Situation Update: Bu Tho Township, January to March 2013," Karen
    Human Rights Group, June 18, 2013, http://www.khrg.org/khrg2013/khrg13b35.pdf.

35 Back Pack Health Worker Team, *Chronic Emergency: Health and Human Rights in
    Eastern Burma* (Thailand: Back Pack Health Worker Team, 2006),
    http://www.ibiblio.org/obl/docs3/Chronic_Emergency-links.html.

36 Maureen Lynch, "Futures Denied: Statelessness among Infants, Children and
    Youth," *Refugees International*, 2008,
    http://www.icyrnet.net/UserFiles/File/Publication%20Resources/Research%20
    Reports/Stateless_Children_FINAL.pdf.

37 Royal Thai Government, Child Protection Act 2003, trans. Pornchai Danvivathana
    (Bangkok: Royal Thai Government, September 24, 2003),
    http://www.law.yale.edu/rcw/rcw/jurisdictions/asse/thailand/Thai_Child_Prot
    _Eng.pdf.

38 CPPCR, *Feeling Small*, 29–30.

39 Committee for Protection and Promotion of Children's Rights (Burma) (CPPCR), *Recognise Us! CPPCR Working to Protect Children—10th Anniversary* (Mae Sot, Thailand: CPPCR, 2012), 14.

40 Ibid., 16.

41 LT and Y, community child protection workers, in discussion with the author, August 19, 2012.

42 Margaret Green-Rauenhorst, Karen Jacobsen, and Sandee Pyne, *Invisible in Thailand: Documenting the Need for International Protection for Burmese* (Thailand: International Rescue Committee 2008), 31, http://www.fmreview.org/FMRpdfs/FMR30/31-33.pdf; "World Report 2013," 1, 6.

43 CPPCR, *Feeling Small*, 28.

44 Royal Thai Government, "Labor Protection Act of 1998," http://www.ilo.org/dyn/natlex/docs/WEBTEXT/49727/65119/E98THA01.htm#c5.

45 "Suffer the Little Children," *Bangkok Post*, June 30, 2013, www.bangkokpost.com/news/investigation/357583/suffer-the-little-children.

46 S, in discussion with the author, August 15, 2012.

47 CPPCR, *Feeling Small*, 41.

48 Wietse A Tol, Suzan Song, and Mark JD Jordans, "Annual Research Review: Resilience and Mental Health in Children and Adolescents Living in Areas of Armed Conflict: A Systematic Review of Findings in Low- and Middle-Income Countries," *Journal of Child Psychology and Psychiatry* 54 no. 4 (2013): 9, doi: 10.1111/jcpp.12053.

49 International Rescue Committee, *Concepts of Child and Family Wellbeing among Burmese Migrant and Displaced Communities in Tak Province* (Thailand: IRC, 2011), 19.

50 Jonathan Gruber, Nathaniel Hendren, and Robert M. Townsend, "The Great Equalizer: Health Care Access and Infant Mortality in Thailand," *American Economic Journal: Applied Economics* 6, no. 1 (January 2014):15, http://scholar.harvard.edu/files/hendren/files/the_great_equalizer_vaejv130318.pdf.

51 "Stateless Minorities Seek Healthcare at Thai-Myanmar border," *Bangkok Post*, cited in *Mizzima*, June 24, 2013, http://www.mizzima.com/news/health/9575-stateless-minorities-seek-healthcare-at-thai-myanmar-border.

52 "Mae Tao Clinic History," http://maetaoclinic.org/about-us/history/.

53 Verena Carrara, Sara Canavati, and Francois Nosten, *Nutritional Assessment of Children 0–12 Years Enrolled in the SMRU Vaccination Campaign for Migrant Population* (Bangkok, Thailand: Shoklo Malaria Research Unit [SMRU], 2009), 3.

54 World Health Organization (WHO), *Mental Health and Psychosocial Well-Being among Children in Severe Food Shortage*, WHO (2006), 2, http://www.who.int/nutrition/publications/emergencies/WHO_MSD_MER _06.1/en/.

55 Green-Rauenhorst et al., *Invisible in Thailand*, 31.

56 "United Nations Declaration of Human Rights Article 26," http://www.un.org/en/documents/udhr/; UNESCO, "After Conflict, Peace-Building through Education," last updated June 28, 2012, http://www.unesco.org/new/en/education/resources/online-materials/single-view /news/after_conflict_peace_building_through_education/; United Nations Convention on the Rights of the Child (1989), http://www.unesco.org/education/pdf/CHILD_E.PDF.

57 Voluntary Services Overseas (VSO), *In School, In Society: Early Childhood Development in Myanmar Migrant Communities in Thailand* (Thailand: VSO, 2013), 9.

58 Ibid., 32–33.

59 Ibid., 34–35.

60 Ibid., 39.

61 Ibid., 25.

62 Jerry Huguet cited in Kerry Richter, Aphichat Chamratrithirong, Sakkarin Niyomsilpa, and Rebecca Miller, "Forward to the Special Issue: Migrants, Minorities and Refugees: Integration and Well-Being," *Journal of Population and Social Studies* 21, no. 1 (July 2012): 2–11, http://www.migrationcenter.mahidol.ac.th/download/JPSS-vol21-No1-chap1.pdf.

63 VSO, *In School, In Society*, 18.

64 Ibid., 24–25.

65 "About Us," Youth Connect Thailand, http://www.youthconnectthailand.org.

66 CPPCR, *Feeling Small*, 35.

67 LT and Y, discussion, August 19, 2012.

68 JF and NT, Room to Grow Foundation program staff, in discussion with the author, August 17, 2012.

69 Weiss et al., "Mental Health in the Aftermath of Disasters," 611.

70 AS, Child Protection Trainer and Coordinator, in discussion with the author, September 12, 2013.

71 Inter-Agency Standing Committee, *IASC Guidelines on Mental Health and Psychosocial Support in Emergency Settings* (Geneva: Inter-Agency Standing Committee, 2007), 9–11. http://www.who.int/mental_health/emergencies/guidelines_iasc_mental_health _psychosocial_june_2007.pdf.

72 Ibid., 12.

73 Ibid., 11.

74 Mae Tao Clinic, *MTC Child Protection Programme Report January–June 2012*, 1, http://www.pureandco.com/ourcompany/ourcauses/docs/MTC%20Child%20 Protection%20Report%20Jan-Jun%202012.pdf.

75 United Nations Convention on the Rights of the Child.

76 Co-Ordinating Team on Displaced Children's Education and Protection (CTDCEP), *Child Protection Policy and Procedures Guidebook (CPP)* (Mae Sot, Thailand, August 2013), 4.

77 IASC, *Guidelines*, 12.

78 International Rescue Committee, *Concepts of Child*, 5.

79 Kumpfer et al., "Cultural Adaptation for International Dissemination of the Strengthening Families Program," *Evaluation & the Health Professions* 31, no. 2 (2008): 226, doi: 10.1177/0163278708315926.

80 IRC, "IMPACT Evaluation of a Family-Based Intervention with Burmese Migrant and Displaced Children and Families in Tak Province, Thailand," http://clinicaltrials.gov/ct2/show/NCT01668992.

81 Presentation of interim findings of IMPACT project in Mae Sot, February 21, 2013.

82 S, discussion, August 15, 2012.

83 World Education, *Creating Opportunities for Psychosocial Enhancement COPE Teacher Training Manual* (Mae Sot, Thailand: World Education, 2009).

84 LT and Y, discussion, August 19, 2012.

85 Ibid.

86 Ibid.

87 IASC, *Guidelines*, 13.

88 Ibid.

89 Pat Dolan and Bernadine Brady, "Child and Youth Mentoring: New Models with New Opportunities" (conference paper at La Tutela dei Minori Conference, Italy, June 28, 2012), 1, http://www.childandfamilyresearch.ie/sites/www.childandfamilyresearch.ie/files /prof__dolan_and_dr_brady_conference_paper_italy__28_june_2012.pdf.

90 DuBois et al., "How Effective Are Mentoring Programs for Youth? A Systematic Assessment of the Evidence," *Psychological Science in the Public Interest* 12, no.2 (2011): 57, doi: 10.1177/1529100611414806.

91 Charles A Rapp, Dennis Saleebey, and W Patrick Sullivan, "The Future of Strengths-Based Social Work," *Advances in Social Work* 6, no. 1 (Spring 2005): 1–82, http://journals.iupui.edu/index.php/advancesinsocialwork/article/view/81.

92 Burma Partnership, *Nothing about Us without Us* (Burma Partnership, December 2012), video.

93 Aung San Suu Kyi, media interview in Mae Sot, Thailand, June 2, 2012 (private recording).

94 "ASEAN Chief Warns Firms of Labour Shortage," *Bangkok Post*, March 10, 2012, http://www.bangkokpost.com/news/local/283696/asean-chief-warns-firms-of -labour-shortage.

95 Malee Sunpuwan and Sakkarin Niyomsilpa, "Perception and Misperception: Thai Public Opinions on Refugees and Migrants from Myanmar," *Journal of Population and Social Studies* 21, no. 1 (2012): 50, http://www2.ipsr.mahidol.ac.th/Journal/index.php?option=com_content& view=article&id=139%3Avol21-no1-issue3&catid=150%3Ajpss-vol21-no1& Itemid=105.

96 Sunpuwan and Niyomsilpa, "Perception and Misperception," 56.

Bibliography

"ASEAN Chief Warns Firms of Labour Shortage." *Bangkok Post*, March 10, 2012. http://www.bangkokpost.com/news/local/283696/asean-chief-warns-firms-of -labour-shortage.

Aung San Suu Kyi. Media interview in Mae Sot, Thailand, June 2012 (private recording).

Back Pack Health Worker Team. *Chronic Emergency: Health and Human Rights in Eastern Burma*. Thailand: Back Pack Health Worker Team, 2006. http://www.ibiblio.org/obl/docs3/Chronic_Emergency-links.html.

The Border Consortium (TBC). *Displacement and Poverty in South East Burma/ Myanmar 2011*. http://www.refworld.org/docid/4ea7e9652.html.

Burma Partnership. *Nothing about Us without Us*. Burma Partnership, December 2012. Video.

Carrara, Verena, Sara Canavati, and Francois Nosten. *Nutritional Assessment of Children 0–12 Years Enrolled in the SMRU Vaccination Campaign for Migrant Population*. Bangkok, Thailand: Shoklo Malaria Research Unit (SMRU), 2009.

"Chance for Change: Ending the Recruitment and Use of Child Soldiers in Myanmar." *Child Soldiers International*, January 2013.

Clarke, Roger. "A Primer in Diffusion of Innovations Theory." Unpublished paper, 1999. http://www.anu.edu.au/people/Roger.Clarke/SOS/InnDiff.html.

Committee for Protection and Promotion of Children's Rights (Burma). *Feeling Small in Another Person's Country: The Situation of Burmese Migrant Children in Mae Sot Thailand*. Mae Sot, Thailand: CPPCR, 2009.

———. *Recognise Us! CPPCR Working to Protect Children—10th Anniversary*. Mae Sot, Thailand: CPPCR, 2012.

Co-Ordinating Team on Displaced Children's Education and Protection (CTDCEP). *Child Protection Policy and Procedures Guidebook (CPP)*. Mae Sot, Thailand, August 2013.

Dolan, Pat, and Bernadine Brady. "Child and Youth Mentoring: New Models with New Opportunities." Conference paper at La Tutela dei Minori conference, Italy, June 28, 2012. http://www.childandfamilyresearch.ie/sites/www.childandfamilyresearch.ie/files /prof__dolan_and_dr_brady_conference_paper_italy__28_june_2012.pdf.

DuBois, David L, Nelson Portillo, Jean E Rhodes, Naida Silverthorn, and Jeffrey C Valentine. "How Effective Are Mentoring Programs for Youth? A Systematic Assessment of the Evidence." *Psychological Science in the Public Interest* 12, no. 2 (2011): 57–91. doi: 10.1177/1529100611414806.

Fries, Elizabeth. "Steps towards Empowerment for Community Healing." *Intervention* 1, no. 2 (2003): 40–46. http://www.interventionjournal.com/downloads/12pdf/1207%20Fries.pdf.

Galappatti, Ananda. "What Is a Psychosocial Intervention? Mapping the Field in Sri Lanka." *Intervention* 1, no. 2 (2003): 3–17. http://www.interventionjournal.com/downloads/12pdf/1204%20Ananda%20 Galappatti.pdf.

Green-Rauenhorst, Margaret, Karen Jacobsen, and Sandee Pyne. *Invisible in Thailand: Documenting the Need for International Protection for Burmese.* Thailand: International Rescue Committee 2008. http://www.fmreview.org/FMRpdfs/FMR30/31-33.pdf.

Gruber, Jonathan, Nathaniel Hendren, and Robert M Townsend. "The Great Equalizer: Health Care Access and Infant Mortality in Thailand." *American Economic Journal: Applied Economics* 6, no. 1 (January 2014): 91–107. http://scholar.harvard.edu/files/hendren/files/the_great_equalizer_vaejv130318.pdf.

Government of the Republic of the Union of Myanmar Ministry of Education. "Education for All: Access to and Quality of Education in Myanmar." Conference on Development Policy Options with Special Reference to Education and Health in Myanmar, Nay Pyi Taw, Myanmar, February 13–16, 2012. http://yangon.sites.unicnetwork.org/files/2013/05/Final-UBW-presentation-12-2-12 -UBW.pdf.

Human Rights Watch. "World Report 2013: Burma (events of 2012)." http://www.hrw.org/world-report/2013/country-chapters/burma.

———. "World Report 2013: Thailand (events of 2012)." http://www.hrw.org/world-report/2013/country-chapters/thailand.

Inter-Agency Standing Committee. *IASC Guidelines on Mental Health and Psychosocial Support in Emergency Settings.* Geneva: Inter-Agency Standing Committee, 2007. http://www.who.int/mental_health/emergencies/guidelines_iasc_mental_health _psychosocial_june_2007.pdf.

International Rescue Committee. *Concepts of Child and Family Wellbeing among Burmese Migrant and Displaced Communities in Tak Province.* Thailand: IRC, 2011.

———. "Impact Evaluation of a Family-Based Intervention with Burmese Migrant and Displaced Children and Families in Tak Province, Thailand." http://clinicaltrials.gov/ct2/show/NCT01668992.

Karen Human Rights Group. "Abuses since the DKBA and KNLA Ceasefires: Forced Labour and Arbitrary Detention in Dooplaya." *Karen Human Rights Group Field Report* (May 7, 2012). http://www.khrg.org/khrg2012/khrg12f2.pdf.

———. "Papun Situation Update: Bu Tho Township, January to March 2013." June 18, 2013. http://www.khrg.org/khrg2013/khrg13b35.pdf.

Karen News. "About Karen News." http://karennews.org/about-us/.

Kumpfer, Karol L, Methinin Pinyuchon, Ana Teixeira de Melo, and Henry O Whiteside. "Cultural Adaptation for International Dissemination of the Strengthening Families Program." *Evaluation & the Health Professions* 31, no. 2 (2008): 226–239. doi: 10.1177/0163278708315926.

Lynch, M. "Futures Denied: Statelessness among Infants, Children and Youth." *Refugees International* 2008. http://www.icyrnet.net/UserFiles/File/Publication%20Resources/Research%20Reports/Stateless_Children_FINAL.pdf.

Mae Tao Clinic. "History." http://maetaoclinic.org/about-us/history/.

———. *MTC Child Protection Programme Report January–June 2012*. Mae Sot, Thailand: MTC, 2012. http://www.pureandco.com/ourcompany/ourcauses/docs/MTC%20Child%20Protection%20Report%20Jan-Jun%202012.pdf.

Naker, Dipak. "Creating Violence-Free Childhoods: What Will It Take?" *Bernard van Leer Foundation Early Childhood Matters* 116 (2011). http://vps.earlychildhoodmagazine.org/wp-content/uploads/2011/06/ECM116_Creating-violence-free-childhoods_13.pdf.

Perrin, Sean, Patrick Smith, and William Yule. "Practitioner Review: The Assessment and Treatment of Post-Traumatic Stress Disorder in Children and Adolescents." *Journal of Child Psychology and Psychiatry* 41, no. 3 (2000): 277–289.

Rapp, Charles A, Dennis Saleebey, and W Patrick Sullivan. "The Future of Strengths-Based Social Work." *Advances in Social Work* 6, no. 1 (Spring 2005): 79–90. http://journals.iupui.edu/index.php/advancesinsocialwork/article/view/81.

Richter, Kerry, Aphichat Chamratrithirong, Sakkarin Niyomsilpa, and Rebecca Miller. "Forward to the Special Issue: Migrants, Minorities and Refugees: Integration and Well-Being." *Journal of Population and Social Studies* 21, no. 1 (July 2012): 2–11. http://www.migrationcenter.mahidol.ac.th/download/JPSS-vol21-No1-chap1.pdf.

Rogers, Everett M. *Diffusion of Innovations*. 5th ed. New York: Free Press, 2003.

Royal Thai Government. Child Protection Act 2003. Translated by Pornchai Danvivathana. Bangkok: Royal Thai Government, September 24, 2003.

http://www.law.yale.edu/rcw/rcw/jurisdictions/asse/thailand/Thai_Child_Prot_
Eng.pdf.

———. "Labor Protection Act of 1998."
http://www.ilo.org/dyn/natlex/docs/WEBTEXT/49727/65119/E98THA01.htm#c5.

Save the Children. "Myanmar." Last updated July 2012.
http://www.savethechildren.org/site/c.8rKLIXMGIpI4E/b.6150543/.

Silove, Derrick, Zachary Steel, and M Psychol. "Understanding Community
Psychosocial Needs after Disasters: Implications for Mental Health Services."
Journal of Postgrad Medicine 52 (2006): 121–125.

"Stateless Minorities Seek Healthcare at Thai-Myanmar Border." *Bangkok Post*, cited in
Mizzima, June 24, 2013.
http://www.mizzima.com/news/health/9575-stateless-minorities-seek-healthcare-at
-thai-myanmar-border.

"Suffer the Little Children." *Bangkok Post*, June 30, 2013.
http://www.bangkokpost.com/news/investigation/357583/suffer-the-little-children.

Sunpuwan, Malee, and Sakkarin Niyomsilpa, "Perception and Misperception: Thai
Public Opinions on Refugees and Migrants from Myanmar." *Journal of Population
and Social Studies* 21, no. 1 (2012): 47–58.

Tol, Wietse A, Suzan Song, and Mark JD Jordans. "Annual Research Review: Resilience
and Mental Health in Children and Adolescents Living in Areas of Armed Conflict:
A Systematic Review of Findings in Low- and Middle-Income Countries." *Journal of
Child Psychology and Psychiatry* 54, no. 4 (2013): 445–460. doi:10.1111/jcpp.12053.

UNESCO. "After Conflict, Peace-Building through Education." June 28, 2012.
http://www.unesco.org/new/en/education/resources/online-materials/single-view
/news/after_conflict_peace_building_through_education/.

———. *United Nations Convention on the Rights of the Child.* UNESCO,
http://www.unesco.org/education/pdf/CHILD_E.PDF 1989.

UNICEF. *Situational Analysis of Children from Myanmar.* Myanmar: UNICEF, July
2012. http://www.unicef.org/eapro/Myanmar_Situation_Analysis.pdf.

United Nations. "Report of the Independent Expert for the United Nations Study on
Violence against Children. Sixty-First Session. UN General Assembly, Item 62A,
Promotion and Protection of the Rights of Children." August 29, 2006.
http://www.unicef.org/violencestudy/reports/SG_violencestudy_en.pdf.

———. "United Nations Declaration of Human Rights Article 26."
http://www.un.org/en/documents/udhr/.

Voluntary Services Overseas (VSO). *In School, In Society: Early Childhood
Development in Myanmar Migrant Communities in Thailand.* Thailand: VSO, 2013.

Watchlist. "Children and Armed Conflict." Watchlist, April 2013.
http://watchlist.org/wordpress/wp-content/uploads/Watchlist-CAC-Update-April
-2013.pdf.

Weiss, Mitchell G, Benedetto Saracerno, Shekhar Saxena, and Mark Van Ommeren. "Mental Health in the Aftermath of Disasters: Consensus and Controversy." *Journal of Nervous and Mental Disease* 191, no. 9 (2003): 611–615. doi: 10.1097/01. nmd. 0000087188.96516.a3.

Wickramage, Kolitha. "Sri Lanka's Post-Tsunami Psychosocial Playground: Lessons for Future Psychosocial Programming and Interventions Following Disasters." *Interventions* 4, no. 2 (2006): 167–172. http://ourmediaourselves.com/archives/42pdf/WTF14.pdf.

World Education. *Creating Opportunities for Psychosocial Enhancement COPE Teacher Training Manual.* Thailand: World Education, 2009.

World Health Organization. "Community Mental Health Services Will Lessen Social Exclusion." Last modified June 1, 2007. http://www.who.int/mediacentre/news/notes/2007/np25/en.

———. "Mental health and Psychosocial Well-Being among Children in Severe Food Shortage." WHO, 2006.

Zerrougui, Leila. Special Representative for Children in Armed Conflict Statement to Security Council Working Group Debate on Children and Armed Conflict. June 17, 2013. http://childrenandarmedconflict.un.org/statements/open-debate-security-council -statement/.

Chapter 6

Gender-Based Violence

Realities, Challenges, and Solutions

from a Refugee Camp Context

Abigail Erikson, Kristin Kim Bart, and Moe Moe Aung

Dor Meh, a 45-year-old woman, lives with her three children in a refugee camp in northwest Thailand. While living in the camp, she and her children escaped from the terror of repeated physical and psychological abuse at home, seeking shelter at the Women's Community Center operated by the International Rescue Committee. Dor Meh had been married for over eighteen years, much of that time living with a husband who was an alcoholic and abusive. She endured repeated violent attacks, and during the last attack, her husband tried to beat his daughters. After receiving legal counseling, Dor Meh made the difficult decision to pursue a divorce. This decision was difficult for Dor Meh because while she wanted the violence to stop, she did not necessarily want to be a divorced woman and carry the stigma this has in the community. Further, Dor Meh was not confident that, even if she were granted a divorce, she would remain safe, as long as her ex-husband could still find her in the camp. In Dor Meh's case, she was granted a divorce from the camp justice committee, yet, because she was still fearful of attacks by her ex-husband, she did not feel safe leaving the shelter. A continual challenge for Dor Meh was how to continue regular community life under ongoing threat of violence from her ex-husband. For example, her children needed to go to school, yet were unsafe walking from the shelter to school every day. As a result, the camp security guards had to accompany the children. While this helped them feel safe, it also created shame and embarrassment in the community. Being escorted to school by camp security is a public admission that they have a family that is not peaceful. In a community that values peaceful family life, this can be very shameful. In this case, Dor Meh and her daughters were accepted into the US resettlement program, ending the uncertainty they faced in this particular situation, yet also opening up a whole new set of uncertainties about life in America.

Violence against Women and Girls: An Overview

Around the world, as many as one in every three women has been beaten, coerced into sex, or abused in some other way.[1] This global epidemic of violence encompasses a wide range of human rights violations, including the sexual abuse of children, rape, sexual exploitation, sexual assault and abuse, sexual harassment and discrimination, physical assault, intimate-partner violence, trafficking of women and girls, forced prostitution, and denial of women's rights. It also encompasses forms of violence that are specific to cultures and societies, such as female genital mutilation and forced and early marriage.[2] Statistics show that most often, a woman is abused by someone she knows, including her husband, another male family member, or a male community leader.[3] Violence against women and girls is not a new phenomenon, nor does it discriminate. Women of all ages, religions, ethnic groups, and social and economic status experience violence.[4]

Gender-based violence (GBV) is defined as any harm perpetrated against a person's will that results from power inequities based on gender roles. The overwhelming majority of cases involve women and girls. The above examples provide a glimpse of the violence that can form the landscape of the lives of women and girls. From infancy to death, girls and women are at risk for all types and forms of violence in ways that boys and men are not. For this reason, the term "gender-based violence" is often used synonymously with the term "violence against women and girls." This is done deliberately, to highlight the gender-based nature of the violence—meaning the relationship between females' subordinate status in society and their increased vulnerability to violence. For the purposes of this chapter, the terms will be used interchangeably.

It is widely recognized that the root causes of gender-based violence lie in a society's attitudes toward and practices of gender roles and the discrimination that women typically face simply because they are women.[5] The World Health Organization characterizes violence against women across the world as an "extreme manifestation of gender inequality" requiring urgent attention and action.[6] Around the world, gender dynamics between men and women maintain that men have authority over women and possess more privileges and entitlements than the women around them. This gender inequality means that women and girls have reduced access to resources and opportunities and, as a consequence, fewer opportunities to determine their own lives and an increased exposure to violence. Women and girls are often considered as resources to be transferred and inherited between men—for example, when a girl is married and is no longer the responsibility or property of her father but becomes that of her husband. This type of social structure and practice upholds and often sanctions the use of violence and discrimination against women and girls. Thus the violence women and girls experience is both an indicator of gender inequality and a means through which that inequality is perpetuated.[7]

Domestic violence, an often hidden form of gender-based violence, is one of the biggest threats to women's health and well-being.[8] Domestic violence, for the purposes of this chapter, is defined as acts of physical, sexual, and emotional violence inflicted against a woman by her intimate partner, whether cohabiting or not. These behaviors also include men refusing to provide money to cover basic necessities and controlling behaviors such as constraining a woman's mobility or access to friends and relatives. Violence may begin with insults or intermittent physical violence—a shove or slap—and over time develop into more severe actions—choking, burning, kicking, using weapons—that put a women's life in grave danger. Perpetrators use threats and physical violence to control the actions and behaviors of female partners and, in the process, diminish their self-worth and isolate them from support networks. If children are involved, perpetrators can use the children against their mothers or threaten to harm the children. This helps perpetrators maintain control over their partners over time. Domestic violence is rarely a one-time event; instead, the violence is a pattern and tends to increase in severity and frequency over time.[9]

Power inequalities derived from gender roles permeate cultures and societies to varying degrees. In contexts of ongoing or recent conflict, inequalities are exacerbated and sometimes even exploited. The general breakdown of law and order caused by conflict, natural disaster, or population displacement can lead to an increase in all types of violence against women and girls.[10] Violence against women and girls in conflict is an effective means of breaking down society. It succeeds in tearing apart families and ripping the social fabric of a community. In the past decade, sexual violence has continued to be used as a tool of war to terrorize and control women, girls, and their communities.[11] This has been seen in the Democratic Republic of the Congo, in the newly established Republic of South Sudan and across the Middle East during the Arab Spring. Furthermore, domestic violence tends to increase during prolonged displacement: as men feel frustrated, powerless, and lose their traditional male roles, they exert their control in the one socially accepted place—their home.

It is important to emphasize that it is not the context of conflict or displacement that causes the violence to occur. The underlying gender inequality between men and women creates a backdrop on which women and girls become targets of violence. The United Nations High Commissioner for

Refugees (UNHCR), the UN agency responsible for assisting and protecting refugees around the world, states the following in their global guidelines on gender-based violence: "The lack of social and economic value for women and women's work and the accepted gender roles perpetuate and reinforce the assumption that men have decision-making power and control over women. Through acts of sexual and gender-based violence, whether individual or collective, perpetrators seek to maintain privileges, power, and control over others."[12] In these contexts, women and girls face threats of violence in all stages of conflict and displacement. The societal upheaval that takes place also means that existing formal and informal mechanisms to protect women and girls have often collapsed or are inaccessible, leaving them more vulnerable to all forms of violence. When fleeing war and conflict, women and girls are at risk for rape and sexual assault by armed members of parties to the conflict or security personnel such as border guards. While seeking refuge or in refugee and internally displaced camps, women and girls continue to be at risk for violence. These risks include sexual attack, coercion or extortion by those in positions of authority, trafficking, domestic violence, and increases in harmful traditional practices such as early or forced marriage. And during repatriation and reintegration, women and girls continue to be at risk for all forms of sexual violence, domestic violence, and denial of or obstructed access to resources or proper legal status.[13]

In short, when the conflict ends, violence against women and girls most often does not. Ann Jones, a leading feminist author, describes this reality in postconflict West Africa:

> When any conflict of this sort officially ends, violence against women continues and often actually grows worse. Not surprisingly, murderous aggression cannot be turned off overnight. When men stop attacking one another, women continue to be convenient targets. Here in West Africa, as in so many other places where rape was used as a weapon of war, it has become a habit carried seamlessly into the "post-conflict" era. Where normal structures of law enforcement and justice have been disabled by war, male soldiers and civilians alike can prey upon women and children with impunity. And they do.[14]

Effects of Violence on Women and Girls

The effects of violence for women and girls is far-reaching and results in adverse effects on an individual's physical, intellectual, emotional, and social functioning. Women and girls who are victims of violence often live in a constant state of fear, leading to high levels of stress, anxiety, and posttraumatic stress disorder (PTSD).[15] A study in North America showed that abused women were three times more likely to suffer from posttraumatic stress disorder than non-abused women.[16] A multicountry study by the World Health Organization examining violence against women, particularly intimate-partner violence, found that women in Peru, Brazil, Thailand, and Japan who had been physically and sexually abused by their partners were more than twice as likely as non-abused women to have considered suicide.[17]

Women who have survived violence typically require a variety of services and support to heal and recover. In conflict-affected settings, this is made more difficult as even the most basic services, such as primary health care and public security, do not exist. And yet survivors may require health services to treat wounds, broken bones, sexually transmitted infections, or unwanted pregnancies; psychosocial support to help rebuild self-esteem and social networks; safety mechanisms to access temporary emergency shelter; or legal support to press charges or seek a divorce.[18]

The ongoing safety risks women and girls face can exacerbate the effects of violence on women and girls and has specific implications for how to deliver services. Practitioners in the mental health field must be aware of the myriad effects violence has on women's functioning and understand the fundamental dynamics that underpin violence against women to tailor psychosocial care for survivors of such violence. For example, psychosocial staff requires specialized training in empowerment-based case management, in which a survivor's authority in decision-making and her capacity for self-sufficiency are promoted. In addition, specialized training on how to provide care that emphasizes survivor safety throughout is critical.

Despite evidence and widespread acknowledgement that women and girls who suffer from traumatic abuse need abuse-specific and appropriate mental health interventions to promote healing and recovery, in conflict settings, access to specialized mental health services is scarce.[19] In settings where the UN and nongovernmental organizations (NGOs) have established programs to meet the needs of survivors of violence, psychosocial staff generally provides supportive counseling and case management only. While these interventions are essential, ideally they are delivered within a broader trauma treatment framework to promote sustained health and healing outcomes.

Responding to Violence against Women in Humanitarian Settings

Initial programs developed to respond to gender-based violence in humanitarian settings focused on war-related sexual violence. Most often these were stand-alone projects, not integrated into other humanitarian programs, and ended once the funding was spent. This model has proved ineffective, as programs started and stopped quickly and did not meet the broad needs of sexual-violence survivors, such as ongoing security and health care. The short term of most funding opportunities also severely hindered working on effective prevention strategies, which require long-term and sustained efforts. Further, this model did not meet the needs of survivors of other types of violence against women, who soon started to seek assistance. Once basic services were established for sexual-violence survivors and women heard there was a program to help them, regardless of whether they were raped by a combatant or beaten by their husbands, they started to come forward for assistance. Gradually there was recognition that supporting survivors of any type of violence against women and girls requires the involvement of multiple sectors working within a humanitarian response— from health to protection to food security. Aid agencies now prioritize developing comprehensive, coordinated services for survivors of all types of violence, including health care, psychosocial support and case management, safety and security interventions, and access to justice options.[20]

With multiple agencies and sectors responding to the needs of survivors, it was evident that common ethical standards for all sectors and agencies was critical to ensure a quality continuum of care. Across humanitarian settings, the standard set of guiding principles, initially outlined in the UNHCR Sexual and Gender-Based Violence Guidelines for Prevention and Response, are

- Ensuring safety: All actions taken on behalf of a survivor should be aimed at restoring or maintaining safety.
- Respect and dignity for the survivor: Survivors' opinions, thoughts, and ideas should be listened to and treated with respect.
- Nondiscrimination: All survivors are equal and should be treated the same and have equal access to services.
- Confidentiality: At all times, confidentiality of the affected person(s) and their families should be respected. This means sharing only the necessary information, as requested and as agreed on by the survivor, with those actors involved in providing assistance.[21]

Guidance for implementing a multisectoral, coordinated approach to gender-based violence is outlined in the Inter-Agency Standing Committee's *IASC Guidelines for Gender-Based Violence in Humanitarian Settings.*

These guidelines, finalized in 2005, were developed by leading United Nations agencies and NGOs. The guidelines outline minimum standards of care, how to set up interagency referral networks and information sharing protocols, and how to coordinate, monitor, and evaluate services across multiple sectors. While the document details both response and prevention interventions, it recommends that actors prioritize response services—in particular the establishment of health and psychosocial services for survivors—at the outset of a humanitarian response. When resources are limited, this helps ensure prioritization of the needs of women and girls who have already experienced violence. The guidelines also emphasize the need for effective coordination mechanisms, recognizing that all survivors need a host of services and someone to help them navigate the confusing web of services and options (or lack of options) available.[22]

Presently, gender-based violence programs use these guiding principles and existing standards, adapted to the specific context on the ground, to advocate for an appropriate level of care for survivors. In many settings however, a lack of understanding of the principles and overall resistance to the issue of violence against women creates a significant challenge to holding service providers accountable to these survivor-centered principles. Strategies for overcoming this and other challenges are discussed below.

Domestic Violence in Refugee Camps: Experiences and Lessons Learned from the Thai-Burma Border

In communities ravaged by conflict, violence of all kinds tends to become normalized; this frequently translates into the private sphere, with increased rates of domestic violence in conflict-affected populations. A recent report on domestic violence published by the International Rescue Committee (IRC)[23] reveals that since the end of wars in Liberia, Sierra Leone, Uganda, and Iraq, service providers and police have received increased reports of violence against women and girls, perpetrated by intimate partners. The report states, "In these post-conflict settings, the primary threat to women is not a man with a gun or a stranger. It is their husbands." Over 60 percent of assault survivors whom the IRC assists in West Africa are seeking help because of violence committed by an intimate partner.[24] This is also the case in many protracted refugee camp contexts, where domestic violence is one of the more common forms of violence women and girls report to service providers.[25] UNHCR defines protracted refugee situations as "refugee populations of 25,000 persons or more who have been in exile for five or more years in developing countries."[26]

The root cause of domestic violence is unchanged across cultures—that is, male power and men's control over women—but different contributing factors emerge across settings. In protracted refugee camp contexts, common contributing factors to high levels of domestic violence include the breakdown of family and social structures; the lack of effective protection, including the use of customary and traditional laws and practices that enforce gender discrimination; and difficulty coping with feelings of stagnation and frustration, often coupled with alcohol use/abuse. Moreover, the complex dynamics at play in a domestic violence relationship are difficult to understand for someone outside the relationship and contribute to women staying long after they know it is dangerous. These dynamics include men's use of fear and intimidation to control a women's behavior, women's lack of access to financial and other resources that provide choices to leave relationships, and the emotional bonds that exists in a relationship, even a violent relationship, and keep women hopeful that their husbands can, and will, change.

Along the Thai-Burma border, more than 150,000 refugees displaced from their homes in Burma have been living in refugee camps for almost two decades. In Mae Hong Son Province, in the far northwest of Thailand, two refugee camps house more than 17,000 refugees mostly from the Karenni state. Eighty-five percent of the camp population is ethnically Kayah, while the remainder is made up of the ethnic minorities Kayan, Paku, Kayaw, Manaw, Burman, Shan, Pa-O, and others.[27] As with most camps in Thailand, the camps are quite isolated—one to three hours by vehicle, in the dry season, along a rutted road from Mae Hong Son town. Mae Hong Son town is the capital city of Mae Hong Son Province. It is a sleepy, small border town populated mainly by ethnic Shan residents. Mae Hong Son is the closest town to the two refugee camps in the province, and is where all the local NGO head offices are located.

Refugees from these camps have had minimal opportunity for safe repatriation, local integration or, until recently, resettlement to other countries. Also worth noting is that Thailand, while housing refugees from Cambodia and Burma throughout the past thirty years, is not party to the 1951 United Nations Convention Relating to the Status of Refugees. This landmark international convention outlines who is a refugee, what their legal rights are, and the legal obligations of the states. This means that while the Thai authorities have permitted displaced people to reside in Thailand and cooperate with UN agencies and NGOs providing aid, they are not technically obligated to do so. Despite the decades-long existence of the refugee camps along the Thai-Burma border, the camps are still referred to as temporary shelters, which simply underscores the limited options for refugees in Thailand.

Many camp residents are peaceful, gracious people, but are experiencing high levels of domestic violence as years of stagnation and frustration coupled with cultural beliefs and attitudes that condone violence against women take their toll. According to IRC's service delivery statistics, domestic violence made up 75 percent of all incidents reported to IRC-supported services in 2011, with 62 percent being physical assault.[28] The broader community views domestic violence as a private issue, and it can be dishonorable for a woman to disclose such violence publicly in her community. There is a common belief that domestic violence is "normal," and therefore not as serious as other types of violence to which refugees are exposed, including sexual violence. A phrase casually and commonly used among the Karenni community to describe domestic violence is, "pot and spoon hitting is typical." Domestic violence can therefore go unnoticed and unaddressed if attention is not brought to the issue.

Since 2004, the IRC has worked with the Karenni women's community on developing psychosocial and safety services specifically for women and girls experiencing violence. The Karenni women's community has played a central role in breaking the silence about gender-based violence and, in particular, violence in the home. Women leaders who represent women's interests and help identify and protect those most vulnerable to violence have been critical to developing greater community support for survivors. The refugee-run women's organization leads community dialogues about gender-based violence (i.e., what it is, the effects it can have on survivors, why it is important for survivors to have access to care); runs shelters and psychosocial support services for survivors; and trains health care workers, security officers, teachers, and other community leaders on gender violence–related topics. These efforts are crucial to engendering broader community support not only for survivors of violence seeking assistance, but also for service providers. They have also helped gain necessary support from refugee leaders—mainly men—who influence community norms and practices that affect the comfort and safety of survivors who seek services.

Consistent with the IASC global guidelines, the IRC and its community partners in the camps employ the multisectoral approach to gender-based violence response. This approach—central to effective care for survivors of domestic violence—helps ensure that key services for survivors are developed in the community, including clinical health care, psychosocial support, security and safety, and access to legal justice. To ensure a participatory and community-led approach to addressing violence, a GBV working group was established in 2004 in the camps that helped ensure locally developed approaches rather than the perception that the problem was brought on by actors external to the community. The working group, a cornerstone of the humanitarian response to GBV and the forum to bring the IASC guidelines to life, is made up of community leaders, service providers, NGOs, and United Nations representatives, who meet monthly. The working group is tasked with developing GBV response protocols, addressing ongoing challenges facing women and girls' protection, and leading prevention campaigns in the community.

Intensive dialogue and debate take place during these meetings, as people have differing levels of acceptance and understanding of the issue. In particular, garnering support for implementing the survivor-centered principles outlined in the IASC guidelines requires ongoing deliberation. The principle and practice of confidentiality is one debated topic within the working group. Confidentiality was a fairly new idea to the community, and at first, it was hotly contested and widely misunderstood. In part, this misunderstanding was caused by the challenge of translating the concept into Burmese and Karenni. In Burmese and Karenni languages, there is no one word for confidentiality, which makes explaining the concept—and the importance of it—challenging. The closest words to confidentiality in Burmese and Karenni are *liu wak* and *teb dot teh er*, respectively, meaning "secret," which connotes an entirely different meaning. Use of the word "secret" led community leaders in these camps to misunderstand the intentions of service providers, and they began to blame them for "keeping secrets" from them about their own community members. Service providers, particularly social and health care workers, spent considerable time explaining that they were upholding a survivor's right to decide for herself who she wants informed about her personal situation and not intending to keep secrets from them. In fact, many times, leaders in the security and legal justice sector of the camps are aware of cases of violence because survivors wish for them to know. In these instances, health and psychosocial service providers assist in facilitating the exchange of information about an individual woman's case according to what the survivor wishes to be shared. Through extensive and ongoing dialogue, the working group agreed that a woman has the right to seek services in private and has the right to determine to whom, how, and when information about her situation will be shared, and that service providers should deliver services in a way that upholds this practice. In 2010, community leaders, NGOs, UNHCR, and the Thai authorities signed a GBV response protocol that included the principle of confidentiality. While the term "secret" is still used, it is translated with additional context to help people understand the difference between secrecy and confidentiality.

Despite the challenges, the presence of the GBV working group and interagency GBV protocol has played a key role in upholding best practice standards and ensuring effective service delivery in the community.

SUPPORTING SURVIVORS: INTERVENTIONS AND CHALLENGES

Survivors of domestic violence almost always have varied and multiple needs, and safety is usually top-ranked. In the Karenni community, where the majority of women seeking services are survivors of domestic violence, psychosocial workers are trained on specific approaches to domestic violence case management and psychosocial care. "Psychosocial workers" in this chapter refers to GBV case workers who are working at the Women's Community Centers. In the refugee camp, there is also a psychosocial program, with psychosocial workers who provide counseling and follow-up to clients with general mental health issues, not necessarily specific to gender-based violence.

For example, developing safety plans and skills-building on psychosocial approaches that build women's self-esteem and helps them evaluate danger are critical competencies for psychosocial staff responding to violence against women. Also essential are access to safe shelter and specialized health care services for survivors and training for local security and justice officials on domestic violence. The services for survivors are then coordinated through the community-based protocol, which outlines the referral pathways in the community developed in the GBV working group as outlined above.

WOMEN'S COMMUNITY CENTERS: THE ROLE OF SAFE SHELTER

In the Karenni camp, a key feature of the response is the operation of two safe shelters, referred to as the Women's Community Centers (WCCs). The centers are essentially safe shelters for women and children fleeing violent homes, and while there, survivors are provided with case management and counseling services, food and clothing, and ongoing advocacy with the camp leaders for some sort of resolution of their grievance. In any given month, roughly seven women and eleven children seek safe shelter from violence at home or in the community. The majority of the women are fleeing violent husbands, often returning more than once and usually with several children accompanying them. Many women in the community do not dare to flee a violent relationship; if or when they do, it is because the violence is becoming more and more severe. While the average length of stay at a wcc is two weeks, with survivors most often returning home after their case has been "resolved" in the traditional justice system, for many women the stay is longer, as the fear of returning home is great. Thus, the role of multiple community actors is fundamental in protecting women's safety and security. The wcc shelters are governed by an operational protocol that outlines the rules and regulations of the shelters, including who can stay at the shelters and for how long, rules for staff and residents, an overview of services provided, and guiding principles for working with survivors. These operational guidelines are shared with other community-based organizations.

Although access to safe shelter is a crucial need for women and girls in refugee settings, specific shelters for survivors of gender-based violence are not the norm. Along the Thai-Burma border, however, where refugees have been housed for decades, the construction of shelters for women and girls has been prioritized, acknowledging the length of the refugee context and the need expressed by the refugee women's community. Operating safe shelters in refugee camp settings is a challenge, however. Unlike safe houses in other settings, for example, it is impossible to keep the location of the shelter confidential in a refugee camp. This means survivors and their children at the shelter can be exposed while staying there. The shelter staff therefore goes to great lengths to ensure privacy of clients through locating shelters strategically (in less crowded areas of the camp), building tall bamboo fences around the perimeters, and maintaining confidentiality when communicating about their work with friends and family.

The lack of confidentiality also presents security risks to shelter residents and staff. More than once, an angry perpetrator has shown up at a wcc demanding that his wife and children return home. These visits are terrifying for survivors and other residents and staff, and many women report they are unable to sleep for several weeks after one of these incidents. The value of a multisectoral approach is evident when a safe shelter exists, as multiple actors are responsible and necessary for ensuring effective and ongoing security for survivors and staff who support them. Persistent efforts by the women's community to garner support from the camp leaders for the centers led to an unprecedented alliance between the women's community and the local camp security. In the camps, the camp security, part of the overall local governance structure, supports overall security for the camp residents and is responsible for promoting peace and order in the camp.

The alliance led to enhanced partnership between the centers and camp security, whereby the camp security agreed to provide around-the-clock protection for the residents and staff at the shelters. Prior to this agreement, the only line of defense against angry perpetrators was the tall bamboo fence. The bamboo, shaved at the top to create a razor-like edge, was an attempt to dissuade perpetrators from climbing over into the compound but was frequently unsuccessful. The presence of twenty-four-hour security not only meant increased safety for the residents, it also signaled more broad-based support from leaders for the idea that survivors have a right to safe shelter—and it was their responsibility to help protect women and children experiencing violence. Since then, the security personnel monitoring the centers have expanded their role to assist survivors and children in moving safely in the community while their cases are being handled (e.g., accompanying survivors to medical appointments or walking children to school). The security staff is provided with intensive training on core concepts related to domestic violence, confidentiality protocols, and overall best practices for supporting survivors. Forging this alliance with camp security has resulted in fewer threatening visits to the shelters by perpetrators and has increased women's confidence in the centers as a viable safety option. Now, if a perpetrator arrives at the centers, the camp security staff immediately detains the man and removes him from the premises. This support from the camp security has been vital for the centers, providing more robust security for the survivors and staff at the WCCs.

THE ROLE OF SAFETY PLANNING AND MULTIAGENCY RESPONSIBILITY

A key function of psychosocial services for survivors is to help them navigate the challenging (and sometimes dangerous) family terrain that develops after seeking help, at the same time safely coordinating an array of services for the survivor and her children. To do this, service providers receive specialized case management training on the dynamics of domestic violence (e.g., the cyclical nature of the violence), the crucial link between confidentiality and security in service delivery, and how to support survivors as they work toward strategies for living safely from day to day. As each survivor presents with unique circumstances and drives decision-making in her own case, every safety plan—and overall management for each case—is handled differently.

Safety planning is a critical component in domestic violence case management. Safety plans can range from supporting a survivor as she seeks support from community leaders in holding her violent husband accountable to strategizing how to mitigate harm during a future violent episode. Through the process of discussing and planning out steps, survivors walk through a series of choices, weighing every possible action against the risk for increased violence.

The case of Keh Meh illustrates the key role safety planning plays in working with domestic violence survivors. (All names and other identifying information have been changed to protect the anonymity of survivors.) Keh Meh has been in an abusive relationship for many years, with the violence increasing over time. Keh Meh has two children—both girls, ages 12 and 14. Her daughters have witnessed the violence most of their lives, but have never been struck directly by their father. Keh Meh has cycled in and out of the WCC for more than two years, as well as cycling in and out of the camp leader's office for mediation. After returning home, there was generally a period of calm before the violence would start up again. After helping Keh Meh access medical treatment, the counselor working with Keh Meh explored the consistent factors that present each time violence occurs. In this process, Keh Meh identified that her husband is violent almost every time he returns from a night of gambling. She reported that more recently, upon returning home, he has gone for the knives in the kitchen and has threatened to cut her. Through the process of developing the safety plan, Keh Meh identified that on the nights her husband gambles, she could stay with her sister next door or she could hide the knives in the house that night, so her husband cannot find them.

The psychosocial counselor suggested that her daughters also participate in the safety planning process. Because of the potential for intentional or unintentional harm to them, the counselor discussed with Keh Meh the importance of her daughters also planning steps to take to keep safe. The counselor and Keh Meh decided that having her daughters involved might also help them overcome feelings of helplessness stemming from the chronic exposure to the abuse of their mother. The counselor, having been trained on domestic violence safety planning, knew the extent of children's involvement would depend on their age, developmental stage, comfort level, and the family dynamics. She also knew to communicate to Keh Meh and her children that safety plans involving children should in no way make a child responsible for anyone else's safety. Before returning home, Keh Meh and her daughters had developed a safety plan together.

Once a survivor returns home from the center, psychosocial workers follow up with her, with her expressed permission, to make sure the plan is actually keeping the survivor safe and to monitor whether modifications or adjustments are needed. It can be dangerous for staff to go to a survivor's home, so the safety plan includes methods of contact and communication between the woman and the counselor that are the most discrete. In the case of Keh Meh, during a follow-up visit several weeks after she left the center, the counselor learned the safety plan was not working. In particular the decision to stay next door on the nights when Keh Meh's husband gambles was ineffective, as the sister was also afraid of her husband. Ultimately, the decision was made for Keh Meh and her children to return to the wcc while the psychosocial worker coordinated with camp security, irc, and unhcr for more support in keeping Keh Meh and her children safe.

In addition, as is typical in domestic violence cases, once one risk was resolved for Keh Meh, another arose. After returning to the wcc, Keh Meh reported that she was being harassed by her husband's brother. Many women who report abuse become the target of harassment from the perpetrator's friends or family members. Therefore, monitoring and responding to potential new threats is vital to ensuring medium- and longer-term safety, as is fostering community members' understanding that they will be safe and protected if violence is reported. Once the psychosocial counselor learned about this new threat, she helped Keh Meh report the perpetrator to the camp security. Reporting new safety risks to the camp security is necessary to secure additional support from other key actors in the community to help women stay safe after seeking help. Psychosocial staff cannot operate independently in response to safety and security risks and concerns; therefore, it is critical to work with the camp security staff and, often, unhcr and NGOs that provide legal aid and protection services.

SPECIALIZED HEALTH CARE: RESPONSE TO CRISIS TEAMS

As more and more women reported to the wcc, the women's organization recognized the need for specialized health care to respond to their needs. Women who experienced sexual violence needed access to confidential treatment and physical stabilization while they waited to be transferred outside the camp for comprehensive clinical care for sexual assault. As more cases of domestic violence were presented, it became evident that the health staff were not properly equipped to provide quality care in these sensitive cases. Many health staff members preferred not to get involved in situations deemed private family matters or in sensitive cases such as rape—and so provided the minimum level of care without asking any further questions.

Primary health care is provided in the camp by the Karenni Health Department, which has received years of capacity building and support from international NGOs, primarily irc. The health staff is from the refugee community and often has attitudes and beliefs similar to those of community members about the acceptability of violence against women, including domestic violence: for example, the belief that a woman causes violence by not being a good enough wife or that, if she is experiencing violence, she should remain quiet about it. Specialized health teams consisting of a medic (typically a man) and a reproductive health worker (typically a woman) were formed to meet the specialized needs of survivors of domestic and sexual violence. The specialized teams, referred to as response-to-crisis teams—or RCTs—received training on domestic and sexual violence and how to provide care to survivors. Specialized care included how to conduct referrals to other agencies, how to provide confidential, compassionate care to women, and how to document injuries, particularly in domestic violence cases, as forensic evidence collection for rape and sexual assault must be done at the Thai hospital. The members of the RCT care about women in the community, but they have been hesitant to take on this additional work, primarily because of security concerns health workers have as key service providers to a survivor of gender-based violence. For example, the health worker may be the neighbor of the women coming in for care and afraid to document injuries or refer the women to the safe shelter, for fear the perpetrator will target his anger at the health worker. In addition, with limited resources and an already busy workload, some RCT staff members feel the extra responsibilities are burdensome and feel too much additional pressure being part of the team. Despite these challenges, however, the RCTs have remained a survivor-centered service for several years, with many women seeking confidential treatment for all forms of gender-based violence. Moreover, out of the efforts to support survivors of violence, a domestic violence screening program was developed in the prenatal clinic to support women who may be at risk for or already experiencing violence. Women are screened for violence, educated on the health risks to a pregnant woman if she is in a violent relationship, and offered referrals and support to help increase her safety.

RESOLVING DOMESTIC VIOLENCE USING TRADITIONAL JUSTICE: REALITIES AND CHALLENGES

Most cases of domestic violence are resolved through the traditional justice system led by male leaders from the community. In refugee camp settings along the Thai-Burma border, including the Karenni camps, traditional justice approaches such as mediation are commonly offered to survivors of violence. Mediation is available for a variety of disputes and offenses that happen in the camp, with the exception of very serious crimes such as murder. Mediation had been practiced by the refugees back in their villages and remains a key dispute resolution practice in the camp. Despite recognition that mediation is not an effective dispute resolution mechanism for domestic violence,[29] it remains the most common mechanism used in the Karenni camps. The IRC has consistently witnessed the ineffectiveness of mediation in domestic violence cases in the community. Examination of cases solved through mediation has found that they rarely result in an end to the violence and frequently hold the survivor at least partly responsible for the violence.

Mediation is practiced in a fashion similar to the way it was practiced in Burma. The camps are divided into sections and each section is managed by a section leader, who is most often a man. Every section leader is also a mediator for his/her section. The camp also has a camp justice office. Similar to camp security, camp justice is part of the local governance structure in the camp. The camp justice office is presided over by three people who act as mediators and arbitrators for more serious matters or matters referred from the sections when section mediation is unsuccessful or requested by both parties. After receiving the report of an incident of domestic violence either directly from the survivor, or from her family or witnesses, the mediator calls the survivor and perpetrator to a meeting along with their support persons, such as family or friends. Often, mediation is conducted at the section leader's office, with all participants sitting in a circle. With the permission of the mediator they discuss the solution to the issue. Although the setting of the process looks like a family conference, the process is mediation. When lack of confidence or feelings of intimidation prevent the survivor from expressing herself, or if she prefers the support persons to speak on her behalf, the mediator allows them to do so. In the Karenni refugee camps, mediation is the only resolution mechanism other than divorce. A survivor will often have her case mediated many times because, as noted above, mediation rarely ends the violence. Despite intensive efforts to improve perpetrator accountability in mediation, husbands are often simply asked to "promise" not to be violent again. In some cases during mediation, a survivor may be encouraged to have a hot meal ready when her husband comes home or to stop nagging, in an effort to keep her husband happy and less prone to resorting to violent behavior— which wrongly places blame on the survivor. Another common community reaction that places blame on a survivor is talk that the wife is "lazy" and does not do household chores such as laundry and sweeping the house. A survivor has little choice but to agree to be "less" lazy and complete household chores, or whatever the charge may be that led her husband to abuse her, given the lack of other dispute resolution mechanisms. Pressure from the women's community group has resulted in camp justice, with the support of international NGOs, working toward using more structured processes for mediation, especially for domestic violence cases. Mediators have received training on the mediation process, options for survivors, and ways to hold perpetrators more accountable for violence.

In some cases, the violence is closely related to alcohol abuse. Through GBV work with Karenni Women's Organization and IRC Women's Protection and Empowerment, it is observed that in such a case, the mediation outcome would be for the husband to stop drinking alcohol. However, this kind of agreement is usually violated at some point. Other common outcomes of mediation are the parties issuing a formal apology and/or a traditional cleansing ceremony. Traditional cleansing ceremonies are reserved for more specific issues, such as adultery or violence that occurred at someone else's house. For example, if a person commits adultery, it is believed that he/she brings bad luck on his/her spouse. Similarly, if violence takes place at someone's house, it is believed that those involved have brought bad luck to the house owner. In these situations, the person concerned about bad luck will call for a cleansing ceremony to clean the evil spirit brought upon him/her. The camp officials order the wrongdoer to pay for the ceremony. However, this remedy is typically not available to domestic violence survivors.

Survivors who experience severe and/or repeated violence may remain in the shelter until their case is heard by the camp justice if they are seeking a divorce. Divorce is often viewed by survivors as an unfortunate, yet necessary, option to enable a life free from violence. It is not common for divorce to be sought—and granted—unless the violence has reached severe levels. In these cases, even with divorce granted, it is not unusual for a survivor to stay for a prolonged period of time at the shelter, sometimes up to a year or more, because she does not feel safe at home—or anywhere else—in the camp.

SUPPORTING THE SUPPORTERS: SUPERVISION OF PSYCHOSOCIAL STAFF

Survivors' repeated stays at the shelter demonstrate the challenge of stopping domestic violence in the community. However, they also indicate that the shelter service is accessible to survivors and considered a place of safety and support. In the end, there are few options for escaping the violence, and this reality take its toll on both survivors and staff. One of the primary complaints by psychosocial staff is their sense of helplessness in these cases.

While they recognize their contribution to survivors' well-being through the counseling, encouragement, and advocacy they offer, seeing women and children come back to the shelter because of repeated episodes of violence can be discouraging and even frustrating. In conflict settings especially, women face great barriers to escaping from violence. Husbands threaten violence and other punishments, such as hurting the children, if a women attempts to leave. In conflict and displacement settings, women have very limited options for moving to a different location. Moreover, with families uprooted to refugee camps, women are even more dependent on their husbands for access to basic needs such as food, clothing, and shelter, which are distributed in humanitarian aid settings. Or maybe the husband has destroyed a woman's sense of self-worth and isolated her to the point that she feels she does not deserve a better, violence-free life. Whatever the reason, understanding the dynamics of domestic violence is crucial for service providers who watch women return to abusive husbands many times before considering whether a final break is possible.

Psychosocial staff and other direct service providers responsible for providing care to survivors require close supervision, as responding to these cases can be highly complex and emotionally draining. Staff needs to be monitored for signs of secondary trauma and to ensure interventions are implemented appropriately. Secondary trauma is the stress that helpers can carry as a result of helping people in very difficult situations. IRC's model of support in the Karenni camps includes regular case supervision, both individual and group supervision, to help staff manage these complex cases. Supervision also functions as a time to provide emotional support to the workers, who are often deeply affected by the violence they bear witness to daily. In addition, technical support to the shelter staff was provided as they developed the operational protocol for the shelters.

Conclusion

Conflict, displacement, and ongoing insecurity create the perfect storm in which all forms of violence against women and girls can escalate. This includes domestic violence, which has historically received less attention in humanitarian settings than sexual violence. However, particularly in post-conflict settings, one of the biggest threats to women's safety is violence perpetrated by intimate partners. Similar to what is necessary in stable settings, services for survivors of gender-based violence in humanitarian contexts are crucial, and standards of ethics and care specific to these settings have been established. The multisectoral approach is essential, as responding to violence against women requires an array of services to ensure survivors can fully heal and recover. In addition, international organizations working on programs for survivors must collaborate with the local women's community, which knows best how to develop and run care for women in the community. Despite the challenges in developing services for survivors in conflict settings, the efforts of the women's organization in the Karenni refugee camps in Thailand provide a picture of what is possible. This work indicates that it is possible to overcome the security challenges, the capacity deficits across all sectors in the camps, and the vastly imperfect and patriarchal structure, to provide quality services and support to survivors of domestic violence in particular. Each day, women arrive at the WCC or seek support from a trained psychosocial caseworker. This program and others like it prove that it is possible to effectively support and care for survivors of domestic violence, even in the most complex of environments.

Notes

1 "Ending Violence against Women," *Population Reports*, Series L, no. 11 (Baltimore: Johns Hopkins University School of Public Health, Population Information Program, December 1999).

2 Ibid.

3 Claudia Garcia-Moreno, Henrica AFM. Jansen, Mary Ellsberg, Lori Heise, and Charlotte Watts, *WHO Multi-Country Study on Women's Health and Domestic Violence against Women* (Geneva: World Health Organization, 2005), http://www.who.int/gender/violence/who_multicountry_study/en/index.html.

4 "Ending Violence against Women," *Population Reports*.

5 Inter-Agency Standing Committee. *Guidelines for GBV Interventions in Humanitarian Settings: Focusing on Prevention of and Response to Sexual Violence in Emergencies* (Geneva: Inter-Agency Standing Committee, 2005), http://humanitarianinfo.org/iasc/pageloader.aspx?page=content-subsidi-tf _gender-gbv.

6 Garcia-Moreno et al., *WHO Multi-Country Study*.

7 Susan Schechter, *Women and Male Violence: The Visions and Struggles of the Battered Women's Movement* (Boston: South End Press, 1982).

8 Garcia-Moreno et al., *WHO Multi-Country Study*.

9 Ibid.

10 "Burma's Displaced People," *Forced Migration Review* 30 (Oxford: Refugee Studies Centre, April 2008).

11 Jeanne Ward and Mendy Marsh, "Sexual Violence against Women and Girls in War and Its Aftermath: Realities, Responses and Required Resources," *United Nations Population Fund Briefing Paper*, 2006,

http://www.unfpa.org/emergencies/symposiumo6/docs/finalbrusselsbriefing
paper.pdf.

12 United Nations High Commissioner for Refugees, *Sexual and Gender-Based
    Violence against Refugees, Returnees, and Internally Displaced Persons: Guidelines
    for Prevention and Response* (United Nations High Commissioner for Refugees,
    May 2003).

13 Elizabeth Rehn and Ellen Johnson Sirleaf, "Violence against Women," in *Women,
    War and Peace: The Independent Expert's Assessment on the Impact of Armed
    Conflict on Women and Women's Role in Peace Building* (New York: United
    Nations Development Fund for Women [UNIFEM], 2002), 9–18,
    http://www.unifem.org/attachments/products/213_chaptero1.pdf.

14 Ann Jones, *War Is Not Over when It's Over: Women Speak Out from the Ruins of
    War* (New York: Metropolitan Books, 2010).

15 JC Campbell, "Health Consequences of Intimate Partner Violence," *Lancet* 359, no.
    9314 (April 2002): 1331–1336.

16 Ibid.

17 Garcia-Moreno et al., *WHO Multi-Country Study*.

18 United Nations High Commissioner for Refugees, *Sexual and Gender-Based
    Violence*.

19 World Health Organization and Mental Health Gap Action Programme, *mhGAP
    Intervention Guide for Mental, Neurological and Substance Use Disorders in
    Non-specialized Health Settings* (Geneva: World Health Organization, 2010).

20 United Nations High Commissioner for Refugees, *Sexual and Gender-Based
    Violence*.

21 Ibid.

22 Inter-Agency Standing Committee, *IASC Guidelines for Gender-based Violence
    Interventions in Humanitarian Settings: Focusing on Prevention and Response to
    Sexual Violence in Emergencies* (Geneva: Inter-Agency Standing Committee,
    2005),
    http://humanitarianinfo.org/iasc/pageloader.aspx?page=content-subsidi-tf
    _gender-gbv.

23 International Rescue Committee, *Let Me Not Die before My Time: Domestic
    Violence in West Africa* (New York: International Rescue Committee,
    2012), 3.

24 International Rescue Committee, *Gender Based Violence Information
    Management System Report* (International Rescue Committee, 2012).

25 Ibid.

26 United Nations High Commissioner for Refugees, "Protracted Refugee Situations,"
    *Executive Committee of the High Commissioner's Programme, Standing Committee,
    30th Meeting* (UN Doc. EC/54/SC/CRP.14, 10 June 2004), 2.

27 "Karenni Overview," http://www.karennirefugees.com.

28 International Rescue Committee, *Gender Based Violence Information.*

29 Anita Vestal, "Domestic Violence and Mediation: Concerns and Recommendations," May 2007, http://www.mediate.com/articles/vestala3.cfm.

Chapter 7

Substance Use, Conflict, and Displacement

Lucinda Lai, Naw Dah Pachara Sura, and Kenneth Curry

An escalation of problems related to alcohol use among residents of refugee camps on the Thai-Burma border prompted one organization to distribute a special health bulletin on the topic of alcoholism.[1] "Why do people drink alcohol in the camp?" asked the article written by community health educator Win Win Yi of Nu Poh camp:

> There are several causes for using alcohol. Because some people feel depressed or confused and are in a state of utter desolation, to overcome fright or shyness, after successfully accomplishing some tasks, for relaxation or as a custom. Some people consider that the rules and regulations of the camp are too strict. They cannot go and work outside the camp causing economic problems in the family. Consequently they feel depressed and confused. As an outlet they consume alcohol. People drink alcohol to forget temporarily their miseries and losses they faced in the past. The loss of property or families and relatives give them too much pain.[2]

In the article, Win Win Yi criticized people who fail to support their families because they spend all their time drinking with other men and at times become violent toward their wives and children. She called on camp authorities to crack down on lawbreakers and for women's affairs organizations to provide support to affected women and children. She hoped that some of the problems caused by alcohol could be prevented with greater education about the disadvantages of consuming alcohol.

Introduction

Alcohol problems in refugee camps are just one facet of the complicated relationship of substance abuse, conflict, and displacement. Burma, one of the world's largest producers of opium, gained notoriety over the past century as a cornerstone of the famously lawless "Golden Triangle" of Burma, Thailand, and Laos. According to a 2013 report by the United Nations Office on Drugs and Crime, Burma is currently a major source of methamphetamine and opiates in Southeast Asia and stands second only to Afghanistan for the size of its opium production, which is used to make heroin and trafficked globally.[3] Between 2012 and 2013, opium production in Burma rose 26 percent to an estimated 870 tons—the highest level recorded since these assessments began ten years ago.[4]

The majority of the opium cultivation occurs in eastern Burma in the states of the Shan and Kachin ethnic minorities.[5] Far from being a peripheral issue, however, the thriving opium trade in Shan State of northeast Burma is inextricably tied to the political economy of Burma as a whole. As political economist Catherine Brown argues, "The expansion of the drugs trade can be seen as both a cause and a consequence of the wider economic and social dislocation of Burmese society after decades of military rule and civil war."[6] Eastern Burma has been the arena for decades of armed conflict between the minority groups' armies and the central government's military.[7] Even as the country experienced years of economic decay and authoritarian rule, the opium industry grew as Burma's single financial success.[8]

The material profits of the drugs trade go a long way to accounting for the persistence of conflict and complex emergencies in these areas. Regional instability, while exposing the population to exploitation and human rights abuses, is conducive to the success of the drugs trade. Violence follows the spread of opium cultivation in a vicious cycle of impoverishment, human rights violations, and population displacement, in which large numbers of the area's ethnic minorities are forced to flee as refugees.[9]

With cruel irony, refugees fleeing from conflict in Burma reach the refugee camps on the Thai side of the border to find themselves confronted by another set of drug-related dangers: refugee camps in Thailand have become a fertile breeding ground for drug and alcohol addiction. Individuals turn to drugs and alcohol as a way to cope, however dysfunctionally, with the stress of protracted confinement in a place devoid of the basic freedoms and opportunities for meaningful living.

Substance Use in Situations of Conflict and Displacement

Problems with substance use are prevalent in a variety of conflict-affected situations, including camps for refugees and internally displaced people.[10] The World Health Organization's Mental Health Gap Action Programme (mhGAP) has identified alcohol use and drug use disorders as conditions of high priority because they represent a large burden of mortality, morbidity, or disability,[11] have high economic costs, and are associated with violations of human rights.[12] Both the United Nations High Commissioner for Refugees (UNHCR) and the World Health Organization (WHO) affirm that a rise in alcohol and other substance use is among the many health and social concerns related to conflict and displacement.[13]

Substance use can quickly reach epidemic proportions in response to posttraumatic stress, disruption of socioeconomic situations, and prolonged instability or hardships of a society or government.[14] Problems related to substance use can develop at any stage of displacement: in the country of origin, in transit, in temporary refuge, or in resettlement. Forcibly displaced persons commonly experience a high number of traumatic events related to the armed conflict and persecution they have fled. This past exposure to trauma may explain why some turn to harmful substance use as a coping and response strategy.

The process of adaptation to new cultural and physical environments can be extremely stressful.[15] Displaced persons are faced with decreased social support, austere living conditions, impoverishment, and socioeconomic challenges. Upheaval from their home countries can mean losing family, friends, possessions, and employment, with associated losses of livelihoods, cultural and social supports, and self-esteem.[16] A systematic review of the evidence of harmful alcohol use following from forced displacement indicates high rates of psychiatric disorders such as depression, anxiety, and generalized psychological distress in post-displacement conditions.[17]

The most visible health problems associated with alcohol and other substance use are injuries caused by acute intoxication or life-threatening overdose. In these populations, a wide range of legal and illegal substances may be used, including alcohol, cannabis, hypnosedatives, inhalants, opioids, and psychostimulants.[18] Dependent users can also suffer withdrawal symptoms during interruptions to the drug supply. Though some studies have detected elevated or excessive substance use in populations displaced by conflict,[19] most studies are limited by a lack of comparative data to populations that have not been displaced (but for whom substance-related health problems are well documented).[20] Problems specific to conflict-affected populations include alcohol-related suicides;[21] gender-based violence;[22] injection drug use–related risks; and disruptions to the household economy that exacerbate already high levels of poverty.[23] In some long-term displaced populations, the local economy may become dependent on the commercialization of psychoactive substances, including alcohol, khat, cannabis, and opium, which is also associated with commercial sex work.[24]

A transition to injected drug use has been observed in conflict settings, where there may be a disruption of harm reduction interventions or increased access to injecting equipment.[25] Conflict and displacement increase HIV and other blood-borne virus transmission via an increase in unsafe injected drug use and unsafe sexual practices while under the influence of addictive substances.[26] Injected drug use can introduce HIV into already vulnerable communities, leading to explosive HIV epidemics in areas of previously low prevalence.[27]

Several humanitarian institutions have highlighted substance abuse as a major challenge to public health. The Sphere Project's *Humanitarian Charter and Minimum Standards in Humanitarian Response* considers the minimization of harm related to alcohol and drugs to be a key action in the provision of essential health services.[28] The UNHCR and the WHO Department of Mental Health and Substance Abuse have jointly published a field guide for the rapid assessment of the causes and patterns of substance use in conflict-affected and displaced populations.[29] In addition, the Inter-Agency Standing Committee (IASC) "Action Sheet 6.5" calls attention to the far-reaching psychosocial, mental health, medical, and socioeconomic problems, and the threats to protection, related to alcohol and other substance use.[30]

The IASC recognizes that conflict and natural disasters create situations in which people, in an attempt to cope with the stress of emergency situations, may experience severe problems related to substance use. The committee urges humanitarian emergency response programs to realize that communities will have difficulties recovering from the effects of emergencies when substance use inhibits individuals and communities from addressing problems; finite family and community resources are spent on alcohol and other substance use; and substance use promotes violence, exploitation, neglect of children, and other protection threats. As such, harm related to substance use is increasingly recognized as an important public health and protection issue that requires a multisectoral response in emergency settings.[31]

Diagnosing Substance Use Disorders

There are two commonly used systems for classifying substance-use disorders: the International Classification of Diseases (ICD-10) and the Diagnostic and Statistical Manual of Mental Disorders (DSM-5). The core syndromes are hazardous use, harmful use, substance use, substance dependence, and substance withdrawal.

"Harmful use" is defined as a pattern of substance use that causes damage to health. The damage may be physical (as in cases of hepatitis from the self-administration of injected drugs) or mental (such as episodes of depressive disorder secondary to heavy consumption of alcohol).[32] "Substance use disorder" in the DSM-5 combines the previous DSM-4 categories of substance abuse and substance dependence into a single disorder, measured on a continuum from mild to severe. Overall, the diagnosis of a substance-use disorder is characterized by a pattern of continued pathological use of a substance: impaired control over the use of the substance; social impairment (failure to fulfill major obligations at work, school, or home); risky use (recurrent substance use in situations in which it is physically hazardous); and pharmacological criteria (developing an increased tolerance to the substance).[33]

The ICD-10 defines "dependence syndrome" as "a cluster of physiological, behavioral, and cognitive phenomena in which the use of a substance or class of substances takes on a much higher priority for a given individual than other behaviors that once had greater value."[34] A diagnosis of dependence can be made if three or more of the following have been present together at some time during the previous year: a strong desire to take a substance, impaired control over its use, a higher priority given to substance use over other activities and obligations, increased tolerance, symptoms of withdrawal, or continued use despite clear evidence of overtly harmful consequences (such as harm to the liver through excessive drinking, depressive mood states consequent to periods of heavy substance use, or drug-related impairment of cognitive functioning).[35]

Withdrawal is a syndrome that occurs when blood or tissue concentrations of a substance decline in an individual who had maintained prolonged heavy use of the substance.[36] After developing withdrawal symptoms, the individual is likely to consume the substance to relieve the symptoms. Withdrawal symptoms vary greatly across the different classes of substances, so the DSM-5 provides separate criteria for the drug classes. For example, features of alcohol withdrawal appear following the cessation of heavy alcohol consumption, typically between six hours and six days after the last drink. Things to look for and ask about include a tremor in the hands, sweating, vomiting, increased pulse and blood pressure, agitation, headache, nausea, and anxiety.[37]

Substance Use in the Thai-Burma Camps

In her research, addiction medicine specialist Dr. Nadine Ezard compared patterns of substance use in six different settings of protracted displacement: three in Africa (Kenya, Liberia, and northern Uganda) and three in Asia (Iran, Pakistan, and Thailand). Despite the geographical and cultural diversity of the six study sites, common experiences of deprivation of land and property, changing social norms and networks, restricted livelihoods, hopelessness, and profound uncertainty about the future were shown to make these communities particularly vulnerable to harmful patterns of substance use.[38] For a variety of reasons, religious belief may be a protective factor from substance-related harms. The question of whether humanitarian responses to populations displaced by conflict have served to protect people from problem substance use or promote it showed mixed results.[39]

Ezard et al.'s (2011) interviews with culturally representative samples of refugee camp residents revealed that widespread use of alcohol in Kenya, Liberia, Uganda, and Thailand and opiates in Iran and Pakistan were believed to be linked to a range of health, social, and protection problems, including illness, injury (intentional and unintentional), gender-based violence, behavior at higher risk for HIV and other sexually transmitted infection and blood-borne virus transmission, and effects detrimental to household economy.[40] Furthermore, limited access to services (including health services) and exclusion from relevant population programs in the host country may exacerbate substance use–related harms for displaced persons.[41]

In the Thai-Burma camps, Ezard et al. (2011) determined that alcohol is the most commonly abused drug.[42] It is cheap and readily available in the form of home-brewed distilled rice liquor (costing about 5 to 10 baht, or 16 to 32 cents in U.S. currency at 2009 rates, for the equivalent of approximately 10 grams of ethanol). These home brews can be toxic, with brewers adding pesticides, fertilizers, rubber, and other substances in an attempt to accelerate the fermentation process and/or enhance potency.

Beer, wine, and spirits can be obtained at nearby bars and shops, although their sale is not officially permitted inside the camp. A number of other substances were mentioned, including *ya ba* (a tablet form of methamphetamine and caffeine), diazepam, cough syrup, cannabis, and opiates (predominantly available in a smokable form). Inhalant use of glues by young people was reported in Mae La and Ban Mai Nai Soi camps. Use of these other substances was still considered less important than that of alcohol.

In interviews, the Burmese refugees spoke about the link between dispossession and alcohol use.[43] A resident of Ban Ma Nai Soi camp explained, "We have lost our traditions, our property, our belongings and our country. Here we have a restricted limited life, so we drink." Dispossession promoted alienation, idleness, and loss of traditional gender roles among men. "Men have nothing to do, now many even choose not to work in the fields, they have too much time on their hands. Their other responsibilities have been eliminated by camp life and they have become idle," observed one female camp resident. Restricted opportunities for movement, education, and employment were seen to drive a sense of hopelessness and idleness among men. This, coupled with the ready availability and social acceptability of alcohol consumption for men, was believed to result in the disproportionately high levels of alcohol use among male residents.

The interviewees shared the dominant belief that the pressures of displacement and of life in a refugee camp promoted alcohol use.[44] Some men said that they resort to substance abuse because they feel deprived of their typical means of livelihood: "We have only alcohol. It's like being in a farm . . . surrounded by a fence." Many of these disenfranchised young men felt they had no other avenues for expressing their frustration: "There is only alcohol to get release." One characterized peoples' constrained options, saying, "Some people stay here and they feel trapped. If they go back to Burma, they will be arrested. Living like that, they don't know what to hope for. So they just drink alcohol." Another resident directly attributed his drinking to his pervasive sense of hopelessness: "I have no goal. I don't know the future. At that time, I drank only alcohol. . . . When does the UN call me? By waiting like this, I lost my goal. So I drank alcohol. After that, time flies by a day at a time."

Another study by Ezard et al. in 2009 looked at gender differences in alcohol use among refugees living in Mae La camp, the largest of the nine camps on the Thai-Burma border.[45] The interview data suggest a number of features of life in displacement that promote high-risk drinking in Mae La, such as a sense of powerlessness and hopelessness. The interviewees estimated that the majority of adult men in the camp drink alcohol. Alcohol use among men was described as culturally acceptable and an appropriate response to the stressors of displacement. The negative health effects, which many participants thought were made worse by the addition of adulterants to the alcohol, included dependence, high-risk sexual behavior (associated with in- and out-of-camp mobility), family and neighborhood disruption, and gender-based violence. Population surveys in Mae La camp confirm that alcohol use is viewed as an important security concern in the camp, where service provider data listed alcohol as an important cofactor in recorded incidents of gender-based violence, physical assault, and suicide.

Despite the prevalence of substance-related problems in refugee populations on the Thai-Burma border, limited research and few practical resources exist on the subject. One exception is the *Substance Abuse, Drugs and Addictions Guidebook*, published by the international nongovernmental organization Aide Médicale Internationale (AMI).[46] The guidebook is meant to serve as a practical resource for health and social workers in the field. It presents a compendium of the most commonly abused substances, how they are used, their street names, and their intoxicating and health effects.

The AMI guidebook advises fieldworkers that the signs and symptoms of alcoholism vary depending on the person, their tolerance for the drug, and the consequences of their use. Sometimes ashamed of their dependence, people with alcohol dependence may find themselves drinking in secret to hide from friends and family the fact that they are drinking or how much they are drinking. This can make it more difficult to find out about their dependence. The guidebook suggests being aware of the signs of abuse, including intoxicated or erratic behavior, combative and aggressive behavior related to disinhibition of thinking and emotions, passive behavior that is uncharacteristic, and incoordination of movement. This may result in injuries and bruising that people cannot adequately explain, or that they pass off without explanation, perhaps because they do not remember. Craving is commonly a symptom of alcohol dependence: the insatiable thirst for an alcoholic drink. Physical and psychological withdrawal symptoms can occur if an alcohol dependent individual goes too long without a drink.[47]

Alcoholism as a "Social Disease"

In settings of conflict and displacement, as elsewhere, the social problems associated with alcohol and other substance abuse are significant. These include interpersonal and gender-based violence, organized crime, and the serious neglect of children.[48] The locally-distributed *Health Messenger* bulletin describes why alcoholism should be considered a "social disease":

> Alcoholism not only affects the physical and mental health of the person, but also his familial and social life. It has been found that many partners of alcoholics suffer anxiety, insomnia, tension and depression. They often feel a strong sense of guilt or anger and want to punish the addict, which they may take out on their children or colleagues at work. Social problems, such as domestic violence, sexual assault, and childhood abuse and neglect are often related to alcoholism.[49]

The health bulletin emphasizes, "What is important to understand is that alcoholism is not a disease that only affects one person but also everyone around them, and it is the responsibility of both the individual and society to support efforts of overcoming alcoholism."[50] One camp resident put it another way: "The majority of addicts are men. Because of this, women are mentally ill."[51]

Current patterns of alcohol and drug use should be considered in the context of how these substances were used in the past. While the various ethnic communities that make up the Burmese refugee population differ in their traditional uses of drugs, the Karen people have produced and used alcohol for many generations. Alcohol is incorporated in many important ceremonies, such as weddings, social gatherings, and funerals, as well as used for medicinal purposes.[52] Tobacco and betel nut are used for personal consumption. Cannabis has traditionally been used as an animal feed and occasionally as treatment for intestinal worms. Opium production and heroin use has existed at least since British colonial rule, primarily among ethnic Wa communities, though to a lesser extent among Karenni, Shan, PaO, and Lahu populations. It had limited use as a ceremonial intoxicant and was primarily a commodity for sale.[53]

While addictive substances have been available to Karen and other ethnic communities for many generations, the use of these substances was generally kept under control by the social stability of communities. For men, occasional alcohol use was considered a culturally appropriate aid to socialization and perhaps even a normal part of the transition to adulthood.[54]

Drinking to intoxication or dependence, and any kind of drinking by women, were strictly prohibited. Ezard's study of Mae La camp showed that in the Karen culture alcohol use by men was subject to a number of social controls that predate displacement.[55] Alcohol use was a social activity, and it was often referred to in Karen as "happy water." One man, 56 years old, who had been living in and out of camp since the camp was first established, said: "It is like we drink alcohol in order to make us happy, but I do not know how to explain it. . . . As for me I have a lot of friends, sometimes we buy a bottle of alcohol and drink together with friends and come back to eat after drinking, but I do not continue to have more. I just drink it in moderation." In addition to aiding in socialization and mood, there was a commonly held belief that a small amount of alcohol use is beneficial for physical health. The researchers were repeatedly told that "alcohol is good to eat rice" (improves appetite) and "alcohol is like medicine" (improves health). The concept of "drinking in moderation" appeared to be a core tenet of culturally acceptable use, while intoxication and dependence were stigmatized. Another man, 43 years old and a long-term resident, explained: "[If alcohol is drunk] within limits, it is like medicine. If it is over the limit, it is dangerous."

In this community, drinking behaviors and norms are heavily gendered.[56] A literature review of substance use among populations displaced by conflict suggests that cultural controls against women's drinking and against men drinking to intoxication can remain strong despite the chronic and disruptive nature of displacement.[57] Abstinence is seen as a virtue for women, who are expected to exert more self-control than men. A 24-year-old male resident of Mae La thought that fewer women drink than men because, "Women can control themselves if they get upset. Usually, men have no self-control." This "self-control," however, is driven by strong normative

pressures against women's use of alcohol and a fear of exclusion for contra-
vening social norms. "They are afraid that the neighbors will gossip about
them," said one 20-year-old man. Religious norms were sometimes invoked
to explain the prohibition of women's drinking. Women should not drink
"because they are females. It is not suitable for our [Muslim] religion, it is
not accepted. It's not good to see," explained one male resident, who is
22 years old and a regular drinker. Ezard et al. (2009) conclude that alcohol
use by women was seen as aberrant, and the shame and stigma associated
with public drinking, drunkenness, and dependence for women far outweighed that for men.[58]

Traditional social controls on drinking have been eroding under the
pressures of displacement and refugee camp life. Ezard et al.'s (2009) assessment highlighted responses from residents who thought that young
people and women now drink more often and more prominently than in
the past.[59] Alcohol was used not only more frequently, but also more often
to the point of intoxication or dependence: "Now more and more people
are drinking alcohol," said one 80-year-old man who had been a resident of
Mae La for seventeen years. Various explanations were given, including
exposure to new cultures and alcohol-use behaviors, ongoing population
movements, increased social diversity in the camp, increased economic resources coming from third country remittances, and changing social networks. The man continued, "Before, there were not so many people in the
camp and there are fewer cases [of alcohol and drug problems] happening
in our community . . . but now more and more people are coming into the
camp with different ethnic backgrounds and different characteristics and
more fighting, more drugs, and more problems happen in the camp."

The notion that abrupt socioeconomic change can have adverse effects
on population health is not a new idea. Émile Durkheim, one of the found-
ers of modern social science, coined the term "anomie" to describe the unfolding situation in which existing social and moral norms no longer seem
to apply.[60] For Durkheim, dramatic change results in a temporary disruption of the normal mechanisms through which society imposes limits on
behavior, which in turn results in increased rates of self-destructive behavior. This self-destructive behavior frequently involves the immoderate use
and abuse of substances.

Changing cultural norms were thought to be linked to increased substance use among young people and women in Mae La camp, according
to Ezard et al.'s (2009) rapid assessment.[61] Remarking on the changing cultural norms, one woman said, "Now there are no rules for drinking alcohol." Changing cultural norms also promoted disrespect toward male clan

elders and leaders. As one youth said, "How can I respect these older men when I see them becoming drunk and falling down in the dirt?" The net effect of these adverse consequences may be a disruption to community cohesion, possibly impeding the community's capacity to recover.

Ezard et al. (2011) draws several conclusions about the challenges of transition that they observed across the six study sites of the rapid assessment.[62] Factors that mediate these observed transitions—why, when, and under what conditions populations and subgroups change patterns of substance use—are still not clearly understood. Proximal facilitators may include the ready availability of alcohol and other substances, and psychological triggers such as alleviation of emotional reactions associated with loss and adjustment. Changing social networks and cultural controls of substance use may also promote change. In addition, the studies suggest that a number of underlying elements of the displacement context may be important, such as restricted movement, limited livelihood, dispossession, and a sense of hopelessness. In particular, the findings suggest that substance-use problems exploit the underlying power fault lines in the community, including gender, ethnic, and economic power differences. For example, many of the studies traced gender-based violence to alcohol intoxication (usually by men directed toward women). Cultural expectations and patterns of behavior of men who drink to intoxication play an important role, along with situational and individual factors.

Indeed, the various models that have been applied to explain how the features of life in displacement might promote high-risk drinking in Mae La camp, such as the social stress model, whereby social stressors may promote individual substance use, and the "self-medication" hypothesis, whereby drugs are thought to be used in order to relieve individual suffering, do not explain why the observed prevalence of high-risk drinking is *lower* than would be expected.[63] In the past, qualitative data had suggested that the relative geographical and social isolation of the camps was partially protective against unsafe behaviors, such as sexual behaviors risky for sexually transmitted infections, but even this situation is changing with the growth of the camp, increased contact with populations outside the camp, and more people moving in and out of the camp to look for work.[64]

Future efforts to prevent transition to more harmful use can be guided by investigation into why the prevalence of high-risk alcohol use in the camp is not as high as would be predicted. One promising line of investigation explores the role of community resilience. For example, tight social networks have been suggested to be partially protective against problem substance use in some conflict-affected populations. Furthermore, a sense of hopefulness provided by access to education and resettlement was seen as preventive for problem alcohol use. Strong social controls on high-risk drinking, wherein drinking by women, intoxication, drinking by young people, and solitary drinking are all proscribed, may act to limit the spread of problem alcohol use in Mae La camp.[65] That the level of risky alcohol use among displaced Burmese populations may be lower than that of other displaced populations with alcohol-drinking cultures highlights the complexity and context-specificity of the relationship between alcohol and displacement.

Interventions

Despite the high prevalence of mental, neurological, and substance-use disorders and the large portion of the global burden of disease they represent, resources to tackle these problems are insufficient, inequitably distributed, and inefficiently used. The majority of people with these disorders receive no care at all. Even when treatment and care is available, it is seldom based on evidence or of high quality. In an effort to reduce the large treatment gap, the WHO launched the Mental Health Gap Action Programme (mhGAP) to scale up services for people in low- and middle-income countries. mhGAP recommendations have been incorporated into an integrated package of interventions called *mhGAP Intervention Guide for Mental, Neurological and Substance Use Disorders in Non-specialized Health Settings.*[66] The guide translates the evidence-based recommendations into simple clinical protocols and algorithms to facilitate decision-making by busy non-specialists in low- and middle-income countries. For example, in clinical scenarios of alcohol dependence, the guide suggests explaining the short-term and long-term risks of continuing use at the current level, discussing the person's motivations for their alcohol use, facilitating alcohol cessation if the person is willing, arranging detoxification and medical management if necessary and available, considering referral to a self-help group or a residential therapeutic community, providing information and support to caregivers and family members, and following up. A detailed evidence profile can be accessed through the mhGAP Evidence Resource Centre (http://www.who.int/mental_health/mhgap/evidence/en/index.html). The reader is referred to the sections on "Alcohol Use and Alcohol Use Disorders" and "Drug Use and Drug Use Disorders" for step-by-step guides for the assessment and management of these conditions.

Rapid Assessments

The research literature on interventions among conflict-displaced populations is sparse. This reflects an overall lack of research on mental health in low-resource settings in general, and on harmful alcohol use in particular.[67] Intervention research among displaced populations is limited by ethical considerations and methodological difficulties such as ongoing population movements, short time frames, and limited funding sources.[68]

One way to both improve information regarding conflict-displaced populations and build experience developing interventions is to promote the conduct of rapid assessments.[69] The UNHCR and WHO have jointly published a field guide to conducting rapid assessments in conflict-affected and displaced populations.[70] The guide takes a public health approach and prioritizes harm- and risk-reduction (including the reduction of HIV transmission risks) for individuals, families, and communities. The purpose of conducting a rapid assessment is to describe the current substance-use and harms situation in the target population and to identify a range of interventions that could be feasibly implemented to minimize harms. The reader is referred to the field guide for full instructions and operational guidance on the conductance of rapid assessments.[71]

Screening and Brief Intervention

In 1980, a WHO expert committee stressed the need for efficient methods to identify persons with harmful and hazardous alcohol consumption in primary health care settings, before the health and social consequences become pronounced.[72] This led to the development of the Alcohol Use Disorders Identification Test (AUDIT), a ten-item questionnaire that provides a simple method for screening for excessive drinking and assisting in brief assessment with a minimum of time and resources. Screening can help identify excessive drinking as the cause of the presenting illness, since the majority of excessive drinkers are undiagnosed and present in clinic with symptoms or problems that would not normally be linked to their drinking. AUDIT provides a framework for intervention to help risky drinkers reduce or cease alcohol consumption, as well as personal feedback that these patients can use as motivation to change their drinking behavior. Brief interventions range from five minutes of simple advice about how to reduce hazardous drinking to several sessions of brief counseling to address more complicated conditions. Elements of brief interventions include presenting screening results, identifying risks and discussing consequences, providing medical advice, soliciting patient commitment, giving advice and encouragement, and identifying the goal, whether it is reduced drinking or abstinence.[73]

Screening for alcohol consumption among patients in primary care carries many potential benefits. Primary care health workers are in an ideal position to use their expertise, knowledge, and respected role as gate-keepers to refer alcohol dependent patients to the appropriate type of care. Furthermore, screening provides an opportunity to educate patients about low-risk consumption levels and the risks of excessive alcohol use and thus has the capacity to change norms in the community through education. Information about the amount and frequency of alcohol consumption may inform the diagnosis of the patient's presenting condition, and it may alert clinicians to the need to advise patients whose alcohol consumption might adversely affect their use of medications and other aspects of their treatment. Of utmost importance for screening is the fact that people who are not dependent on alcohol are capable of stopping or reducing their alcohol consumption with the appropriate assistance and effort.

A number of effective interventions exist for problem substance use,[74] but little attempt has been made to adapt these interventions to populations displaced by conflict.[75] Although addressing substance use requires a concerted effort involving multiple sectors and several levels of engagement, it is not often seen by either humanitarian workers or donors as an integral component of the relief response, even in the postacute period. This problem is compounded by the lack of adequate and comprehensive information on the harmful consequences of substance use in these settings, as well as lack of training of humanitarian workers in dealing with substance use problems. Humanitarian efforts should include advocacy for national health data collection efforts and prevention strategies that include displaced populations. Substance use should not be seen as an isolated stand-alone issue: substance-use interventions need to be considered as essential components of general health services (including tuberculosis control and chronic disease management), mental health and psychosocial support, HIV and sexually transmitted infections interventions, and gender-based violence prevention.[76]

Interventions will need to incorporate systematic human resources capacity–building efforts with an emphasis on practical skills–based training programs. Changing population dynamics, such as movements in and out of camps, are the norm in most humanitarian settings and must be taken into account. Although it is indeed difficult to make recommendations on future planning for border communities given uncertainty about the future (e.g., camp closures, repatriation), incorporation of substance use interventions into return, resettlement, and repatriation planning is an important response.[77]

Complex interventions include access to comprehensive treatment services for mental health problems as both a cause and consequence of substance use.[78] Examples include drug therapy and cognitive behavioral therapy for alcohol withdrawal and dependence, relapse prevention,[79] and opiate agonists for opiate dependence.[80] Mental health assessments should include information on substance use. As far as possible, substance use and HIV and other blood-borne virus prevention, treatment, care, and support should be integrated into primary health and community-based services. Despite their popularity among many service providers and community groups, general public information campaigns and school-based education for primary prevention programs have not been shown to be effective in reducing alcohol-related harm.[81]

PROGRAM DESCRIPTION: DARE NETWORK

Despite the gravity and scale of substance abuse problems in the Thai-Burma camps, one camp-based recovery program, Drug and Alcohol Recovery and Education (DARE) Network, has had remarkable success in the treatment of addicts. DARE Network finds hope in the work they do because they subscribe to the belief that "A free mind cannot be destroyed." Widespread addiction to drugs takes away people's ability to think, plan, and resist a regime that is bent on destruction. DARE Network, however, envisions the ethnic people of Burma using the power of recovery from addiction to resist oppression by the former military dictatorship without the use of violence. Recovery from drug and alcohol addiction returns people to their communities, which makes communities more resilient in dealing with the political and economic changes to come: "Even though everything else has been taken from them, as long as they keep their minds they are free people."[82]

DARE Network was the first organization to comprehensively address substance abuse problems within the refugee and migrant populations along the Thai-Burma border, having gotten their start as a grassroots organization in 2000 in response to the urgent need to bring an end to alcohol and drug problems in the community. DARE Network uses Burmese herbal medicines, acupuncture, herbal saunas, traditional massage, and culturally appropriate therapies in their detoxification and rehabilitation programs, in addition to providing prevention education for the reduction of substance abuse and associated social problems within the communities of the displaced ethnic people from Burma along the Thai-Burma border. The reader is referred to www.darenetwork.com for a fuller description of DARE Network's programs.

Conclusion

Considerable evidence now exists for what does and does not work to reduce the hazardous use of alcohol and drugs.[83] Although research in the field of mental, neurological, and substance-use disorders has significantly advanced in recent years, most of these advancements have been driven by the health care needs of the richest countries. To appropriately translate research findings into clinical and public health practices, it is critical to accelerate implementation research to evaluate interventions beyond the controlled conditions of research settings, in the type of populations that suffer the largest proportion of the global burden of morbidity and mortality.[84]

At the individual level, addiction is directly related to feelings of powerlessness. But there is also the growing realization of addiction's role in the bigger story of Burmese refugees: persecution, armed conflict, instability, a profitable drugs trade, and undemocratic rule. It is only by supporting those who are trying to break free from the cycles of addiction that full and inclusive participation in the creation of a free Burma will be possible for all.

Notes

1   DARE Network, *Health Messenger* 11, Special Issue: *Alcoholism*, 2000,
    http://www.ibiblio.org/obl/docs3/PdF%20FINAL%20ISSUES/ISSUE%2011.pdf.

2   Ibid.

3   UNODC, *Southeast Asia Opium Survey 2013* (Vienna: United Nations Office on Drugs and Crime, 2013),
    http://www.unodc.org/documents/southeastasiaandpacific/Publications/2013/SEA _Opium_Survey_2013_web.pdf.

4   Ibid.

5   UNODC, *Patterns and Trends of Amphetamine-Type Stimulants and Other Drugs: Asia and Pacific* (Vienna: United Nations Office on Drugs and Crime, 2012),
    http://www.unodc.org/documents/scientific/Patterns_and_Trends_of _Amphetaime-Type_Stimulants_and_Other_Drugs_-_Asia_and_the_Pacific _-_2012.pdf.

6   Catherine Brown, "Burma: The Political Economy of Violence," *Disasters* 23, no. 3 (September 1999): 234–256.

7   UNODC, *Patterns and Trends.*

8   Brown, "Political Economy of Violence."

9   Ibid.

10 United Nations High Commissioner for Refugees and World Health Organization, *Rapid Assessment of Alcohol and Other Substance Use in Conflict-Affected and Displaced Populations: A Field Guide*, 2008,
    http://www.who.int/entity/hac/network/unhcr_al_eng2.pdf.

11 World Health Organization, *The Global Burden of Disease: 2004 Update* (Geneva: World Health Organization, 2008), http://www.who.int/healthinfo/global_burden_disease/2004_report_update/en/.

12 Tarun Dua et al., "Evidence-Based Guidelines for Mental, Neurological, and Substance Use Disorders in Low- and Middle-Income Countries: Summary of WHO Recommendations," *PLoS Med* 8, no. 11 (November 15, 2011): e1001122, doi:10.1371/journal.pmed.1001122.

13 United Nations High Commissioner for Refugees and World Health Organization, *Field Guide*.

14 Steffanie A Strathdee et al., "Complex Emergencies, HIV, and Substance Use: No 'Big Easy' Solution," *Substance Use & Misuse* 41, no. 10/12 (January 2006): 1637–1651, doi:10.1080/10826080600848116.

15 Matthew Porter and Nick Haslam, "Predisplacement and Postdisplacement Factors Associated with Mental Health of Refugees and Internally Displaced Persons: A Meta-Analysis," *JAMA: Journal of the American Medical Association* 294, no. 5 (August 3, 2005): 602–612, doi:10.1001/jama.294.5.602.

16 Manuel Carballo and Aditi Nerukar, "Migration, Refugees, and Health Risks," *Emerging Infectious Diseases* 7, no. 3 (Suppl 2001): 556–560; Kenneth E Miller and Lisa M Rasco, "An Ecological Framework for Addressing the Mental Health Needs of Refugee Communities," in *The Mental Health of Refugees: Ecological Approaches to Healing and Adaptation*, ed. Kenneth E Miller and Lisa M Rasco (Mahwah, NJ: Lawrence Erlbaum Associates, 2004).

17 Heather Weaver and Bayard Roberts, "Drinking and Displacement: A Systematic Review of the Influence of Forced Displacement on Harmful Alcohol Use," *Substance Use & Misuse* 45, no. 13 (November 2010): 2340–2355, doi:10.3109/10826081003793920.

18 United Nations High Commissioner for Refugees and World Health Organization, *Field Guide*.

19 D Kozarić-Kovacić, T Ljubin, and M Grappe, "Comorbidity of Posttraumatic Stress Disorder and Alcohol Dependence in Displaced Persons," *Croatian Medical Journal* 41, no. 2 (June 2000): 173–178; Gloria Puertas, Cielo Ríos, and Hernán del Valle, "Prevalencia de trastornos mentales comunes en barrios marginales urbanos con población desplazada en Colombia" [The Prevalence of Common Mental Disorders in Urban Slums with Displaced Persons in Colombia], *Revista panamericana de salud pública [Pan American Journal of Public Health]* 20, no. 5 (November 2006): 324–330.

20 Robin Room, Thomas Babor, and Jürgen Rehm, "Alcohol and Public Health," *Lancet* 365, no. 9458 (February 2005): 519–530, doi:10.1016/S0140-6736(05)17870-2; Allan W Graham, Terry K Schultz, and Michael F Mayo-Smith, *Principles of Addiction Medicine*, 3rd ed. (Chevy Chase, MD: American Society of Addiction

Medicine, 2003); World Health Organization, *ICD-10: International Statistical Classification of Diseases and Related Health Problems*, 10th ed., 2007, http://www.who.int/classifications/icd/en/; Jürgen Rehm et al., "The Relationship of Average Volume of Alcohol Consumption and Patterns of Drinking to Burden of Disease: An Overview," *Addiction (Abingdon, England)* 98, no. 9 (September 2003): 1209–1228.

21 Alan Bosnar et al., "Suicide Rate after the 1991–1995 War in Southwestern Croatia," *Archives of Medical Research* 35, no. 4 (August 2004): 344–347, doi:10.1016/j.arcmed.2004.03.001; Alan Bosnar et al., "War and Suicidal Deaths by Explosives in Southwestern Croatia," *Archives of Medical Research* 37, no. 3 (April 2006): 392–394, doi:10.1016/j.arcmed.2005.06.007.

22 Claudia Catani et al., "Family Violence, War, and Natural Disasters: A Study of the Effect of Extreme Stress on Children's Mental Health in Sri Lanka," *BMC Psychiatry* 8 (2008): 33, doi:10.1186/1471-244X-8-33; Roselidah Ondeko and Susan Purdin, "Understanding the Causes of Gender-Based Violence," *Forced Migration Review* 19 (2004): 30.

23 Joseph Westermeyer, *Poppies, Pipes, and People: Opium and Its Use in Laos* (Berkeley: University of California Press, 1983); Kamaldeep Bhui and Nasir Warfa, "Drug Consumption in Conflict Zones in Somalia," *PLoS Med* 4, no. 12 (December 11, 2007): e354, doi:10.1371/journal.pmed.0040354.

24 United Nations High Commissioner for Refugees and World Health Organization, *Field Guide*.

25 Steffanie A Strathdee et al., "Rise in Needle Sharing among Injection Drug Users in Pakistan during the Afghanistan War," *Drug and Alcohol Dependence* 71, no. 1 (July 20, 2003): 17–24; Tariq Zafar et al., "HIV Knowledge and Risk Behaviors among Pakistani and Afghani Drug Users in Quetta, Pakistan," *Journal of Acquired Immune Deficiency Syndromes (1999)* 32, no. 4 (April 1, 2003): 394–398; United Nations High Commissioner for Refugees and World Health Organization, *Field Guide*.

26 Tim Rhodes et al., "The Social Structural Production of HIV Risk among Injecting Drug Users," *Social Science & Medicine (1982)* 61, no. 5 (September 2005): 1026–1044, doi:10.1016/j.socscimed.2004.12.024.

27 Irene Kuo et al., "High HCV Seroprevalence and HIV Drug Use Risk Behaviors among Injection Drug Users in Pakistan," *Harm Reduction Journal* 3, no. 1 (August 16, 2006): 26, doi:10.1186/1477-7517-3-26.

28 Sphere Project, *Humanitarian Charter and Minimum Standards in Disaster Response* (Geneva: Sphere Project, 2004).

29 United Nations High Commissioner for Refugees and World Health Organization, *Field Guide*.

30 Inter-Agency Standing Committee, "Action Sheet 6.5: Minimise Harm Related to Alcohol and Other Substance Use," in *Interagency Guidelines on Mental Health and Psychosocial Support in Emergencies (IASC Guidelines)* (Geneva: Inter-Agency Standing Committee, 2007).

31 Ibid.

32 World Health Organization, *ICD-10*.

33 American Psychiatric Association, *Diagnostic and Statistical Manual of Mental Disorders: DSM-5*, 5th ed (Washington, DC: American Psychiatric Association, 2013).

34 World Health Organization, *ICD-10*.

35 Ibid.

36 American Psychiatric Association, *Diagnostic and Statistical Manual.*

37 World Health Organization and Mental Health Gap Action Programme, *mhGAP Intervention Guide for Mental, Neurological and Substance Use Disorders in Non-specialized Health Settings* (Geneva: World Health Organization, 2010).

38 Nadine Ezard et al., "Six Rapid Assessments of Alcohol and Other Substance Use in Populations Displaced by Conflict," *Conflict and Health* 5, no. 1 (December 1, 2011): 1–15, doi:10.1186/1752-1505-5-1.

39 Ibid.

40 Ibid.

41 Ibid.

42 Ibid.

43 Ibid.

44 Ibid.

45 Nadine Ezard et al., "Risky Alcohol Use among Reproductive-Age Men, Not Women, in Mae La Refugee Camp, Thailand, 2009," *Conflict and Health* 6, no. 1 (September 11, 2012): 7, doi:10.1186/1752-1505-6-7.

46 Aide Médicale Internationale, *Substance Abuse, Drugs & Addictions Guidebook* (Aide Médicale Internationale and UNHCR, 2009), http://www.burmalibrary.org/docs07/DrugGuidebook-LowReso-red.pdf.

47 Ibid.

48 United Nations High Commissioner for Refugees and World Health Organization, *Field Guide.*

49 DARE Network, *Health Messenger* 11, Special Issue: *Alcoholism.*

50 Ibid.

51 Ibid.

52 Ibid.

53 DARE Network, *Annual Report*, 2011, http://www.darenetwork.com/images/documents/2011dare_annual_report.pdf.

54 Ezard et al., "Risky Alcohol Use."

55 Ibid.

56 Ibid.

57 Nadine Ezard, "Substance Use among Populations Displaced by Conflict: A Literature Review," *Disasters* 36, no. 3 (July 2012): 533–557, doi:10.1111/j.1467-7717.2011.01261.x.

58 Ezard et al., "Risky Alcohol Use."

59 Ibid.

60 Emile Durkheim, *Le Suicide*, trans. John A Spaulding and George Simpson (New York: Free Press, 1958).

61 Ezard et al., "Risky Alcohol Use."

62 Ezard et al., "Six Rapid Assessments."

63 Ezard et al., "Risky Alcohol Use."

64 Ibid.

65 Ibid.

66 World Health Organization and Mental Health Gap Action Programme, *mhGAP Intervention Guide.*

67 Weaver and Roberts, "Drinking and Displacement."

68 Ezard, "Substance Use among Populations."

69 Ezard et al., "Six Rapid Assessments."

70 United Nations High Commissioner for Refugees and World Health Organization, *Field Guide.*

71 Ezard et al., "Six Rapid Assessments."

72 Thomas F Babor et al., *The Alcohol Use Disorders Identification Test: Guidelines for Use in Primary Care* (Geneva: World Health Organization, 2001), http://whqlibdoc.who.int/hq/2001/who_msd_msb_01.6a.pdf.

73 Thomas F Babor and John C Higgins-Biddle, *Brief Intervention for Hazardous and Harmful Drinking: A Manual for Use in Primary Care* (Geneva: World Health Organization, 2001), http://whqlibdoc.who.int/hq/2001/who_msd_msb_01.6b.pdf.

74 Peter Anderson, Dan Chisholm, and Daniela C Fuhr, "Effectiveness and Cost-Effectiveness of Policies and Programmes to Reduce the Harm Caused by Alcohol," *Lancet* 373, no. 9682 (June 27, 2009): 2234–2246, doi:10.1016/S0140-6736(09)60744-3; Wendy Loxley et al., *The Prevention of Substance Use, Risk and Harm in Australia: A Review of the Evidence* (Sydney: The National Drug Research Centre and the Centre for Adolescent Health, 2004); Wayne Hall et al., "Illicit Opiate Abuse," in *Disease Control Priorities in Developing Countries*, ed. Dean T Jamison et al., 2nd ed. (Washington, DC: World Bank, 2006), 907–932, http://www.ncbi.nlm.nih.gov/books/NBK11797/.

75 Inter-Agency Standing Committee, "Action Sheet 6.5: Minimise Harm Related to Alcohol and Other Substance Use."

76 Ezard et al., "Six Rapid Assessments."

77 Ibid.

78 Ibid.

79 Anderson, Chisholm, and Fuhr, "Effectiveness and Cost-Effectiveness of Policies."

80 Hall et al., "Illicit Opiate Abuse"; Richard P Mattick et al., "Methadone Maintenance Therapy versus No Opioid Replacement Therapy for Opioid Dependence," *Cochrane Database of Systematic Reviews* no. 3 (2009): CD002209, doi:10.1002/14651858.CD002209.pub2.

81 Anderson, Chisholm, and Fuhr, "Effectiveness and Cost-Effectiveness of Policies."

82 DARE Network, *Annual Report.*

83 Room, Babor, and Rehm, "Alcohol and Public Health"; Royal Australasian College of Physicians, Royal Australian and New Zealand College of Psychiatrists, and GROW (Australia), *Illicit Drugs Policy: Using Evidence to Get Better Outcomes* (Sydney: RACP, 2004).

84 Dua et al., "Evidence-Based Guidelines."

Bibliography

Aide Médicale Internationale. *Substance Abuse, Drugs & Addictions Guidebook.* Aide Médicale Internationale and UNHCR, 2009. http://www.burmalibrary.org/docs07/DrugGuidebook-LowReso-red.pdf.

American Psychiatric Association. *Diagnostic and Statistical Manual of Mental Disorders: DSM-5.* 5th ed. Washington, DC: American Psychiatric Association, 2013.

Anderson, Peter, Dan Chisholm, and Daniela C Fuhr. "Effectiveness and Cost-Effectiveness of Policies and Programmes to Reduce the Harm Caused by Alcohol." *Lancet* 373, no. 9682 (June 27, 2009): 2234–2246. doi:10.1016/S0140-6736(09)60744-3.

Babor, Thomas F, and John C Higgins-Biddle. *Brief Intervention for Hazardous and Harmful Drinking: A Manual for Use in Primary Care.* Geneva: World Health Organization, 2001. http://whqlibdoc.who.int/hq/2001/who_msd_msb_01.6b.pdf.

Babor, Thomas F, John C Higgins-Biddle, John B Saunders, and Maristela G Monteiro. *The Alcohol Use Disorders Identification Test: Guidelines for Use in Primary Care.* Geneva: World Health Organization, 2001. http://whqlibdoc.who.int/hq/2001/who_msd_msb_01.6a.pdf.

Bhui, Kamaldeep, and Nasir Warfa. "Drug Consumption in Conflict Zones in Somalia." *PLoS Med* 4, no. 12 (December 11, 2007): e354. doi:10.1371/journal.pmed.0040354.

Bosnar, Alan, Valter Stemberga, Miran Coklo, Emina Grgurevic, Gordana Zamolo, Tamara Cucic, and Nunzio di Nunno. "War and Suicidal Deaths by Explosives in

Southwestern Croatia." *Archives of Medical Research* 37, no. 3 (April 2006): 392–394. doi:10.1016/j.arcmed.2005.06.007.

Bosnar, Alan, Valter Stemberga, Drazen Cuculic, Gordana Zamolo, Sanja Stifter, and Miran Coklo. "Suicide Rate after the 1991–1995 War in Southwestern Croatia." *Archives of Medical Research* 35, no. 4 (August 2004): 344–347. doi:10.1016/j.arcmed.2004.03.001.

Brown, Catherine. "Burma: The Political Economy of Violence." *Disasters* 23, no. 3 (September 1999): 234–256.

Carballo, Manuel, and Aditi Nerukar. "Migration, Refugees, and Health Risks." *Emerging Infectious Diseases* 7, no. 3 (Suppl. 2001): 556–560.

Catani, Claudia, Nadja Jacob, Elisabeth Schauer, Mahendran Kohila, and Frank Neuner. "Family Violence, War, and Natural Disasters: A Study of the Effect of Extreme Stress on Children's Mental Health in Sri Lanka." *BMC Psychiatry* 8 (2008): 33. doi:10.1186/1471-244X-8-33.

DARE Network. *Annual Report*, 2011. http://www.darenetwork.com/images/documents/2011dare_annual_report.pdf.

———. *Health Messenger* 11, Special Issue: *Alcoholism*, 2000. http://www.ibiblio.org/obl/docs3/PdF%20FINAL%20ISSUES/ISSUE%2011.pdf.

Dua, Tarun, Corrado Barbui, Nicolas Clark, Alexandra Fleischmann, Vladimir Poznyak, Mark van Ommeren, M. Taghi Yasamy, et al. "Evidence-Based Guidelines for Mental, Neurological, and Substance Use Disorders in Low- and Middle-Income Countries: Summary of WHO Recommendations." *PLoS Med* 8, no. 11 (November 15, 2011): e1001122. doi:10.1371/journal.pmed.1001122.

Durkheim, Emile. *Le Suicide*. Translated by John A Spaulding and George Simpson. New York: Free Press, 1958.

Ezard, Nadine. "Substance Use among Populations Displaced by Conflict: A Literature Review." *Disasters* 36, no. 3 (July 2012): 533–557. doi:10.1111/j.1467-7717.2011.01261.x.

Ezard, Nadine, Edna Oppenheimer, Ann Burton, Marian Schilperoord, David Macdonald, Moruf Adelekan, Abandokoth Sakarati, and Mark van Ommeren. "Six Rapid Assessments of Alcohol and Other Substance Use in Populations Displaced by Conflict." *Conflict and Health* 5, no. 1 (December 1, 2011): 1–15. doi:10.1186/1752-1505-5-1.

Ezard, Nadine, Supan Thiptharakun, François Nosten, Tim Rhodes, and Rose McGready. "Risky Alcohol Use among Reproductive-Age Men, Not Women, in Mae La Refugee Camp, Thailand, 2009." *Conflict and Health* 6, no. 1 (September 11, 2012): 7. doi:10.1186/1752-1505-6-7.

Graham, Allan W, Terry K Schultz, and Michael F Mayo-Smith. *Principles of Addiction Medicine*. 3rd ed. Chevy Chase, MD: American Society of Addiction Medicine, 2003.

Hall, Wayne, Chris Doran, Louisa Degenhardt, and Donald Shepard. "Illicit Opiate Abuse." In *Disease Control Priorities in Developing Countries*, edited by Dean T

Jamison, Joel G Breman, Anthony R Measham, George Alleyne, Mariam Claeson, David B Evans, Prabhat Jha, Anne Mills, and Philip Musgrove, 907–932. 2nd ed. Washington, DC: World Bank, 2006. http://www.ncbi.nlm.nih.gov/books/NBK11797/.

Inter-Agency Standing Committee. "Action Sheet 6.5: Minimise Harm Related to Alcohol and Other Substance Use." In *IASC Guidelines on Mental Health and Psychosocial Support in Emergencies*. Geneva: Inter-Agency Standing Committee, 2007.

Kozarić-Kovačić, D, T Ljubin, and M Grappe. "Comorbidity of Posttraumatic Stress Disorder and Alcohol Dependence in Displaced Persons." *Croatian Medical Journal* 41, no. 2 (June 2000): 173–178.

Kuo, Irene, Salman ul-Hasan, Noya Galai, David L Thomas, Tariq Zafar, Mohammad A Ahmed, and Steffanie A Strathdee. "High HCV Seroprevalence and HIV Drug Use Risk Behaviors among Injection Drug Users in Pakistan." *Harm Reduction Journal* 3, no. 1 (August 16, 2006): 26. doi:10.1186/1477-7517-3-26.

Loxley, Wendy, John W Toumbourou, Tim Stockwell, Ben Hains, Katie Scott, Celia Godfrey, Elizabeth Waters, et al. *The Prevention of Substance Use, Risk and Harm in Australia: A Review of the Evidence*. Sydney: The National Drug Research Centre and the Centre for Adolescent Health, 2004.

Mattick, Richard P, Courtney Breen, Jo Kimber, and Marina Davoli. "Methadone Maintenance Therapy versus No Opioid Replacement Therapy for Opioid Dependence." *Cochrane Database of Systematic Reviews* 3 (2009): CD002209. doi:10.1002/14651858.CD002209.pub2.

Miller, Kenneth E, and Lisa M Rasco. "An Ecological Framework for Addressing the Mental Health Needs of Refugee Communities." In *The Mental Health of Refugees: Ecological Approaches to Healing and Adaptation*, edited by Kenneth E Miller and Lisa M Rasco. Mahwah, NJ: Lawrence Erlbaum Associates, 2004.

Ondeko, Roselidah, and Susan Purdin. "Understanding the Causes of Gender-Based Violence." *Forced Migration Review* 19 (2004): 30.

Porter, Matthew, and Nick Haslam. "Predisplacement and Postdisplacement Factors Associated with Mental Health of Refugees and Internally Displaced Persons: A Meta-Analysis." *JAMA: Journal of the American Medical Association* 294, no. 5 (August 3, 2005): 602–612. doi:10.1001/jama.294.5.602.

Puertas, Gloria, Cielo Ríos, and Hernán del Valle. "Prevalencia de trastornos mentales comunes en barrios marginales urbanos con población desplazada en Colombia" [The Prevalence of Common Mental Disorders in Urban Slums with Displaced Persons in Colombia]. *Revista panamericana de salud pública [Pan American Journal of Public Health]* 20, no. 5 (November 2006): 324–330.

Rehm, Jürgen, Robin Room, Kathryn Graham, Maristela Monteiro, Gerhard Gmel, and Christopher T Sempos. "The Relationship of Average Volume of Alcohol Consumption and Patterns of Drinking to Burden of Disease: An Overview." *Addiction* (Abingdon, England) 98, no. 9 (September 2003): 1209–1228.

Rhodes, Tim, Merrill Singer, Philippe Bourgois, Samuel R Friedman, and Steffanie A Strathdee. "The Social Structural Production of HIV Risk among Injecting Drug Users." *Social Science & Medicine (1982)* 61, no. 5 (September 2005): 1026–1044. doi:10.1016/j.socscimed.2004.12.024.

Room, Robin, Thomas Babor, and Jürgen Rehm. "Alcohol and Public Health." *Lancet* 365, no. 9458 (February 2005): 519–530. doi:10.1016/S0140-6736(05)17870-2.

Royal Australasian College of Physicians, Royal Australian and New Zealand College of Psychiatrists, and GROW (Australia). *Illicit Drugs Policy: Using Evidence to Get Better Outcomes.* Sydney: RACP, 2004.

Strathdee, Steffanie A, Julie A Stachowiak, Catherine S Todd, Wael K Al-Delaimy, Wayne Wiebel, Catherine Hankins, and Thomas L Patterson. "Complex Emergencies, HIV, and Substance Use: No 'Big Easy' Solution." *Substance Use & Misuse* 41, no. 10/12 (January 2006): 1637–1651. doi:10.1080/10826080600848116.

Strathdee, Steffanie A, Tariq Zafar, Heena Brahmbhatt, Ahmed Baksh, and Salman ul Hassan. "Rise in Needle Sharing among Injection Drug Users in Pakistan during the Afghanistan War." *Drug and Alcohol Dependence* 71, no. 1 (July 20, 2003): 17–24.

Sphere Project. *Humanitarian Charter and Minimum Standards in Disaster Response.* Geneva: Sphere Project, 2004.

United Nations High Commissioner for Refugees and World Health Organization. *Rapid Assessment of Alcohol and Other Substance Use in Conflict-Affected and Displaced Populations: A Field Guide.* Geneva: United Nations High Commissioner for Refugees Public Health and HIV Section and World Health Organization Department of Mental Health and Substance Abuse, 2008. http://www.who.int/entity/hac/network/unhcr_al_eng2.pdf.

UNODC. *Patterns and Trends of Amphetamine-Type Stimulants and Other Drugs: Asia and Pacific.* Vienna: United Nations Office on Drugs and Crime, 2012. http://www.unodc.org/documents/scientific/Patterns_and_Trends_of _Amphetaime-Type_Stimulants_and_Other_Drugs_-_Asia_and_the_Pacific _-_2012.pdf.

———. *Southeast Asia Opium Survey 2013.* Vienna: United Nations Office on Drugs and Crime, 2013. http://www.unodc.org/documents/southeastasiaandpacific/Publications/2013/SEA _Opium_Survey_2013_web.pdf.

Weaver, Heather, and Bayard Roberts. "Drinking and Displacement: A Systematic Review of the Influence of Forced Displacement on Harmful Alcohol Use." *Substance Use & Misuse* 45, no. 13 (November 2010): 2340–2355. doi:10.3109/10826081003793920.

Westermeyer, Joseph. *Poppies, Pipes, and People: Opium and Its Use in Laos.* Berkeley: University of California Press, 1983.

World Health Organization. *ICD-10: International Statistical Classification of Diseases and Related Health Problems.* 10th ed. Geneva: World Health Organization, 2007. http://www.who.int/classifications/icd/en/.

———. *The Global Burden of Disease: 2004 Update.* Geneva: World Health Organization, 2008.

http://www.who.int/healthinfo/global_burden_disease/2004_report_update/en/.

World Health Organization and Mental Health Gap Action Programme. *mhGAP Intervention Guide for Mental, Neurological and Substance Use Disorders in Non-specialized Health Settings.* Geneva: World Health Organization, 2010.

Zafar, Tariq, Heena Brahmbhatt, Ghazanfar Imam, Salman ul Hassan, and Steffanie A Strathdee. "HIV Knowledge and Risk Behaviors among Pakistani and Afghani Drug Users in Quetta, Pakistan." *Journal of Acquired Immune Deficiency Syndromes (1999)* 32, no. 4 (April 1, 2003): 394–398.

Chapter 8

Vulnerable Populations

Chronically Ill Individuals, People Living with HIV, Women with Reproductive Health Concerns, Land Mine Victims, and Former Political Prisoners

Meredith Walsh, Aung Khaing Min, Saw Than Lwin, and Saw Ku Thay

Introduction

The Thai-Burma border's unique ethnic, linguistic, and religious diversity creates an environment appropriate for a variety of approaches to addressing myriad needs. The varying levels of legal status among border populations (i.e., migrants with and without documentation, refugees living in and out of camps, internally displaced persons, and villagers who have lived their entire lives in conflict-affected settings) weave an even more complicated tapestry of needs based on access to service. All this diversity creates a multilayered mosaic of vulnerability in areas of security, discrimination, isolation, and displacement.

Along the border, chronic disease and disability are exacerbated by displaced persons' precarious status and by security constraints. Living in fear day-to-day creates a new paradigm for stress management and coping skills and sets a new bar for normative stress levels. Lack of sanctioned mobility for those who are undocumented creates social isolation, as some are restricted to the confines of housing arranged for migrant laborers while others are not permitted to leave the refugee camps. Even inside Burma, villagers often cannot travel safely to the next village because of nearby offensives or because the government requires a permit to pass checkpoints along the road. Yet the population in Burma crosses the national border anonymously with remarkable fluidity every day, refugees do regularly leave the camps in search of work, and villagers in Burma will walk through the mountain jungles to get where they need to be. This is a population of survivors.

Burma's total yearly expenditure on health care per capita is twenty-eight US dollars, or 2 percent of the gross domestic product,[1] which leaves a dearth of services in the country. Few hospitals have enough medicine, diagnostic instruments, and trained medical professionals to provide proper health services. In the eastern parts of Burma, where the ethnic resistance armies have been fighting the government's military regime, health care services are limited to those established by local ethnic authorities, often fueled by cross-border efforts from groups based in Thailand. International aid agencies provide health services in refugee camps in Thailand, and many people in Burma face great challenges traveling to the camps solely in search of such services. Those with chronic illnesses such as cancer, tuberculosis (TB), and human immunodeficiency virus (HIV) often suffer a slow death after receiving one rejection after another seeking treatment that is not locally available or financially feasible.

Women who face unwanted pregnancies on the Thai-Burma border have few choices, and as a result they often take great risks to end their pregnancies in isolation, endangering their lives. These women risk morbidity and mortality and spend the rest of their lives carrying secrets while struggling to keep their families alive. Unsafe abortion and postpartum hemorrhage are the leading causes of maternal death in Burma. In longstanding conflict areas of eastern Burma, maternal mortality is the highest in Southeast Asia, on par with countries in Sub-Saharan Africa. Although the reported maternal mortality ratio for Burma as a whole has stayed relatively constant over the last decade, at 320 deaths per 100,000 live births,[2] the rate in eastern Burma is thought to be significantly higher, at approximately 1,000 deaths per 100,000 live births.[3] The national contraceptive prevalence rate in Burma is just 34 percent[4] and is estimated to be even lower in eastern states.[5] To address the unmet need for contraception and to reduce the morbidity and mortality associated with unsafe abortion, Mae Tao Clinic (MTC) has offered contraceptive services and postabortion care services for women from Burma for over twenty years.

Land mine injuries are all too common along the Burma border. Land mine victims' lives change dramatically in a matter of seconds, and the immediate and long-term support they need is significant. Around the world, 800 deaths each month are caused by land mines[6] or, by other estimates, 15,000–20,000 deaths each year.[7] Rehabilitation for victims includes both physical and emotional healing, which can be achieved with medical treatment and physical therapy, as well as counseling and social support. These services are challenging to deliver in a conflict setting with an unstable, migrant population.

Many people start new lives and take on new identities when they cross the border from Burma to Thailand, as in the case of former political prisoners. Many escape the fear of rearrest only to find new fears living without documentation in Thailand. A new life in a new country does not erase the suffering of the past but does create an environment that local organizations have adapted to facilitate a healing process. Though nearly one thousand political prisoners have been released since May 2011, there are still 122 languishing in prisons in Burma and approximately 100 former political prisoners living in exile on the Thai-Burma border.[8]

Addressing Myriad Mental Health Needs

The challenges to providing psychosocial support and mental health counseling for high-risk subgroups are significant, but many organizations and individuals are dedicated to offering such services in a meaningful context that is culturally appropriate, safe, and feasible within this protracted conflict setting. All quotes in this chapter are from personal communication with key actors working with organizations in this setting.

One such organization detailed in this chapter is the Mae Tao Clinic, a community-based health center on the Thai-Burma border. MTC was founded in 1989 by Dr. Cynthia Maung, a newly trained ethnically Karen doctor who, like many of her student counterparts, was fleeing the oppressive military regime in Burma. The health facility has grown from a one-room clinic serving exiled political activists to a burgeoning hospital with thirteen departments serving over 100,000 patients each year. Tucked away from view off the main road in Mae Sot, a Thai border town in Tak Province, MTC provides free care to all. Half the patients live in Burma and cross the border (two kilometers down the road) to seek care, and half the patients live in Thailand as migrants from Burma. Many travel for weeks across Burma, not able to access health care in their own country, to receive care at the free clinic in Thailand they have heard about through word of mouth.

Though MTC is not registered as a health facility in Thailand and none of the medical staff have licenses to practice medicine in Thailand, the clinic has gained local, national, and international recognition for providing health care services to hundreds of thousands of people flowing across the Thai-Burma border over the past twenty years. Dr. Cynthia Maung, known affectionately as Dr. Cynthia, has won numerous international awards, including nomination for the Nobel Peace Prize in 2005. MTC has become a hub of health care services and medic training along the border, and as such has developed strong collaborations with the Thai Ministry of Public Health, international nongovernmental organizations, and a plethora of community-based health care organizations. Over three hundred medics at MTC offer a range of clinical services, including pediatric and adult outpatient and inpatient care, reproductive health care, dental and eye care, acupuncture, surgery and trauma care, prostheses, and mental health care.

MTC's vision focuses on building capacity not only to provide health care for patients at their facility, but also to improve the health care system in the ethnic areas of Burma, where decades of civil war and military rule have decimated the health infrastructure. Over one hundred medics from Burma are trained at MTC each year, about one-third of whom will return to their villages in Burma to provide health services once they have finished their practical training. The medics and patients at MTC share the same communities of origin; as such, the services are culturally appropriate and are offered in multiple languages. The most common languages spoken at MTC are Burmese and Karen. The clinic's community-based model of health care allows medics to treat patients who share a common history of struggling for survival in a country riddled by conflict. Sharing this common history fosters empathy and trust, but can also trigger vicarious trauma for medics who have experienced particular hardship.

As the clinic grew during the 1990s, Dr. Cynthia recognized the need to offer psychological therapy for medics facing routine retraumatization during patient care. In 2006, after several years of extensive trainings provided by mental health professional consultants, MTC opened its counseling center, now called the Mental Health Counseling Center (MHCC), to provide psychotherapy and psychosocial support for medics and patients.

CHRONIC ILLNESS
Moe Khaing is a 42-year-old Muslim woman with diabetes and hypertension who presented to the Mental Health Counseling Center at Mae Tao Clinic complaining of headaches, drowsiness, nausea/vomiting, anger when confused, and severe anxiety. She has had diabetes since childhood and goes to Mae Sot General Hospital (Thai government hospital) for monthly insulin injections with her daughter, who is also diabetic and takes insulin. Moe Khaing lives with her family on the Burma side of the border in the town of Myawaddy. Her eldest daughter married eight years ago, and her son-in-law manages a plant shop where the family sells orchids they find in the forest. Moe Khaing's husband moved away three years ago to work in Thailand. Three years ago Moe Khaing's son went to the forest to find orchids but did not come back. Since then she has had economic and emotional problems. She can no longer afford her insulin injections. Eight months ago she heard that her son had become a soldier for the Karen National Union. Then her neighbor told her that he had seen her son's dead

body in the forest. Initially she did not believe her neighbor; she believed in
her heart that her son was alive. She has not heard any more information
about her son. A counselor from MTC goes to Moe Khaing's home in
Myawaddy once or twice a month to provide counseling. Moe Khaing says
that the people close to her do not listen to her and do not understand her.
She feels that her husband does not care about her and that she must face
her mental and physical problems alone. She wants to receive insulin at
MTC, but she has been told that MTC does not have insulin in the pharmacy.
The counselor's goal is to reduce her stress, explaining to her that the more
stress she has, the more her diabetes will be exacerbated. "I teach her how to
relax her muscles and her mind," the counselor says.

Prevention and treatment of chronic diseases that require basic primary
care and public health infrastructures pose a major challenge to resource-
poor countries and displaced communities, highlighting the greatest global
health disparity of our time. In Burma, this reality is further compounded
by political instability, human rights abuses, and lack of political will to
invest in primary and secondary health prevention services over the past
several decades. MTC is beginning to address this service gap, and the MHCC
focuses on the psychosocial needs of patients affected by chronic illness.

The MHCC is a single-story building nestled in the back of the clinic
compound, hidden from view, where staff members provide counseling for
patients with diverse mental health needs. Patients with chronic illness
such as cancer, TB, or diabetes are referred from the medical inpatient and
outpatient departments, or they are identified when the counselors visit the
medical departments to inquire whether there are any patients who might
want counseling. Three male and two female counselors are available to
provide counseling, both in the clinic and in patients' homes.

Many patients prefer that counselors meet them in their homes. Home
visits are also more suitable than clinic visits because patients risk arrest
and deportation when traveling to and from the clinic. Counselors visit
patients two to three times each week, and each counselor's caseload may
include over twenty patients at one time. Patients are assigned to counselors
depending on the type of case and who is available at the counseling center
at the time of referral. There is one senior female counselor who manages
all cases involving domestic violence and unwanted pregnancy. Counseling
techniques include psycho-education, cognitive coping, and progressive relaxation. Medication is provided when needed.

Though essential mental health services are available at the MHCC, the
former director, coauthor Saw Ku Thay, explains there are barriers for

patients seeking care there. He says many patients do not come for counseling services, despite being referred from other departments. "Some patients say they do not have time, as they need to get back to work, and some do not understand the purpose of counseling." Sometimes "only the people who have severe cases like extreme weight loss or prolonged insomnia will come to us."

The staff also discovered that the sign in front of the MHCC influenced access to care. Rather than encouraging people to seek services, the sign initially deterred them. The sign read "Mental Health," which created a perception that services were only for those with severe mental illness. Patients who were offered services declined and said, "We are not mad!" Later the sign was changed to "Counseling and Help," which created the misperception that patients could get help with employment or finances. Patients were disappointed to learn that the counselors could not help them find a job or give them money. Today the sign reads "Mental Health Counseling Center" in English and "Sate Kyan Mar Yay—Nint Theint Sway Nway Pay Chin—Htar Na" in Burmese, meaning "Mental Health Consoling, Discussion Department."

Another barrier to accessing services was the MHCC's location. It was originally located in the heart of the clinic, a two-story building sandwiched between the medical and surgical departments. Though seemingly ideal for convenient referrals and integrated care, this location proved challenging because of the stigma of seeking counseling and psychosocial support. Patients had to walk up a flight of stairs on the outside of the two-story building, which created a stigma because of visibility (i.e., lack of confidentiality) and also created a structural barrier, as amputees had more difficulty using the stairs. When the facility was moved to the back of the clinic compound in 2012, more patients began accessing services.

Aside from counseling services in the MHCC and in the home, counselors also provide support group services in MTC's Patient House, a shelter for those who do not necessarily need a hospital bed but who may be awaiting further treatment, referrals, or labor and delivery. There may be up to thirty people staying in the Patient House at any given time, including adults and children. The Patient House serves as a forum for family support groups for patients and their families once a week. These patients are often undergoing or awaiting treatment or surgery, such as those taking TB medication or pending surgical consultation for malignant tumors.

Typically, three to four patients and their caregivers participate in the support group; however groups can include up to ten people. Group members share problems and conditions while the counselor listens. The counselors offer psycho-education and suggestions for coping skills. As the former director notes, "When I arrive [in the Patient House], the patients come to me because they want to talk about their problems." However, the patients are not always the same every week, which means there is not a consistent way to measure progress. Problems addressed during these sessions include those related to depression, PTSD, schizophrenia, alcohol withdrawal, chronic and acute psychosis (including drug-induced), severe stress or anxiety, amputation rehabilitation, and bipolar disorder. "Patients tell me they don't have coping skills, but when I ask them what they do to resolve their stress, they learn they have coping skills already," says the former director. "So I teach them about the difference between healthy and unhealthy coping skills."

Women with cancer are referred to the MHCC from the Reproductive Health Outpatient Department. Many travel great distances across Burma to seek care at MTC, where they have heard there is free treatment available. Often they have been diagnosed in Burma but could not access treatment because of cost or lack of available treatment in Burmese hospitals. Women who arrive at MTC with cervical, breast, ovarian, or uterine cancer are referred to the Burma Women's Medical Fund, a special program funded by private donations from all over the world to cover the costs of evaluation and/or surgery in the Thai health care system.

While patients wait for evaluation results, treatment, or surgery, counselors provide counseling using relaxation, imagery, and cognitive coping skills. According to one senior female counselor,[9] in these patients "we see severe depression." Symptoms include insomnia, weight loss, loss of appetite, inability to work or function in daily life. "They are very sad, they cry a lot, and some say they want to die."

Some patients arrive when their cancer is already too advanced for treatment. Often they choose to return to Burma to die in the comfort of their home with their families. Once the patient knows she will die, the counselors help her find a positive attitude and teach her relaxation methods. "We remind them that everyone must die," says one of the senior counselors.[10] If they are not considered eligible for treatment with chemotherapy or radiation after being evaluated in the Thai hospital (e.g., if the cancer is in advanced stages), patients are encouraged to use Burmese traditional medicine such as *bara say, shwe man,* or *shwe yin kyaw.* These medicines can include drinking tea made from leaves grown naturally in the forest, or applying herbal balms or salves to the skin.

According to one senior counselor, even if the Burmese medicine does not help cure her cancer, it may reduce her depression, especially if she can use relaxation and meditation as well. "Sometimes I tell them that I used to have a cough in Burma and when I took Western medicine (antibiotics) it didn't get better. Then my neighbor gave me a *besat* leaf to pound. She told me to drink the water from the leaves, and then I got better. In this way I explain that sometimes if we take both Western medicine and traditional Burmese medicine, it can help," says the senior counselor.[11] Though there are no Burmese traditional healers, or *bain-doh*, practicing at MTC, patients are encouraged to seek services from those they know in their communities. Some people from Burma also practice a ritual of summoning the spirit of a dead person to remove a curse that causes disease.

In this setting, the lack of culturally appropriate evaluation tools and the challenge of developing them, as well as lack of follow-up caused by patients' migration patterns, makes it difficult to measure success in counseling. According to one counselor, "We don't know if we are successful, but when the patients tell us they are hopeful after talking to us, we know that we are doing something right. We see them happier, and that's all we can do. But sometimes I think I am not successful."[12] Patients may go to the clinic for medical care, but when they are asked about their mental health or the psychological effects of their illness, the stresses and trauma of their lives in Burma (or at the border) are revealed and may become the primary focus of care.

PEOPLE LIVING WITH HIV

Julia is a 15-year-old female initially brought to Mae Tao Clinic at age 12 when her family decided to no longer care for her. Julia was born in Mae Sot, Thailand, to Burmese migrant workers who died when Julia was young. She lived with her elderly grandmother in the border town of Myawaddy, Burma, but they struggled financially and often got their meals from a nearby monastery. A family member brought Julia to MTC with the intention of leaving her permanently, reporting that she believed Julia had HIV and the family no longer wanted Julia to stay with them. A counselor at the MTC Voluntary Counseling and Testing Department provided counseling to both the family member and Julia upon their arrival, and Julia was subsequently referred to a residential community-based organization in Mae Sot, where Julia now lives. The family member reported bringing Julia to MTC, rather than seeking services in Burma, because of MTC's free health care and its coordinated services with other organizations that could further support Julia. Julia began receiving primary care, HIV care, and social support from both MTC and the community-based organization where she lives. After a year and a half,

Julia's mood at school and at home became depressed, and she often looked sad. Her academic progress dropped and she began refusing to attend school, reporting that she hated learning. She became isolated from friends at school and at the shelter and communicated less with everyone. She ran away from the shelter multiple times, reporting that she was attempting to find her grandmother. Other shelter residents reported distress about Julia's behavior and concern for everyone's security. MTC *staff recognized developmental changes in Julia and acknowledged that her behavior may be caused by shame associated with being an adolescent in a first-grade class because of her lack of prior formal education. They recognized that this may be contributing to her desire to quit school. To ensure Julia's safety, caregivers at the shelter began to monitor her more closely to prevent her from running away. The community organization staff collaborated with* MTC *in counseling Julia and the guardian of the shelter. Counseling sessions at* MTC *were irregular because transportation was not always available. The treatment team mitigated this by having frequent meetings by phone about Julia. Gradually they observed a shift in Julia's behavior, and she has since exhibited fewer behavioral problems and seemed happier. She continues to report loneliness and longing for her grandmother and her parents, so staff at the shelter and at* MTC *continue to try to help her cope.*

Over the past three decades, HIV and the clinical manifestation of Acquired Immunodeficiency Syndrome (AIDS) have served to mold and evolve our understanding of global health, sexual health, stigma and discrimination, and inequality in health care systems and in cultural and medical ethics. The HIV/AIDS epidemic in Burma further highlights the sociopolitical inertia that must be surmounted to provide basic comprehensive care (i.e., preventive, medical, and psychosocial support) for some of the most affected vulnerable populations, most of whom were marginalized prior to a diagnosis of HIV/AIDS.

Within Burma, there is a vacuum in our understanding of the precise disease burden of HIV/AIDS. While UNAIDS 2011 national estimates put the adult prevalence of HIV around 0.6 percent among the adult population, the incidence of AIDS-related admissions or visits to border hospitals and clinics suggests the prevalence in particular subpopulations is very much higher.[13]

HIV treatment in Burma has relied heavily on outside donors for resources and clinical management. Médecins Sans Frontières (MSF) of France has historically shouldered much of the burden of care of the HIV-positive populations in Burma through operating medical clinics in several regions. Because of severe resource limitations, however, only a minority of patients who need antiretroviral therapy (ART), even by conservative estimates, have access to necessary medications.[14] The situation is further exacerbated by the most recent World Health Organization (WHO) guidelines, which call for earlier initiation of ART, effectively expanding the number of people who are clinically eligible to take medications but will not receive them.[15]

Yet to focus on access to medications for HIV/AIDS and its associated opportunistic infections, such as TB, is to detract from the fundamental issues that define the tragedy of the HIV/AIDS epidemic in Burma. The key determinants for how individuals contract the disease, how a small fraction of those individuals will learn of their HIV status, and finally how an even smaller fraction of those who know will have access to counseling, medications with continued medical attention, and social support suggest, overwhelmingly, a structural issue. This reflects the larger lack of health and social infrastructure in Burma today. While many of Burma's neighboring countries are now initiating community-based prevention and treatment programs after decades of aggressive public education and awareness campaigns regarding HIV/AIDS, Burma still has communities that have never heard of the disease. Lacking the foundation for awareness-building and advocacy for affected vulnerable groups that has been implemented to varying degrees in most areas of the world affected by HIV/AIDS today, those at risk for HIV in Burma must overcome immense cultural and structural barriers to reach medical or psychosocial support.

MTC's HIV services are one example of a community health clinic–based program for displaced people living with HIV that promotes patient and community awareness of the disease, provides needed medical assessment and intervention, and addresses associated psychosocial issues. MTC's HIV program includes voluntary counseling and testing (VCT) services, antiretroviral (ARV) treatment, preventing-mother-to-child-transition interventions, and peer counseling, including home visits, psychosocial support, and a strong network of community agency partnerships. The MTC HIV program was one of the first clinic programs along the Thai-Burma border to integrate understanding the necessity of mental health treatment into its conceptualization of patient needs and treatment.

MTC actively collaborates with hospitals and community-based organizations to address the myriad needs, including mental health treatment, of the HIV-positive community living inside Burma and in Thailand. In 2003, the MTC's VCT department officially opened, welcoming patients already diagnosed with HIV and those seeking testing for HIV status. Peer counselors provide pre- and post-test counseling and support to patients who are often overwhelmed with anxiety and fear when faced with learning their HIV status. Before this, patients had received all services at a Thai government hospital that provided health services at a cost to the patient and in the Thai language. The opening of the MTC VCT department enabled care at a familiar health care facility, in the patient's preferred language, by an HIV-positive peer counselor with experience living with HIV in the displaced Burmese community, and at no cost to the patient. In 2001, MTC initiated its preventing-mother-to-child-transmission program for its HIV-positive pregnant patients, which included ARV treatment, labor and delivery support, and supplemental feeding for up to one year after delivery. In 2006, the MTC Mental Health Counseling Center opened, offering supportive counseling to all patients including the HIV-positive community. The MHCC and VCT departments, initially located in the same building and jointly managed, had smooth referral processes, and all counselors were familiar with common psychosocial issues faced by HIV-positive individuals, such as fear, anxiety, and discrimination. VCT peer counselors address many of the patients' psychosocial needs while the MHCC counselors provide specialized psychological support, such as addressing imminent suicide risk, psychotic symptoms, domestic violence, and substance abuse. In 2007, MTC moved closer to providing holistic HIV services by initiating provision of ARVs. Before being made available to the general patient population, ARVs were provided to peer counselors to ensure they would be healthy and capable of providing services to the HIV-positive community. Until 2012, MTC also had a supplemental nutritious-food program for all HIV patients; however, this program was discontinued after funding cuts. The HIV services of MTC have evolved over time in response to the evolving needs of this community. Psychosocial care has been incorporated into service provision since the beginning, and staff working with this community recognizes the broad psychological effects of contracting this chronic illness that continues to be stigmatized and hidden in communities along the Thai-Burma border.

Most MTC patients receive the majority of their HIV care on-site, including mental health counseling and psychiatric medication management when indicated. For some patients, such as pregnant women and those with critical care issues, the partnership with Thai hospitals remains necessary and invaluable. MTC has strengthened its collaboration with other health centers to ensure that patients receive high quality health care from these institutions despite linguistic, cultural, and financial obstacles. Patients sometimes experience overwhelming psychological distress when receiving HIV health care in an unfamiliar setting outside the Burmese community, so MTC counselors help facilitate patients' care at these hospitals.

In 2013, MTC supported more than three hundred HIV-positive individuals. Peer counselors, home visitors, and MTC's partner programs are the primary source of psychosocial support for this HIV community. MTC's bimonthly discussion groups also provide social support and encouragement to patients who feel isolated and who struggle daily. MTC facilitates community outings with patients and their family members, providing a day of fun and relaxation with healthy-living didactics and supportive discussions. For some patients, supportive family and caregivers join in their treatment at MTC and for others, family and community members provide encouragement to patients at home. The VCT staff also understands the value of providing appropriate referrals for services in the community, especially for patients who do not have family support. Counselors assess patients' community life and living conditions in Mae Sot or in Burma to determine appropriate recommendations for shelter, nutrition, and intensive medical care such as tuberculosis treatment. In Mae Sot, some men, women, and children receive adjunctive care, including housing, from MTC's community partner programs such as Social Action for Women and Men's Health Center. Partner programs have less training in working with HIV populations, so MTC staff offers training, support, and encouragement to staff at partner agencies.

The clinic's HIV patients report a range of mental health and psychosocial struggles associated with their HIV status, including fears related to their HIV status being known in the community, shame and blame, depressed mood, and environmental stressors affecting access to health care. Many patients worry about disclosure of their HIV status in the community and often do not want to disclose their status even to their partners. Some young women do not come for health appointments because they do not want to be seen seeking services, some market workers miss treatment because they do not want workers from neighboring stalls asking why they are always going to medical appointments, and some sex workers continue to work without using protection because they worry that customers will no longer come if they suspect HIV. For patient confidentiality, VCT signage is not posted on the department; however, the modest offices sit along a main thoroughfare of the clinic, so patients report not wanting to even wait in the chairs opposite the department for fear of people assuming they have HIV or sexually transmitted infections.

While there is now general understanding of HIV and AIDS across most communities of Burma, there is still extensive misinformation, stigmatization, and misunderstanding of transmission. MTC staff recognizes the need for more basic education about HIV, and it is also faced with the challenge of addressing misinformation about psychosocial factors sometimes associated with contracting and living with HIV, such as discrimination, interpersonal violence, shame, guilt, blame, and denial.

At the VCT department, depression is often observed after patients begin antiretroviral treatment and do not notice marked health improvement. Severe depression sets in when patients realize that they will die from HIV or HIV-related illness. Those coping without a family support system sometimes exhibit poor treatment compliance, including discontinuing ARVs. At these times when patients' psychological distress and isolation threatens their health and healing, peer counselors offer more intensive support, understanding, and encouragement.

Both MTC staff and patients struggle with a range of psychosocial and environmental factors that affect HIV patient care. Some patients live in Burma and so do not meet the criteria of living in Mae Sot, Thailand, to receive ARVs. Some begin ARV treatment but discontinue when they cannot find a job in Mae Sot; they choose employment in Burma over ARV treatment in Thailand. Patients who are employed in Thailand are sometimes not permitted by employers to attend health appointments. Many patients fear that reporting their HIV status to their employers will lead to job termination, which has been reported by MTC patients. In fact, there are no cases of HIV-positive patients telling employers their status and subsequently keeping their jobs. Staff members report challenges such as insufficient funding to support HIV services and patients coming to MTC at a late stage of the disease when available interventions will no longer help. Patients' death from HIV-related illnesses is part of weekly life at the HIV program of MTC, with approximately five people dying from HIV-related illnesses every month.

Over time, displaced and transient community members from Burma have developed the structure, design, and services of MTC's HIV services, and through this have identified important and necessary criteria to providing robust HIV prevention and treatment services. The community setting, the strengths of the community, cultural practices, and obstacles to providing care must be considered when developing HIV services in any context. In stable environments with established community and agency systems, HIV services and ARV treatments may not face the challenges of MTC's program, such as risk of arrest for both patient and counselor because of undocumented immigration status, challenges to accessing medications, and inability to locate patients for follow-up because of high rates of migration. Dedicated, compassionate, and knowledgeable peer counselors are necessary in this work.

Ongoing training and support for HIV services staff is imperative to ensure best practices and the well-being of the service providers. Service provider code of conduct adherence is important to maintain appropriate patient-counselor boundaries, high quality care, and respect for the treatment team and the health care facility in the community. ARV treatment is critical as well and serves multiple functions, including significantly decreasing transmission rates and enabling stronger social functioning for people living with HIV, which affects the individual, family, community, and nation.

Home-based care and psychosocial work are strongly recommended to address daily living needs and support system needs and to counter dissemination of misinformation and discrimination. Mental health services for individuals experiencing overwhelming distress are especially important at the time they learn their HIV status, at significant transition times during the illness, and when others in the HIV community develop AIDS or die. An interdisciplinary approach to addressing the plethora of biopsychosocial health issues that the HIV community struggles with promotes an understanding of the patient as a whole being and an understanding of HIV as a chronic disease that can be managed.

REPRODUCTIVE HEALTH ISSUES

Ma Htwe was 18 years old when she arrived at MTC at twenty weeks gestation with a high fever and a foul odor. She had induced an abortion by inserting a stick in her uterus and had taken misoprostol that she had bought in the market. Her uterine membrane had ruptured, and she had been leaking amniotic fluid for several days. She had strong contractions, low blood pressure, and was nearly in septic shock. She was admitted to MTC's reproductive health inpatient department, where she was given intravenous fluids and antibiotics. Fetal heart sounds were detected on ultrasound, but because the membrane had ruptured and because she was septic, she needed to deliver the baby immediately. It took several hours to deliver the baby by breech presentation. The baby weighed 0.5 kilograms (1.1 pounds). The baby's buttocks had been injured by the stick. Initially Ma Htwe told the staff that she had miscarried spontaneously, and when the staff asked her what had happened, she would not answer. After Ma Htwe heard the baby cry, she felt very upset. The baby survived only one day. Ma

Htwe's fever went down and her blood pressure went up. Slowly she regained physical strength. She had come to MTC alone and had no one to support her. Once she was calm and physically stable, the staff asked her why she had induced an abortion. Ma Htwe explained that she lived with her boyfriend, but they were not married. She and her boyfriend wanted a baby, and she thought if she got pregnant she could get married and everything would be okay. However, her boyfriend's older sister did not want them to marry, so the boyfriend's sister forced Ma Htwe to induce an abortion. Because his sister was older than they were, according to cultural tradition they had to follow her orders. While at MTC Ma Htwe received counseling about the complications of unsafe abortion, how to use family planning to prevent future pregnancies, and general encouragement and support. She was discharged with oral contraceptive pills and returned to her home in Burma.

The sixty-year civil conflict in Burma and the consequent population dislocation, disruption of services, and shortage of trained health service personnel has significantly affected reproductive health outcomes. The risk of unintended pregnancy and subsequent unsafe abortion among women in eastern Burma and refugees and migrants in Thailand is considerable. The national contraceptive prevalence rate in Burma is just 34 percent[16] and is estimated to be even lower in eastern states.[17] One of the greatest markers of unmet contraceptive need in eastern Burma is the prevalence of unsafe abortion and the associated mortality and morbidity. Under Burmese law, abortion is only legally permitted to save the life of the woman, and this legal exception is narrowly interpreted.[18] These restrictions on abortion, which are among the most stringent in the world, combined with heightened unintended pregnancy risk, have devastating health consequences: the best available evidence suggests that unsafe abortion is a leading cause of maternal death and may account for as much as 50 percent of maternal mortality in eastern Burma.[19]

It has been well documented that populations from Burma living on the Thai-Burma border face significant barriers to accessing services in Burma and Thailand, including family planning services, and are at increased risk for rape and sexual exploitation.[20] Further, although abortion is legally permissible in Thailand under a broader array of circumstances than in Burma, women from Burma residing in Thailand are generally unable to access safe abortion care even for legal indications because of their precarious legal status and providers' unwillingness to offer the service. Consequently, the rates of both unintended pregnancy and unsafe abortion are high, and the need for postabortion care (PAC) and strategies to reduce unintended pregnancy is pronounced.[21]

Identifying avenues for reducing unplanned pregnancy within this especially vulnerable population has been widely recognized as a public health, service delivery, and research priority.

MTC operates one of the largest and most comprehensive PAC services along the Thai-Burma border. In 2012, the reproductive health departments at MTC provided PAC services for 650 women, attended 3,500 deliveries (an average of ten deliveries each day), and served nearly 10,000 family planning clients.[22] Women presenting for PAC include those who experience spontaneous abortions and those who induce abortions using various methods including drinking traditional herbal remedies and medicines, abusing alcohol, inserting foreign objects, pummeling, and massage. Some women acquire misoprostol, a prostaglandin approved for medication abortions in Western countries, sold in markets on both sides of the Thai-Burma border.

Recognizing that women seeking PAC services are at risk for unintended pregnancy and are also willing to go to great lengths to terminate an unwanted pregnancy, contraceptive counseling and family planning service delivery are proactively incorporated into PAC services. Acceptance of postabortion contraception among PAC patients at MTC is near universal; in 2009 over 99 percent of the nearly five hundred PAC clients adopted a contraceptive method.[23] Nearly all the PAC clients at MTC opt for a hormonal method of contraception, with approximately 65 percent choosing Depo-Provera and roughly one-third electing to use oral contraceptive pills.[24] In 2011, because women from Burma on both sides of the Thai-Burma border face structural, physical, logistical, and service-delivery barriers that impede consistent access to these short-term hormonal contraceptives, MTC began efforts to increase utilization of highly effective long-acting reversible contraceptives, including both hormonal implants and the copper intrauterine device (IUD). Staff members were trained in counseling, insertion, and removal, and as a result, the number of IUD insertions increased dramatically from fourteen in 2010 to ninety in 2012.[25]

While the physical consequences of unsafe abortion are severe and are treated with PAC services at MTC, women with unintended pregnancies who induce abortions in this setting also face grave social, emotional, and mental health challenges. Even if the women do not share their stories, the staff observes they are distressed and often depressed. According to the reproductive health outpatient supervisor, "We can see in their faces, their furrowed brows, and their depressed eyes that they are not only in physical pain. She cries when we ask her to share her situation. Some women feel they cannot tell us their stories because they fear arrest, deportation, or reprisal from their husband or families if they find out what she has done."[26]

According to one former counselor at MTC, "Most women love their baby and they do not want to induce abortion if they can afford to take care of the baby. They never forget their decision, and they will always feel guilty and ashamed. They need assurance that they are doing the right thing at that moment, and they need to feel that they are not guilty. If they feel they are doing the right thing, then they feel better and it is not so painful for them. It's a very difficult decision for them to lose something."[27] Some women deliver their babies at MTC and then return to Burma, leaving the baby behind. Faced with multiple challenges in Burma, the women feel this decision is best for the baby's future.

Although the reproductive health departments at MTC provide clinical and counseling services, staff members are often either limited by time or are not as skilled in counseling. In some cases, women are referred for counseling and support at the Mental Health Counseling Center, where counselors are able to focus on helping the women find peace and accept what has happened. "[The counselors] need to consider the woman's feelings more and relax. They should not think so much about cultural and religious beliefs; they need to think about the health of the patients," says a former counselor at MTC.[28] "We try to compare the situation to a stomach-ache for which one takes medicine. An unwanted pregnancy is a health issue that is natural, and even though religious beliefs may say you will go to hell and cultural beliefs say you are a bad woman, the woman needs to know that abortion is a natural process to take care of her body."[29]

For women who are uncomfortable coming to MTC for counseling, or for whom structural barriers prevent them from coming, many counselors offer counseling by phone. While this is not ideal, says one former counselor, "we are able to adapt to the woman's needs. The choice is hers whether to seek counseling or not."[30]

Aside from counseling services at MTC, women with reproductive health issues may also seek services at Mae Sot General Hospital, the Thai government hospital under Thailand's Ministry of Health. The hospital's One Stop Crisis Center (OSCC) promotes services for women who experience rape, domestic violence, and unwanted pregnancies. One staff member in the OSCC is both Thai and Karen, and she provides culturally appropriate counseling to patients from Burma.

In 2007, an international research collaboration funded by the Safe Abortion Action Fund under International Planned Parenthood Federation and implemented by Darwin University aimed to improve the cross-cultural skills of Thai nurses at the Mae Sot General Hospital providing PAC services to women from Burma.[31] According to one of the bicultural workers involved in this project, while several Thai staff became more empathetic toward women from Burma by the end of the project, overall the services are still not equal.[32] Patients from Burma still experience discrimination when they are unable to pay for services, women are not given proper family planning counseling after an abortion, and the hospital only has funds to hire translators rather than bicultural health workers.

In 2011, a pilot project funded by the New Zealand Women's National Abortion Action Campaign and implemented by Ibis Reproductive Health began to improve referrals from MTC to Mae Sot General Hospital for safe abortion under Thai law.[33] MTC staff members in the reproductive health department were trained in options counseling for unwanted pregnancy and in Thai abortion law. As a result, patients who experience unwanted pregnancy and who are eligible according to Thai law are referred to the Thai hospital for safe abortion. This project is ongoing, and over twenty-five women have been referred to date, only three of whom were not approved, according to the hospital's legal eligibility determination.[34] "When we are able to successfully refer women for safe abortion in the Thai hospital, we can say we prevent the stress and suffering that accompany unwanted pregnancy and unsafe abortion," says the reproductive health outpatient supervisor.[35]

LAND MINE VICTIMS

Maw Ker was a soldier in the Karen National Liberation Army. In 1986 he stepped on a land mine in the jungle, ending his career as a soldier and beginning his career in prosthetics. After receiving a prosthetic limb, he was trained in prosthetics by Handicap International (HI). Over the course of fifteen years with HI, he set up prosthetics workshops in Karen State in Burma and in four refugee camps in Thailand. Because of increasing security challenges both in Karen State and in the refugee camps, in 2000 he approached Dr. Cynthia Maung, director of the MTC, about setting up a prosthetics workshop at her clinic. Since then Maw Ker has trained numerous prosthetic technicians at MTC. Staff turnover is high as some are resettled to third countries and some decide to take their skills back to Burma and provide services there. As a land mine victim and prosthetics recipient, Maw Ker understands the unique perspective he brings to his work. He has carried this forward by hiring and training other disabled technicians in his workshop. He currently supervises five technicians, three of whom are land mine victims with prosthetic limbs. "They can understand very well how to make the sandals fit the prosthesis, and they can understand that the men are feeling bad when they can no longer support their family," says Maw Ker. "When the patients come to the prosthetics workshop, we treat them very carefully and make the prosthetics precisely to fit them. We ask them how they are feeling and ask where the pain is so we can adjust the alignment. When they come back for follow-up and they are earning a living again . . . they feel happy because they say they have regained their normal life."

People who step on land mines in Burma are either civilians—often farmers foraging for wood or food in the forest—or soldiers for the Burmese army or ethnic resistance armies. Occasionally land mine victims are teenagers or children who were either walking to school or looking for bamboo in the forest. Some of those injured in Burma are treated at government hospitals in Burma. The majority of cases that occur in the eastern states of Burma are triaged by backpack medics trained in trauma care and are then carried across the border to Thailand to receive care in refugee camp clinics with services run by international nongovernmental organizations (such as Handicap International), in Thai government hospitals, or at MTC. Several organizations train and support backpack medics in Burma's eastern border states. These medics risk their lives to carry essential medicines and provide lifesaving health services to remote villages and mountain areas where there is no health infrastructure.

At MTC, amputees receive a range of coordinated services, including surgical or postoperative care, psychosocial treatment, prosthetic care, rehabilitation, and pain management with traditional Chinese medicine. This holistic model of care for amputees is unique to MTC within the borderwide community.

Each year, MTC's surgical department sees two hundred patients requiring new and replacement prostheses necessitated by land mine injuries.[36] Though MTC's surgical team has the capacity to perform amputations for most medical conditions, patients with land mine injuries are referred to the Thai government hospital about two kilometers from MTC because of their higher risk for infection. Land mine victims arriving at MTC have often been treated initially by backpack medics and carried by hammock for several days through the jungle to the nearest road. At least one family member often accompanies them to the clinic. MTC staff contact the International Committee of the Red Cross (ICRC), an international nongovernmental organization that arranges transportation and covers the costs of the amputation at the Mae Sot General Hospital. The patient returns to

MTC after ten days for postoperative care, and then again six months later for the prosthesis. Eh Ta Mwe, the director of the MTC surgical department, notes that even though the postoperative patients are sad when they arrive, they are reassured when they see others like them who can still work: "If they are sad when they arrive, we show them the other people who have prosthetics that are strong and can work. We show them one woman (on staff) who has two prosthetic legs, and they feel better because at least they have one leg. They chew betel nut and laugh together. We reassure them they will be able to carry heavy things after they recover."

At times, soldiers from the Burmese army present for care at MTC, though most Burmese soldiers are treated at Burma's government hospitals. Sometimes patients who have received amputations in Burmese hospitals present to MTC with pain from postoperative complications. MTC's surgical team repairs the amputation and provides prostheses for these patients as well.

MTC's prosthetics workshop (highlighted in the case study above) was established in 2000, and currently sees two hundred cases each year, including new and replacement prostheses. According to Maw Ker, the director of the prosthetics department, 80 percent of MTC's prosthetics cases are from land mine injuries, the vast majority of patients are male and over age 20, and about 60 percent are civilian.[37] The rest are soldiers from the Burmese army who need follow-up care after receiving initial treatment in a government hospital or soldiers from one of the ethnic resistance armies who have been carried to Thailand after receiving initial treatment by trauma medics trained by local ethnic health departments in Karen State. Unless they are high-ranking military personnel, Maw Ker notes, Burmese soldiers have to pay high fees for treatment in Burma. As a result, many former soldiers find their way to MTC for follow-up care and replacement prostheses. Even if they are from the Burmese army, says Maw Ker, "We tell them we do not discriminate. Even if you are my enemy, my obligation is to help you."

Rebuilding morale through physical rehabilitation is one of the goals of the technicians in the prosthetics workshop. The staff recognizes that patients feel the immediate burden of not being able to support their family anymore. Sometimes their community forgets about them, or stigmatizes them, assuming they are no longer active participants in community life. They can become destitute if they are unable to reintegrate into society. It is not easy for the patients to find the words to express how they feel to their family or their friends. Maw Ker puts this in perspective by offering, "In Burma we don't have access to human rights. So mostly [land mine victims] don't know how to express their problems. If they step on a land mine, they don't see this as a human rights abuse. They just see something bad has happened to them."

The prosthetics staff take care to precisely measure sockets for casting and monitor the patients closely as they begin to walk for the first time with their new legs. When patients come back for follow-up after several months staff members ask questions such as, "How far are you able to walk?" and "How much weight can you carry?" Once the patients are able to resume their livelihoods, they are more comfortable about talking and sharing how they are feeling. Maw Ker elaborates, "At first they do not want to speak; they want to be alone and do not want to interact with other people. Only they are thinking, thinking. All human beings will feel upset about what happened to them. They will think, 'Even if I get a prosthesis, I cannot walk like I did before' or 'I cannot lead my family.' But after they get their prosthesis, they feel more comfortable to speak. They do not think positively until they are comfortable to walk and work." Once they have received their prosthesis, patients are invited to the Mental Health Counseling Center for further support.

For individuals who have experienced a disabling injury or amputation, MTC's MHCC provides individual, family, and group counseling, support groups, coordinated physical therapy, yoga, and case management. Counselors are trained to help patients find healthy coping skills, develop a strong support network, build resiliency, regain as much independence as possible, and understand, accept, and adjust to environmental and life changes. Patients who are being treated for an amputation are invited to attend a support group for amputees. Family, friends, and caregivers are encouraged to attend support groups as well.

The MHCC began offering support groups for amputees, recognizing the important healing role of peers following an amputation. Depending on the number of amputees in the surgical or prosthetics department or in the Patient House, the support group often consists of three to seven participants. The group takes place once every two weeks, and most members are men between the ages of 16 and 40. Facilitated by mental health counselors from the MHCC, the group often invites a Burmese doctor or one of the medical staff to participate as a resource for medical questions that may arise. Because of the specific context surrounding land mine injuries, participation has been limited to land mine amputees.

The groups are designed to create a safe space for people to share how they are feeling, what they are thinking, and to ask questions. Each group begins with participants sharing their names and where they come from. The facilitator provides translation as needed for Karen and Burmese, the two languages most commonly spoken by patients. Participants are invited to share their experiences and feeling. The facilitator gives encouragement and empowers the patients to recognize their strengths. "We try to focus on what they *can* do, not what they *cannot* do," says Saw Ku Thay, the former director of the Mental Health Department. Some are able to identify things they can do, such as climbing trees, cooking, cutting bamboo, and looking after cows or other livestock. Those who say they cannot do anything are often reminded of many things they can still do when asked about what they can do at home.

The groups are made up of new and old amputees, which allows a peer exchange of coping strategies. Patients at the clinic for follow-up care can share ways they have adjusted to life with prostheses; this gives hope to those still struggling to walk with their new limbs. The facilitator offers examples of healthy coping skills, such as meditating, praying, watching films, or talking to someone who can give encouragement, and discourages unhealthy coping skills such as drinking alcohol. The participants tell jokes, laugh together, play guitar, sing their favorite songs, and request other group members to sing for them.

In 2008, a series of rehabilitative stretches was developed by an American physical therapist and posted in the surgical and prosthetics department to help guide patients in self- and family-directed strength rehabilitation. Support groups also encourage physical therapy techniques to reinforce the need to stretch and move the legs to build physical strength.

Amputees typically join the support group several months after the land mine explosion. The group, combined with support patients receive in the prosthetics department, helps patients feel less detached or isolated because they see other people from their community with amputations. Though initially many say they want to die after stepping on the land mine, later they say, "If other amputees can work, so can I." Soldiers often want to return to the army, so they take administrative positions; others return home to farm.

While staying at MTC in the Patient House, either postoperatively or for follow-up at six months or beyond, patients are invited to attend the support group but attendance is voluntary. At the beginning of the recovery process patients comment that the group helps them to recover their energy. When they return to MTC after reintegrating in their village community, most patients report that they are not depressed and have regained a sense of normalcy. They receive transportation costs to return home after follow-up visits, and blankets and food while staying in the Patient House. Many patients ask the facilitator to help them find a job; however, there is nowhere to refer the patients for employment. The counselor explains that he can only offer encouragement in the job search, which can leave both the patient and the facilitator disappointed and unfulfilled. According to Saw Ku Thay, it is difficult to document whether the amputee support group has made a difference. Measuring the success of such interventions presents a challenge in this setting where the majority of patients are lost to follow-up.

Handicap International is a nongovernmental organization that provides prostheses, physical therapy, psychosocial support, and land mine risk education in five refugee camps on the Thai-Burma border. Among all five camps, approximately fifteen new prosthetic limbs are provided annually, nearly all of which are a result of land mine injuries. Sixty percent of amputees are from Karen State, with the vast majority not registered as refugees. They live in Burma and return to the refugee camp in Thailand for prosthetic care. As of 2012, there were 350 land mine survivors living in the three refugee camps in Tak Province.[38]

HI provides psychosocial support, including peer support, storytelling, goal-setting, and income generation services. The peer support program matches new land mine survivors with a peer who visits them while they are admitted in the camp-based clinic to listen and share stories. HI staff consists of members of the Karen refugee community trained by international and Thai staff to conduct interviews with new land mine survivors to document their experiences and to provide psychological support for survivors to tell their story. Staff members also conduct a three-month assessment to help new land mine survivors set goals, identify barriers to achieving goals, and plan how to earn income. Income generation activities provide material support for amputees to manage small market stalls in the camps.

FORMER POLITICAL PRISONERS

In 2002, Mr. N was arrested for carrying concealed weapons at the house of his sister, Ms. M. Although the authorities did not find any weapons, Mr. N and his sister were arrested under Burma's Unlawful Association Act, Emergency Act, and Immigration Act. In an account of Mr. N's interrogation, Ms. M recalls how authorities from military intelligence handcuffed her brother behind his back with roughly made wooden shackles. According to Ms. M, "[the authorities] also pushed his face into human excrement to force him to talk." She reported that his hands and feet were always shackled; only one hand was freed from time to time to allow him to eat. They used every possible means of torture, including electric shocks when they were not pleased with his answers. Mr. N was given a thirty-eight-year sentence for his alleged crimes. His sister was sentenced to twenty-five years for aiding and abetting, but was released unconditionally in 2005. During his ten years in captivity, Mr. N developed tuberculosis, nervous system ailments, mental disorders, and liver cancer. During his detention, he was admitted to the Rangoon General Hospital for frequent blackouts. He also received treatment at a psychiatric hospital on two occasions. He was confined to a cell in a special ward of the Insein Prison hospital until his release. The general secretary of the Assistance Association for Political Prisoners (AAPP) says that the ward was used for inmates suffering from everything from mental illness to communicable diseases such as leprosy, tuberculosis, and HIV/AIDS. Although Mr. N was suffering mental and physical illness because of torture and ill-treatment during interrogation and imprisonment, he was also kept in solitary confinement and generally denied medical treatment. On one occasion a prison medic did see him following a seizure, and finally in late 2011, Mr. N was admitted to the Rangoon Hospital because of his deteriorating liver condition. Mr. N was so ill that he did not remember his sister when she visited him at the Rangoon Hospital. Organizations and individuals, including Ms. M herself, appealed to the current semi-civilian government and its predecessor to release Mr. N on humanitarian grounds because of his serious condition, but he was not released until the amnesty program on January 13, 2012. Upon release, he could barely walk on his swollen feet. He hardly recognized his sister, the last of his living family members. Nine days after being released from Insein Prison, Mr. N was dead.

Founded in 2000 by former political prisoners living in exile in Thailand, the Assistance Association for Political Prisoners is a human rights organization based in Mae Sot, Thailand that works for the release of all political prisoners in Burma and for the improvement of prison conditions in Burma.[39] AAPP documents and reports human rights abuses carried out by the Burmese military regime against political prisoners and prodemocracy activists, and as such is widely recognized by the United Nations, international governments, Amnesty International, Human Rights Watch, and respected media outlets around the world as a reliable and credible source of information on political prisoner issues in Burma.[40] In addition to providing basic necessities such as food and medicine to current political prisoners and their families in Burma, AAPP offers counseling, encouragement, moral support, and educational opportunities to former political prisoners based in Mae Sot.[41] Mental health issues identified by staff members of AAPP, many of whom are former political prisoners, are described below.

Depression and/or Anxiety
Former political prisoners show symptoms of depression and anxiety such as increased susceptibility to crying, sighing heavily, abusing alcohol and drugs, being easily angered and irritable, feeling lonely and hopeless about the future, worrying about things outside their control, being reticent, having difficulty concentrating, and feeling that there is no one they can rely on. While there are no formal or systematic assessments of mental health among current political prisoners, anecdotal evidence from former political prisoners speaking about their experiences indicates current prisoners suffer similar symptoms.

Nightmares or Difficulty Sleeping
Often, political prisoners wake up in the middle of the night in a sweat. They think often about their future and feel hopeless when they cannot solve problems that are beyond their control. Recurring thoughts or memories of the most hurtful or terrifying events plague political prisoners at night, as well as the feeling that there is no positive future.

Difficulty Coping with Daily Life
Problems that make coping with daily life difficult include difficulty controlling temper, feelings of insecurity, and high levels of tension, stress, and suspicion.

Family Problems
Problems between family members often arise because of misunderstandings surrounding the situation, feelings, and identity. Most political prisoners were breadwinners for their families before their imprisonments, but when they are released from prison, other family members have already filled that role. Also, while some political prisoners think of themselves as having sacrificed a lot to be an important agent of change by fighting against the unjust regime, some family members, friends, or people in the community do not recognize this role. Former political prisoners feel a loss of identity when they are not valued for what they have sacrificed.

Some former political prisoners experience a loss of sexual interest or pleasure, which creates tension in their marital life. A common feeling for former political prisoners is that others do not understand their experiences and thus cannot comprehend how their perspective differs from that of their families or friends. Some former political prisoners are blamed by family members for not considering family matters over their political activism. Most political prisoners were the family breadwinners before their arrest, so while they are imprisoned families suffer economic hardship, which families attribute to the political prisoner and his actions. Families also have difficulty visiting their loved ones to bring them food and other items while in prison, and this separation compounds the tension and suffering.

Difficulty "Fitting In" with Society or Readjusting to Life Outside Prison

Often, fear of harassment, social exclusion, and pressure by authorities causes friends, relatives, and community members to be afraid of engaging with former political prisoners. Authorities often exclude political activists and their families from society by offering them as examples of those who are punished with harsh treatment and imprisonment. Authorities will even punish those who hire, support, or communicate with political activists, especially former political prisoners. As a result, former political prisoners are often isolated from society.

Living in Fear of Reprisal or Retribution from Others

Sometimes, former political prisoners feel like misfits in society because of the situation they encounter after their release. Former political prisoners are denied employment and education opportunities and are not able to return to the normal life they had before prison. Moreover, they feel insecure with the constant threat of rearrest and harassment by authorities.

Difficulty with Relationships

Former political prisoners sometimes speak of using a "different language" in conversations with friends or acquaintances. Often others do not understand what former political prisoners had to go through, and similarly, some former political prisoners do not understand or cannot keep up with popular trending topics. After spending many years in prison, former political prisoners have a hard time catching up with the times, including new technology, economic trends, social media, and the current political situation.

To address these mental health concerns, AAPP aims to create solidarity through a self-sustaining support network for former political prisoners so they never have to feel alone or feel there is no one for them to rely on. AAPP has a rehabilitation program for former political prisoners in Burma.

Over the years AAPP has provided for the medical needs of 363 former political prisoners. In 2010, AAPP began a counseling program in collaboration with Johns Hopkins University entitled Mental Health Assessment Project or MHAP (see chapter 11 for a description of this project). This collaboration provided training in psychotherapeutic techniques for AAPP counselors. Since MHAP training, AAPP has counseled around one hundred former political prisoners along the Thai-Burma border and inside Burma. According to one senior staff member at AAPP, "Overall the way to ease problems [of former political prisoners] is to listen to what former political prisoners say."

Notes

1 "Myanmar Country Profile," World Health Organization, http://www.who.int/countries/mmr/en/.

2 "At a Glance: Myanmar," UNICEF, http://www.unicef.org/infobycountry/myanmar_statistics.html.

3 Back Pack Health Worker Team, *Chronic Emergency: Health and Human Rights in Eastern Burma* (Mae Sot, Thailand: Back Pack Health Worker Team, 2006), http://burmalibrary.org/docs3/ChronicEmergencyE-ocr.pdf.

4 "At a Glance: Myanmar"; Suzanne Belton, "Unsafe Abortion and Its Prevention: Who Cares?," *Health Messenger* (2003): 46–53, http://www.burmalibrary.org/docs/post-abortion-care.htm.

5 United Nations Population Fund, *Cross-Border Migration and Reproductive Health Study* (Yangon: Department of Population, United Nations Population Fund, 2002); UNFPA Myanmar, *Country Report on 2007 Fertility and Reproductive Health Survey* (Myanmar: Union of Myanmar, Ministry of Immigration and Population, Department of Population 2009).

6 "Landmines: Hidden Killers," UNICEF, http://www.unicef.org/sowc96pk/hidekill.htm.

7 "Demining," United Nations, http://www.un.org/en/globalissues/demining/.

8 Release List," Association for the Assistance of Political Prisoners, Mae Sot, Thailand, July 2013.

9 Thandar Shwe, personal interview by Meredith Walsh, Mae Sot, Tak Province, Thailand, April 6, 2012.

10 Ibid.

11 Ibid.

12 Ibid.

13 "HIV and AIDS Estimates," UNAIDS, http://www.unaids.org/en/regionscountries/countries/myanmar/.

14 "Myanmar," *MSF Activity Report 2011*,
    http://www.msf.org.uk/sites/uk/files/MSF_Activity_Report_2011_lowres
    _201208200807.pdf.

15 World Health Organization, "Clinical Guidance across the Continuum of Care:
    Antiretroviral Therapy," in *Consolidated Guidelines on the Use of Antiretroviral
    Drugs for Treating and Preventing HIV Infection, World Health Organization*,
    September 2013, 91–154,
    http://www.who.int/hiv/pub/guidelines/arv2013/art/arv2013_chapter07_low.pdf.

16 "At a Glance: Myanmar"; Belton, "Unsafe Abortion."

17 United Nations Population Fund, *Cross-Border Migration*; UNFPA Myanmar,
    Country Report.

18 Katherine Ba Thike, "Abortion: A Public Health Problem in Myanmar,"
    Reproductive Health Matters 9 (1997): 94–100; Representative from Marie Stoppes
    Myanmar and UNFPA-Myanmar, personal communication with the author,
    Yangon, Myanmar, February 2010.

19 Cynthia Maung and Suzanne Belton, *Working Our Way Back Home: Fertility and
    Pregnancy Loss on the Thai-Burma Border* (Mae Sot, Thailand: Mae Tao Clinic,
    2005); Representative from Mae Tao Clinic (presentation at abortion policy
    meeting, Mae Sot, Thailand, January 2010).

20 Maung and Belton, *Working Our Way Back Home*; Suzanne Belton and Cynthia
    Maung. "Fertility and Abortion: Burmese Women's Health on the Thai-Burma
    Border," *Forced Migration Review* 10 (2004): 36–37; Chris Beyrer, "Shan Women
    and Girls and the Sex Industry in Southeast Asia: Political Causes and Human
    Rights Implications," *Social Science Medicine* 53 (2001): 543–550.

21 Maung and Belton, *Working Our Way Back Home*; Suzanne Belton and Andrea
    Whittaker, "Kathy Pan, Sticks and Pummelling: Techniques Used to Induce
    Abortion by Burmese Women on the Thai Border," *Social Science Medicine* 65
    (2007): 1512–1523.

22 Mae Tao Clinic, *Annual Report*, 2012.

23 Mae Tao Clinic, unpublished data (Mae Sot, Thailand: Mae Tao Clinic, 2010).

24 Ibid.

25 Mae Tao Clinic, unpublished data (Mae Sot, Thailand: Mae Tao Clinic, 2013).

26 Naw Ree, personal interview by Meredith Walsh, Mae Sot, Tak Province, Thailand,
    July 17, 2012.

27 Sweet, personal interview by Meredith Walsh, Mae Sot, Tak Province, Thailand,
    July 21, 2012.

28 Ibid.

29 Ibid.

30 Ibid.

31 Ibid.

32 Ibid.

33 Sophia Hla, personal interview by Meredith Walsh, Mae Sot, Tak Province, Thailand, July 21, 2012.

34 Ibis Reproductive Health, unpublished data, 2013.

35 Naw Ree, personal interview by Meredith Walsh, Mae Sot, Tak Province, Thailand. July 17, 2012.

36 Maw Ker, personal interview by Meredith Walsh, Mae Sot, Tak Province, Thailand, July 20, 2012.

37 Ibid.

38 Alexandre Baillat, personal interview by Meredith Walsh, Mae Sot, Tak Province, Thailand, June 20, 2012.

39 Assistance Association for Political Prisoners, *Annual Report* (Thailand: Assistance Association for Political Prisoners, 2011).

40 Ibid.

41 Ibid.

Part IV.

Managing, Supervising, and Evaluating Programs

Chapter 9

Vicarious Traumatization and
Resilience of Health Workers

Andrew George Lim and Eh Kalu Shwe Oo

> *[The medics] had to [move] together with the soldiers [to help a village]. And*
> *[my friend] saw there a lot of bodies . . . they had gunshot [wounds] . . . many*
> *people were dead. And then he ran. At the time he saw one man lying down and*
> *saying "help me, help me" because he was shot. [He tried to carry] this man, but*
> *when he heard the [troops] again, he . . . he was afraid and he left the person,*
> *and ran away from there. . . . [Since] he came back, he thinks of [this often]. . . .*
> *When he hears a whistle, he lies down immediately. . . . Even in the car, if he*
> *hears a whistle, he lies down in the car. And [this was] always in his mind, he*
> *was always thinking, "If I [could] help that person . . . we both [would be]*
> *dead" . . . he is always thinking about this one . . . for a long time in his mind.*
> —*36-year-old female backpack medic*

Introduction

The critical role first aid responders, relief workers, and other medical personnel play in crisis and disaster settings cannot be understated. Especially in conflict areas, medical personnel face numerous threats to their security and physical well-being, putting them at risk of developing psychiatric symptoms such as depression, anxiety, and posttraumatic stress disorder (PTSD).[1] Because lay medics frequently function as the primary health providers in low-resource conflict situations, their mental health is crucial to the delivery of services to afflicted populations.

In this chapter we examine the experiences of community health workers who serve displaced and war-affected populations in Karen State, eastern Burma. The evidence presented is based on the authors' previous qualitative research with this population.[2] Though it is impossible to neatly deconstruct the myriad experiences of suffering, perseverance, and survivorship intrinsic to these medics' lives into the academic frameworks of psychology and psychiatry, an attempt at finding patterns in their narratives that parallel concepts in mental health literature may be helpful in developing evidence-based interventions. Incongruities are implicit in generalizations, and constant awareness of cultural relativism among widely different societal and linguistic norms must be maintained.

This analysis of the medics' experiences has two goals. The first is to provide concrete narrative examples elucidating mental health concepts as they pertain to victimized populations, and specifically as they apply to service providers in crisis settings. Second, and more important, the authors' aim to provide practical insights for mental health providers working with medics to further understand their stressors and potentially guide interventions to improve provider well-being. The discussion on coping and mental resilience is meant to provide foundational, albeit far from comprehensive, insight into improving individual-focused or group-based interventions for these medics. Ultimately, ensuring the mental health of providers in crisis settings is a long-term investment for populations with limited human resources.

We begin with a brief introduction to the community health organizations responsible for care in Karen State, eastern Burma. Then, local idioms of distress unique to Karen culture and language are introduced as a platform to discuss sources of traumatic stress, other affective disorders, vicarious traumatization, and burnout. Each section begins with a brief review of current psychology and psychiatry literature pertaining to health workers in conflict and/or disaster settings, interspersed with narratives from the medics of Karen State. The chapter ends with a discussion of how concepts of mental resilience, coping, and self-efficacy are relevant to the Karen medics, along with recommendations for improving existing interventions for providers' mental health that might be generalizable to health workers in other conflict and disaster settings.

Community Health Responders in Eastern Burma

Several community-based health organizations based on the Thai-Burma border provide basic primary medical care, disease prevention, and public health education to villages in internally displaced population (IDP) areas of eastern Burma.

The Karen Department of Health and Welfare (KDHW) is the civilian health department of the Karen National Union (KNU). KDHW manages thirty-seven mobile health clinics that can be rapidly relocated in the event of an attack, each providing care to 3,500–5,000 forcibly displaced and war-affected residents of Karen State.[3] Medics can carry small side arms for the purposes of self-defense in the field, but must otherwise remain noncombatants per KDHW protocol.

The Back Pack Health Worker Team (BPHWT) is a multiethnic organization that delivers health care to populations in the eastern ethnic states of Burma—Karen, Karenni, Mon, and Shan states. These mobile teams serve village areas that are the most inaccessible, including populations displaced by conflict who do not have access to even KDHW mobile health clinics.[4] BPHWT consists of approximately 290 health workers working in teams of three to five per unit, providing care for more than 180,000 people.[5] BPHWT medics usually deploy in uninhabited jungle areas, serving clusters of two to four villages and traveling directly to each village or dispensing care from nearby tent "clinics."

A medic's education begins after completing secondary education at the age of 17 to 19 years old. Trainees of both organizations undergo basic community health worker education supplemented by advanced-care topics in trauma life support, obstetrics, and infectious disease prevention, among other skills. These health workers persevere despite perilous security situations, as Burmese soldiers have reportedly destroyed clinics and targeted mobile medic teams, including noncombatant medics, who have been shot and killed.[6]

Local Idioms of Distress

Unsurprisingly, the violence and loss of security experienced by the Karen medics resulted in abundant stressors and, for some, manifestations of psychiatric symptoms. This section examines the idioms of distress used by the medics to describe their mental health, interspersed with anecdotes to illustrate the idioms.

Although Skaw Karen is the predominant language used among these medics, many terms have been co-opted from Burmese to describe mental health. Burmese equivalents for depression (*seik da'kya*), stress (*seik hpizimu*), anxiety (*seik lo'shaa*), and mental trauma (*seik daan yaa*) were often used, although Karen versions of these terms exist. Although these are English transliterations of these psychological concepts, it is important to explore the cultural nuances of these terms. For ease of comprehension, throughout this chapter we use the English terms as proxies for the Burmese or Karen idioms shown in table 9.1.

The definitions of these Karen and Burmese idioms can be imprecise or incongruous to the equivalent Anglo-Western transliterations when describing mental stressors. For example, although the Western concepts of "mind" and "spirit" are arguably distinct, there was much overlap in the understanding and use of the Burmese *seik* (mind) and *seik da'* (spirit). This could be a factor explaining the Karen's somatization of psychology and spirituality; subjects would often point to their chests when speaking of thought processes such as confusion. Other respondents spoke of spiritual reasons or superstitions that compelled them to act, feel, or think in particular ways.

Table 9.1 Local idioms of distress

English	Burmese	Burmese transliteration	Karen	Karen transliteration
Stress	*seik hpizimu*	Mind-spirit suppression	*thar law bwi, thar ba hti tor*	Tired heart
Anxiety	*seik lo'shaa*	Mind-spirit unsteadiness	*thut kot thar gaw*	Liver is hot, heart is red
Depression	*seik da'kya*	Spirit fall	*thar law bwa*	The heart falls down
Mental trauma	*seik daan yaa*	Mind injury	*tha ba doe*	Heart-touch hit

Source: Andrew George Lim et al., "Trauma and Mental Health of Medics in Eastern Myanmar's Conflict Zones: A Cross-Sectional and Mixed Methods Investigation," *Conflict and Health* 7, no. 1 (2013): 15, doi:10.1186/1752-1505-7-15.

In addition to using Burmese terms, respondents commonly described their mental health using Karen terms. The Karen idioms often implied somatic manifestations of mental distress. For example, an approximation of seik lo'shaa (worry or anxiety) in Karen was *thut kot thar gaw*, literally "liver is hot, heart is red." Seik da'kya (depression) translates to *thar law bwa* in Karen, most closely meaning "the heart falls down." Seik hpizimu (stress) translated best to *thar law bwi* or *tha ba hti tor*, literally "tired heart." Finally, seik daan yaa (mental trauma) was *tha ba doe* in Karen, or "heart-touch hit."

Fuertes, in a qualitative study of Karen refugees living in Thailand, described the closest Karen translation of trauma to be "scar of suffering" (*ta tu ba kaw ba er kaw mei law* in Skaw Karen). This term encompasses the idea that the understanding and healing of war trauma cannot be restricted to "the intra-psychic processes of the individual sufferer" but must also include social and cultural contexts and the traditional approaches to spiritual healing.[7] Further, Fuertes stresses the importance of recognizing transgenerational trauma, meaning that trauma can persist "within the family and across generations"—that the children raised in refugee camps carry the legacy of trauma experienced by their parents firsthand.

In the following sections, mental health subjects will be explored using the above idioms as a roadmap to connect pertinent literature with the narratives of the Karen medics.

Traumatic Stress of Health Workers in Emergent Settings

Frequent contact with trauma-afflicted populations causes high levels of occupational stress for physicians, nurses, paramedics, and other health workers, who thus have an increased risk of developing PTSD.[8] A 2003 study of fifty-one emergency department health providers revealed that 12 percent of subjects met the diagnostic criteria for PTSD and 20 percent met the PTSD symptom criteria.[9] A further study of fifty-six paramedics and ambulance technicians revealed that 21 percent of subjects met symptom criteria for PTSD, despite never having experienced trauma personally, with most reporting intrusive thoughts, irritability, sleep disturbance, and detachment from others.[10] Since the Vietnam War, extensive studies have investigated PTSD among combatants and civilians, but relatively few have explored the effects of mental trauma among medics and other health professionals serving in war settings.[11] Although the duty of combat medical personnel is to prevent loss, they likely experience loss more profoundly since they are often present during and after a catastrophe, leading to extraordinary exposure to trauma and intensity of stress.[12]

For the Karen medics, seik hpizimu (stress, or literally "mind suppression" or "spirit suppression") was often characterized in terms of physiologic symptoms such as heart palpitations, the "heart feeling tired," losing appetite, shaking, and losing sleep. Seik hpizimu was also described with psychological or emotional properties, such as wanting to be antisocial, feeling afraid, having a "heaviness" on the mind, "not understanding oneself," or having too many thoughts on the mind.

Medics often referred to seik daan yaa (mental trauma, or literally "mind injury"), caused by physical injury or verbal abuse. Medics recounted traumatic events that left lasting impressions, such as being beaten by Burmese soldiers, witnessing family members abused or killed by soldiers, and seeing dead bodies in the aftermath of destroyed villages. Medics who had been involved in combat (especially former soldiers) manifested symptoms of hypersensitivity to loud noises accompanied by flashbacks and reexperiencing.

Some medics felt that seik daan yaa, if repeated over time, could result in people "losing control of their minds and faces." One respondent talked about having nightmares and persistent, recurring thoughts of death related to the daily vigilance of security issues:

> Before I sleep, I have to think if I heard the Burmese army in our area. I have to plan where, I have to set up the people, the medics, and how many medics, and all [that] we have to do . . . [all] planning in my mind.

I think of this after I sleep, I go to dream, and sometimes I get a night-mare . . . like gunshots and land mine injury.

—*33-year-old male* BPHWT *medic, July 2010*

Another medic alluded to symptoms of dissociation in his inability to determine whether he was awake while in the moment of combat, or whether he was dreaming:

In fighting time, even when I'm shooting . . . it's like a dream. Some-times when I wake up, I know "oh it's fighting." Sometimes I forget—it is like a dream. I just dreamt it.

—*31-year-old male* BPHWT *medic, July 2010*

Inevitably, medics found themselves working in combat situations, be-ing forced to flee by advancing Burmese troops, or being directly threat-ened with violence. Community health organizations often dispatched medics to villages in close proximity to active fighting, where they were subjected to nearby mortar blasts:

The Burmese armies came to attack [our] clinic [in our] area. And we were fighting, nearly seven to twelve days. Every day. Because . . . before they attacked, they use the [rocket] launcher. They use mortar maybe two days, and [after] three days they came to fight.

—*30-year-old male* BPHWT *medic, July 2010*

Medics spoke about a profound sense of powerlessness and futility in their struggle to keep villagers alive and healthy, especially in the face of Burmese troops' superior firepower. Many medics discussed the frustra-tions of being forced to abandon the patients they were treating in the vil-lage because of attacks:

The soldiers came and attack[ed] through the village, and then we had to flee after that time. We saw our patient. . . . We have to help him already, but in case we cannot help him . . . we have to lose them . . . [although] we're willing to help him. Sometimes we feel very bad. And after, if we thought about this patient, then we cannot sleep. We have to realize—all things happen . . . and sometimes it makes us feel bad also.

—*25-year-old male* KDHW *medic, January 2011*

The fear of being attacked while traveling was a significant source of traumatic stress for most medics, who reported feeling unable to relax re-gardless of their location. Whether in villages, or traveling en route, they felt constantly in danger of being ambushed. One medic described constantly searching for escape routes in the forest when stationed at a village, even in times of relative peace. Another medic had to rebuild his clinic five times after it was destroyed repeatedly by Burmese troops.

Additionally, medics traveled long distances through unfamiliar terrain where they were at risk of detonating land mines. In the words of one medic:

> On the road—one of my friends, he stepped on a land mine. At the time, we had to [stop] to control the bleeding. That area [where we stopped] is very close [to an area with fighting between Burmese and Karen armies]. . . . I tore my *longyi* [sarong-like cloth] in order to pack . . . and compress . . . that injury. And we controlled the bleeding like this. But it is too much bleeding. . . .
>
> We arrived [at] the clinic, and gave blood transfusion . . . two bag[s] of blood. And we began an upper knee [amputation]. . . . [*laughs*] I was very worried and so afraid at that time. Because . . . he is my friend—I worry for his family, his home. I worry . . . because he's working with me.
>
> —*30-year-old male* BPHWT *medic, June 2010*

Sometimes medics were forced into hiding in the jungle after an attack; other times, they purposefully moved with displaced populations to provide care until they reached safety. Medics also provided sanctuary to displaced villagers in their clinics.

The constant fear of attack was likely the most palpable source of traumatic stress for the Karen medics. Any discussion of traumatic stress must take into account not only the direct experiences of the medics in their work-related lives, but also of the collective suffering intrinsic to the population that they serve. The next section on vicarious traumatization will explore some of these themes.

Vicarious Traumatization and Burnout

The concept of secondary traumatization has been proposed for health providers who work predominantly with trauma-affected populations, especially in mental health or crisis relief occupations. Professionals who listen to patients' fear, pain, suffering, and narratives of trauma may feel similar pain, fear, and suffering through a process known as vicarious traumatization. It is often accompanied by feelings of burnout and compassion fatigue. Vicarious traumatization is considered a posttraumatic stress reaction experienced by those indirectly exposed to a traumatic stressor, and may lead to symptoms of PTSD.[13]

Many hypotheses have been presented to define vicarious traumatization and the factors of resiliency that are observed in some individuals.

Vicarious traumatization can be understood as the interplay between the painful material presented by the patient or client being served and the provider's "unique cognitive schemas or beliefs, expectations, and assumptions about self and others,"[14] usually framed as a way for the provider to understand and preempt the effects of the mental stressors unique to their job. Researchers have proposed that these professionals can experience a disruption of established views regarding safety and personal vulnerability, resulting in a sense of futility about their benevolent actions.[15] Other studies cite that those who choose to enter a field of rescue work gain resilience to indirect trauma effects from either their inherent personalities or their experiences in handling life-threatening and/or high-stress situations.[16] However, there are likely many social determinants of resilience against vicarious traumatization among hospital workers as well—including the peer support of medical teams.

The term "burnout" describes the emotional exhaustion, cynicism, ineffectiveness, and loss of humanistic compassion, which counters the positive experiences of engagement, caused by exposure to chronic occupational and interpersonal stressors.[17]

The Karen medics were repeatedly exposed to their patients' suffering. Many felt a sense of the futility of their actions in the face of medical illnesses they were unable to diagnose or unable to manage because of a lack of resources.

Medics were often burdened by the social responsibility of patient care and the expectations of the community for the individuals they were unable to help:

> When we are in the field, when we are treating people . . . if we can cure them, they will say thank you. But if [we] cannot, they will swear [at] you. And when I cure twenty people, if ten people are not well, I feel— why [does] it become like this? . . . Men die, and I think because of me, or because of what? [I think about] this a lot, and it becomes troubling for [me].
>
> —28-year-old male BPHWT medic, July 2010

The gap between what medics were able to provide and their inability to fulfill patients' expectations was a common frustration:

> For our medics, even when we know the symptoms and [the] disease, sometimes we don't have enough medicine, so we cannot [treat] perfectly, we cannot help. . . . We cannot reach that image they think of us, they believe of us, so it becomes difficult. [Sometimes] we can only give

knowledge and counseling in that area, so we also see ourselves [as] weak in skill and we cannot help the people as they hope.

—*36-year-old female* BPHWT *medic, July 2010*

Many medics felt the need to hide their self-doubts and insecurities while interacting with patients:

Sometimes I feel depression strike, but I don't want [it] to. . . . Even if something is happening inside of my mind, I always have to smile to patients, because I don't want them to be disappointed. So I always have to pretend [for] myself in front of them. . . . I don't feel anything that is in my body.

—*39-year-old male* BPHWT *medic, July 2010*

For some medics, hearing their patient's narratives of suffering and trauma may have the effect of reinforcing their compassion rather than exhausting it. This was especially true for those who had experienced displacement, violence, or other hardships in their own lives prior to becoming medics. These traumatic memories could be triggered when hearing the parallel life stories of their patients:

This kind of image, this kind of [personally traumatic] memory, it doesn't haunt us—but we cannot ever forget. . . . Usually we're trying to delete this kind of memory, but we still remember sometimes. We will remember when we see patients who got gun injuries. . . . We may remember these feelings [of our own]. . . . If an orphan tells us about their family member [who they witnessed suffering], then we remember and we see those images.

—*24-year-old female* KDHW *medic, January 2011*

Many medics drew on their personal experiences of displacement as a source of empathy for their patients in IDP areas:

[We see] families and our people who escaped and are living, hiding in the [IDP areas]. And when I saw them, I think always—I used to hide like this. I used to move like that.

—*23-year-old female* KDHW *medic, January 2011*

Bearing witness to or being afflicted by a patient's experiences may vicariously traumatize medics but may, conversely, strengthen resilience for those who can draw compassion from their own experiences of victimhood. Later, we will discuss theories of mental resilience and the factors that may contribute to the Karen medics' ability to cope with traumatic stressors.

Other Occupational Sources of Anxiety and Depression

In addition to the effects of traumatic stress, providers' stress is further exacerbated by the increased rates of other anxiety disorders and depressive disorders that can exist among populations affected by war.[18] This is frequently a result of the difficulties intrinsic to delivering health services in a conflict zone—confounded by low resources, strained health infrastructure, loss of medical personnel, transportation hazards, and other barriers to care delivery. Furthermore, the removal of family and community sources of social support while providers work long stretches of time in the field contributes to diminished mental resilience and poor mental health outcomes.

Seik lo'shaa (anxiety, worry or literally "mind unsteadiness" or "spirit unsteadiness") was characterized as "falling," the "inability to stand," faintness, an increased heartbeat, or an inability to breathe. Seik lo'shaa was associated with the same causes as seik hpizimu (security, work-related, and personal stresses) but also included some social sources of anxiety or worry: losing the trust of the community if a patient dies, meeting patients' expectations, revealing weakness to patients or families, hearing that their home community was threatened or attacked, and the general uncertainty about safety in the immediate or long-term future.

Seik da'kya (depression, or literally "spirit fall") was commonly thought of as a "long-term" ailment and "kept in the mind-spirit," not the body. Medics associated it with trembling, loss of appetite, desire to sleep excessively, social isolation, domestic discontent, and "wanting to give up everything." Stories regarding seik da'kya involved reminders of past turmoil, uncertainty of the future, loss of self-control, an inability to reach goals and aspirations, and powerlessness and weakness.

These feelings of inadequacy were underscored most when patients died. Even if a patient's death was unavoidable, many medics expressed a strong feeling of obligation and responsibility to the patient and the patient's family. In some cases, the patients' families accused the medic, blaming them for a death that the medic believed to be inevitable:

> I will give [an] example about two patient[s] that I treat[ed]. They had malaria shock, hypotensive. The two of them are children. So, I know they came to me very late [in symptoms progression]. . . . The first one, I had to treat about five days, and [the child] became better. . . . But, for the other one, after two days [of treatment] . . . they died. . . . I knew [that for the patient who died], before he arrived here, [he was] already [in] shock. So, I knew that the time [was too] late for him.

So, the family [of the dead child] was not happy with me. . . . At that time I felt sad, . . . because the [relatives] told me many things, like I made a mistake. At that time . . . I felt not so good.

—*26-year-old male KDHW medic, January 2011*

Additionally, the constant strain on resources for the medics and clinics was one of the intractable realities of providing health care. Clinics struggled to deal with high patient volume and a broad range of ailments. In many cases, medics felt frustration, stress, and anxiety when they were powerless to treat patients because of a lack of resources or medicines. Sometimes medics struggled to triage and care for multiple casualties at once following land mine blasts or other attacks.

Resource issues were further confounded by the difficulty of transportation between the isolated clinics and the most remote villages. In mountainous jungle areas, winding dirt roads were inaccessible to motor vehicles, trails disappeared under dense overgrowth, and low areas were prone to flooding during rainy months. Because of these transportation barriers, medics struggled to deliver supplies or transport patients by foot. Additionally, these obstructions sometimes prevented villagers from traveling to nearby clinics to solicit care.

While medics struggled to maintain the functioning of under-resourced and understaffed clinics, their efforts were hindered by the frequent turnover of their health workers. Over time, some experienced medics became dissatisfied with their work because of the difficulties (including the significant personal risk) and the lack of contact with their families for long stretches of time. Some medics left their jobs for better financial opportunities. Others resettled with their families in countries such as the United States, Norway, Australia, or the United Kingdom.

One of their greatest challenges was the strain the occupation placed on their family relationships. Although health organizations attempted to place medics in nearby or familiar areas, personnel constraints meant that the majority of medics had to work in villages far from their home communities, often requiring days or weeks of travel by foot along treacherous jungle trails. Some medics communicated with relatives using mobile (or satellite) phones every few months. However, the majority of medics could only contact their families by making the rare trip to their home community:

I came to work here [as a medic], six years already, . . . but I got the chance to stay with my family only two times. The first time was only one hour, the second time, one day.

—*25-year-old male KDHW medic, January 2011*

The physical and emotional distance from their communities had profound effects on the lives of the medics. Many medics felt unable to provide or care for their families and loved ones. Even though medics were able to send money home to their families, they worried about their families' futures should they become disabled, die during service, or be captured by the Burmese military.

Coping

Coping has been defined as an individual's cognitive and behavioral efforts to manage external and internal demands that are appraised as taxing or exceeding the person's resources.[19] Coping habits should be seen as dynamic processes rooted not only in an individual's traits, but also in their social or environmental contexts. For instance, organizational or institutional settings that promote self-efficacy and problem-solving behavior have been found to increase competence, resilience, and the mastery of situations that challenge coping.[20]

Folkman and Lazarus developed a model of psychological stress reaction in which an individual's cognitive appraisal of a stressor determines a process-oriented coping mechanism.[21] In this theory, *cognitive appraisal* is defined as a process through which the person evaluates whether a particular encounter with the environment is relevant to his or her well-being (*primary appraisal*). If a person has something at stake in the encounter, the individual then assesses whether it is primarily threatening (potentially harmful) or challenging (offering the possibility for mastery or benefit) and what can be done to minimize loss or maximize benefit from the event (*secondary appraisal*). The coping mechanisms that arise are categorized as either regulating stressful emotions (*emotion-focused coping*) or altering the source of distress arising from the interaction with the environment (*problem-focused coping*). In reality, coping is usually a combination of both functions. In the following sections, we will discuss how this conceptual framework of coping can be applied to the medics' strategies for dealing with mental stressors.

EMOTION-FOCUSED COPING

For the medics, emotion-focused coping techniques usually centered on social engagement, peer support, and personal time. Many medics acknowledged that conversing with others helped alleviate their suffering. The primary network of support for the medics was their family and relatives, friends, and other respected members of the community (village leaders, teachers, pastors). Group activities, such as sports and singing were common forms of socially engaged coping.

For many, social engagements had strong ties to religious group activities. Though not all Karen communities were Christian, individuals working for the KNU (as medics or otherwise) were more likely to be Skaw Karen-speaking, Baptist Christians.[22] For these communities, the church was closely intertwined with the social organization of the village. Village elders and senior KNU officials were often also sermon leaders at the local church. Many medics cited attending religious services and praying as a major source of stress relief and motivational support:

> I always pray for God as a recreation—we pray, and we [enter] our problems and we [enter] our worries or suffering. Sometimes, we read [the] Bible, and sometimes we pray for God, and [this] can release our suffering.
> —26-year-old female Karen National Liberation Army (KNLA) medic, January 2011

Coping by taking personal recreational time was also common. Medics found solace in meditation or taking walks outside the village. Many would also partake in recreational activities such as fishing, hunting, and swimming.

Some medics admitted to using alcohol or narcotic substances as a mechanism to regulate stress; these activities could also be considered emotion-focused coping. Drinking rice-liquor in moderation was common among the men, for social reasons and to cope with emotional stressors:

> If I have stress, . . . I drink . . . and when I [get] drunk, I sleep. Everything disappears.
> —36-year-old male BPHWT medic, July 2010

One medic described how he coped with a violently traumatic experience by consuming alcohol:

> [I remember] when the Burmese army came to the village, [the people] had to flee from their houses so their little children is [sic] left in their house. . . . When the Burmese soldiers came they killed this baby and later they killed the parents, and [there was] only one child left in the house. Because their baby was left there, [a family] came back to take their baby—then [the soldiers] killed everyone there . . . so when I think of this [memory] it becomes traumatic for me. I think this again, and again, and again and I [feel] very sad for them. . . . So to forget this one, I drank. . . . If I feel like I can't stand the situation, I have to drink. And after drinking I [go to] sleep.
> —28 year-old male BPHWT medic, July 2010

Occasionally, medics used therapeutic drugs they carried such as benzodiazepines, chlorpheniramine, propanolol, and morphine to quell anxiety.

One medic spoke about his use of diazepam as a novice medic to calm his nerves while in stressful security situations.

Some medics were unable to cope with their difficulties. One medic recounted how a member in his team appeared happy, but repressed his distress. Consumed by his depression, he committed suicide:

> Even though [we] know each other very well, he never told [us] about his difficulties. . . . He always [appeared] happier, a happy life, and always smiling. So he didn't say anything. So we [didn't] know what [was] the problem with him.
> —33-year-old male BPHWT medic, July 2010

PROBLEM-FOCUSED COPING

Medics were often motivated by altruism in their community-oriented work. Two medics said that a powerful motivator was "feeling needed" by their leaders and the community. Medics who were able to visit their families with relative frequency spoke of it as a major motivator to continue their work.

Many medics were able to identify realistic work-related goals they were progressing toward, including attaining a leadership role within their organization. They mentioned desires to improve their skills and increase their experience, and that being successful in their work was the most gratifying way to build confidence and relieve their self-doubts. For them, treating patients was the best way to cope with stress or depression:

> I can release my stress [by] talking with the patients. So when I meet with the patient, I'm talking to them, and they respond to me. So we're talking to each other, and I become relaxed, and my depression disappear[s].
> —39-year-old male BPHWT medic, July 2010

Others would problem-solve during work to understand the causes of their work-related stress.

A large factor motivating their work appeared to be the empathetic connection to patients that medics felt when they traveled to war-affected villages, as many had suffered tragedies similar to those of their patients:

> When I go to the IDP place, even some of the villagers, they are very poor, and they don't have the money to go and see the medics [at the clinics near their villages], because of their problems in life. . . . Their life, they have to flee all the time from the Burmese Military and stay in the forest, as well. . . . Sometimes when I see those [people] and I feel pity

for them, and . . . I think it makes me, [it] impacts me, which is why I'm willing to work with them.

—*26-year-old female* KNLA *medic, January 2011*

The medics' ability to express their compassion may have contributed to their personal resilience against mental stressors. The next section will discuss some sources of support that these medics draw on to manage their challenges and mental stressors.

Mental Resilience

One of the most important questions for trauma researchers has revolved around the topic of resilience: given the identical exposure of two individuals to a traumatic stressor, what are the factors that protect and maintain one individual's mental stability, allowing him or her to lead a functionally normal life? Why does another individual develop symptoms of psychiatric distress or become unable to form healthy coping mechanisms, leading to substance abuse or suicide?

Resiliency has been defined as the ability to adapt, cope, or recover successfully despite threatening or challenging situations, such as extreme stress and trauma. Alternatively, resilience has been described as sustained competence in response to demands that tax coping resources.[23] Within the field of trauma studies, resilience is considered to be "efficacious adaptation" despite significant traumatic threats to personal and physical integrity.[24] Many studies have explored the individual and environmental factors that contribute to mental resilience. Resistance to trauma may derive from individuals' physiological or psychological coping processes, or from external risk or protective factors.[25]

It must be emphasized that there is no single model or "type" of resilience. Bonanno suggests there are multiple and unexpected ways to be resilient, often achieved by means that are not fully adaptive under normal circumstances. Furthermore, little is known about the extent to which loss and trauma reactions vary across cultures. Western, independence-oriented societies tend to focus more heavily than collectivist societies (like the Karen) on the personal experience of trauma.[26]

An individual's sense of self-efficacy is a critical factor in determining resilience to trauma. Bandura asserts that individuals make causal contributions to their own functioning through mechanisms of personal agency. The most crucial mechanism of agency is the belief in self-efficacy, described as the capability people have to exercise control over their own levels of functioning and over events that affect their lives.[27] For the Karen medics, the formation of self-efficacy may be a product of successful problem-based coping, as described in the previous section. The ability to take proactive measures to feel capable of making lifesaving decisions for members of their community would certainly contribute strongly to the fulfillment of personal agency.

Community and social factors also played a crucial role in developing medic self-efficacy and promoting positive coping strategies and mental resilience. The individual psychological model of self-efficacy only partially explains this—in the conflict-afflicted areas of Karen State, community well-being must be prioritized above the individual for collective survival. This idea was apparent in the community-oriented language that medics used when discussing mental health, trauma, and goal formation.

In lieu of strong family support and social support, medics' peer groups acted as essential sources of support when dealing with stressful encounters and professional challenges encountered while working in remote villages. In some of these teams, medics described the emotional support they received from their peers after experiencing difficult or potentially traumatic encounters during their work:

> We work together and our friends encourage us. And we also [have to] help each other . . . and sometimes our leader encourages [us] and explains about our future and our work. . . . I always get energy from them. And also when we hug each other—it also makes me motivated.
> —*26-year-old male* KDHW *medic, January 2011*

When conflicts emerged among the teams of medics, teams with increased communication were better able to resolve their issues:

> Sometimes when we work together, some of our coworkers, we misunderstand each other and are not united [or] peaceful. . . . So that makes me lose my confidence. . . . We try to deal with the conflict, and we try to tell each other to make up the misunderstanding. . . . It's not only me—for everyone, we try our best to communicate, to be good communicat[ors] and [promote] good relationships and understanding.
> —*26-year-old male* KDHW *medic, January 2011*

Finally, as mentioned in the section on vicarious traumatization, some medics may have used their personal memories of prior traumatic events as reservoirs of empathy when serving patients. Loss of security was an overarching theme for many Karen individuals living in displaced and/or active conflict areas. These interactions with patients may have facilitated the formation of a *survivor identity* over victimhood, a contributor to both self-efficacy and the reinforcement of resilience against future trauma.

Conclusions and Recommendations

In the past several years, KDHW has begun to implement mental health trainings for their health workers. The trainings educate the medics on mental health topics with an emphasis on coping-mechanism formation. The objectives are to equip the medics with fundamental skills for managing the mental distress of their patients, in addition to providing resources for their own care and that of their peers.

Exploring coping mechanisms is of utmost importance for the development of interventions that seek to improve the mental well-being of the medics. Many of these strategies—such as talking openly about emotions to friends, coworkers, and patients—are the most crucial sources of emotion-focused coping. This is especially true for medics who work far from home communities or on the front lines, given that much of their time is spent together and isolated from traditional sources of support such as community and family networks.

Other forms of coping, such as alcohol and substance use, should be addressed. Alcohol dependency/abuse can lead to serious harm inflicted on the self or to others. The use of narcotics such as benzodiazepines may be a difficult issue to manage, especially since medics and health workers carry these medicines to treat patients. These issues should be explored more in peer discussion groups.

The promotion of mental resilience among the Karen medics can inform interventions for health providers in conflict settings worldwide. The self-disclosure of trauma appears to contribute to positive peer-group interactions.[28] As many medics are deprived of their core community support network, the sense of comfort and bonding they form with their peers is crucial to their mental resilience. The culture of a medic team may be most supportive if it facilitates self-disclosure of traumatic events and emotions.

The sense of group identity can strengthen peer-group interactions. Camaraderie as a medic, in addition to camaraderie as a community, gives rise to a mutual identity and kinship as survivors. Medics' altruistic or pro-social behaviors are exemplified by their motivation to help their patients and communities.

Finally, the capacity to derive meaning from traumatic events is exemplified by some medics' ability to use their experience as a reservoir for empathy when treating patients who have suffered similar tragedies in crisis and/or disaster settings, and may be a means of preventing compassion fatigue.

Despite overwhelming occupational barriers and stressors, the Karen medics exhibited marked resilience in the face of trauma. However, further support is needed to maintain the psychological well-being of these providers. Increased attention to medics' mental health is critical to prevent burnout and retain these essential personnel serving under-resourced populations. As these medics provide the backbone of health for vulnerable communities, their individual needs for physical and emotional support must not be ignored.

Notes

1   Claudia J Dewane, "Posttraumatic Stress Disorder in Medical Personnel in Vietnam," *Hospital & Community Psychiatry* 35, no. 12 (1984): 1232–1234.

2   Andrew George Lim et al., "Trauma and Mental Health of Medics in Eastern Myanmar's Conflict Zones: A Cross-Sectional and Mixed Methods Investigation," *Conflict and Health* 7, no. 1 (2013): 15, doi:10.1186/1752-1505-7-15.

3   "Karen Department of Health and Welfare," *Karen Department of Health and Welfare*, 2012, http://kdhw.org/; Allison J Richard et al., "Essential Trauma Management Training: Addressing Service Delivery Needs in Active Conflict Zones in Eastern Myanmar," *Human Resources for Health* 7, no. 1 (March 3, 2009): 19, doi:10.1186/1478-4491-7-19.

4   Richard et al., "Essential Trauma Management Training."

5   Back Pack Health Worker Team, *Ten Years Report 1998–2009: Life, Liberty, and the Pursuit of Health* (Mae Sot, Thailand: Back Pack Health Worker Team, 2010), http://www.burmalibrary.org/docs11/BPHWT10yearReport_1998-2009.pdf-red.pdf.

6   Karen Human Rights Group, "Enduring Hunger and Repression: Food Scarcity, Internal Displacement, and the Continued Use of Forced Labour in Toungoo District" (2004), http://www.khrg.org/khrg2004/khrg0401d.html; Karen Human Rights Group, "Attacks and Displacement in Nyaunglebin District" (2010), http://www.khrg.org/khrg2010/khrg10b6.html.

7   Al B Fuertes, "In Their Own Words: Contextualizing the Discourse of (War) Trauma and Healing," *Conflict Resolution Quarterly* 21, no. 4 (2004): 491–501.

8   Serena Frank, "The Impact of Working with Trauma: Risk and Resilience Factors Among Health Care Providers," *South African Journal of Psychiatry* 12, no. 4 (2006): 100–104; Rita Giacaman et al., "Mental Health, Social Distress and Political Oppression: The Case of the Occupied Palestinian Territory," *Global Public Health* (2010): 1–13, doi:10.1080/17441692.2010.528443; Lynn E Alden, Marci J Regambal, and Judith M Laposa. "The Effects of Direct versus Witnessed Threat on Emergency Department Healthcare Workers: Implications for PTSD

Criterion A." *Journal of Anxiety Disorders* 22, no. 8 (2008): doi: 10.1016/j.janxdis.2008.01.013.

9   Judith M Laposa and Lynn E Alden, "Posttraumatic Stress Disorder in the Emergency Room: Exploration of a Cognitive Model," *Behaviour Research and Therapy* 41, no. 1 (2003): 49–65, doi: 10.1016/S0005-7967(01)00123-1.

10 Sue Clohessy and Anke Ehlers, "PTSD Symptoms, Response to Intrusive Memories and Coping in Ambulance Service Workers," *British Journal of Clinical Psychology/British Psychological Society* 38, pt 3 (September 1999): 251–265.

11 Kathleen M Palm, Melissa A Polusny, and Victoria M Follette, "Vicarious Traumatization: Potential Hazards and Interventions for Disaster and Trauma Workers," *Prehospital and Disaster Medicine* 19, no. 1 (March 2004): 73–78.

12 Dewane, "Posttraumatic Stress Disorder."

13 Palm, Polusny, and Follette, "Vicarious Traumatization."

14 Lisa McCann and Laurie Anne Pearlman, "Vicarious Traumatization: A Framework for Understanding the Psychological Effects of Working with Victims," *Journal of Traumatic Stress* 3, no. 1 (January 1, 1990): 131–149, doi: 10.1007/BF00975140.

15 Ronnie Janoff-Bullman, *Shattered Assumptions* (New York: Free Press, 2002).

16 Carol S North et al., "Psychiatric Disorders in Rescue Workers after the Oklahoma City Bombing," *American Journal of Psychiatry* 159, no. 5 (May 1, 2002): 857–859, doi:10.1176/appi.ajp.159.5.857.

17 Vicente González-Romá et al., "Burnout and Work Engagement: Independent Factors or Opposite Poles?," *Journal of Vocational Behavior* 68, no. 1 (2006): 165–174, doi:10.1016/j.jvb.2005.01.003; Christina Maslach and Michael P Leiter, "Early Predictors of Job Burnout and Engagement," *Journal of Applied Psychology* 93, no. 3 (May 2008): 498–512, doi:10.1037/0021-9010.93.3.498; Ayala Pines and Christina Maslach, "Characteristics of Staff Burnout in Mental Health Settings," *Hospital & Community Psychiatry* 29, no. 4 (April 1978): 233–237; Maslach and Leiter, "Early Predictors of Job Burnout and Engagement"; Pines and Maslach, "Characteristics of Staff Burnout in Mental Health Settings."

18 Phuong N Pham et al., "Sense of Coherence and Its Association with Exposure to Traumatic Events, Posttraumatic Stress Disorder, and Depression in Eastern Democratic Republic of Congo," *Journal of Traumatic Stress* 23, no. 3 (June 2010): 313–321, doi:10.1002/jts.20527; Patrick Vinck and Phuong N Pham, "Association of Exposure to Violence and Potential Traumatic Events with Self-Reported Physical and Mental Health Status in the Central African Republic," *JAMA* 304, no. 5 (2010): 544–552, doi:10.1001/jama.2010.1065.

19 Susan Folkman et al., "Appraisal, Coping, Health Status, and Psychological Symptoms," *Journal of Personality and Social Psychology* 50, no. 3 (March 1986): 571–579.

20 Michael Rutter, "Competence under Stress: Risk and Protective Factors," in *Risk and Protective Factors in the Development of Psychopathology*, ed. J Rolf et al. (New York: Cambridge University Press, 1990), 181–214.

21 Susan Folkman et al., "Dynamics of a Stressful Encounter: Cognitive Appraisal, Coping, and Encounter Outcomes," *Journal of Personality and Social Psychology* 50, no. 5 (May 1986): 992–1003; Folkman et al., "Appraisal, Coping, Health Status, and Psychological Symptoms"; Richard S Lazarus, "On the Primacy of Cognition," *American Psychologist* 39, no. 2 (1984): 124–129, doi:10.1037/0003-066X.39.2.124.

22 Mikael Gravers, "The Karen Making of a Nation," *Asian Forms of the Nation* (1996): 237–269; Jessica Harriden, "'Making a Name for Themselves': Karen Identity and the Politicization of Ethnicity in Burma," *Journal of Burmese Studies* 7 (2002): 84–144; Ananda Rajah, "A Nation of Intent in Burma: Karen Ethno-Nationalism, Nationalism and Narrations of Nation," *Pacific Review* 15, no. 4 (2002): 517–537; Ashley South, "Karen Nationalist Communities: The 'Problem' of Diversity," *Contemporary Southeast Asia: A Journal of International and Strategic Affairs* 29, no. 1 (2007).

23 John P Wilson and Boris Drozdek, *Broken Spirits: The Treatment of Traumatized Asylum Seekers, Refugees, War, and Torture Victims* (New York: Brunner-Routledge, 2004).

24 Zev Harel, Boaz Kahana, and John P Wilson, "War and Remembrance: The Legacy of Pearl Harbor," in *International Handbook of Traumatic Stress Syndromes*, ed. John P Wilson and Beverley Raphael (New York: Plenum, 1993), 263–275.

25 Michael Rutter, "Implications of Resilience Concepts for Scientific Understanding," *Annals of the New York Academy of Sciences* 1094 (2006): 1–12, doi:10.1196/annals.1376.002.

26 George A Bonanno, "Resilience in the Face of Potential Trauma," *Current Directions in Psychological Science* 14, no. 3 (2005): 135.

27 Albert Bandura, "Perceived Self-Efficacy in Cognitive Development and Functioning," *Educational Psychologist* 28, no. 2 (1993): 117–148.

28 John P Wilson, "Traumatic Events and PTSD Prevention," in *The Handbook of Studies on Preventive Psychiatry*, ed. Graham D Burrows and Beverley Raphael (Amsterdam, the Netherlands: Elsevier North-Holland, 1995), 281–296.

Bibliography

Alden, Lynn E, Marci J Regambal, and Judith M Laposa. "The Effects of Direct versus Witnessed Threat on Emergency Department Healthcare Workers: Implications for PTSD Criterion A." *Journal of Anxiety Disorders* 22, no. 8 (2008): 1337–1346. doi:10.1016/j.janxdis.2008.01.013.

Back Pack Health Worker Team. *Ten Years Report 1998–2009: Life, Liberty, and the Pursuit of Health.* Mae Sot, Thailand: Back Pack Health Worker Team, 2010. http://www.burmalibrary.org/docs11/BPHWT10yearReport_1998-2009.pdf-red.pdf.

Bandura, Albert. "Perceived Self-Efficacy in Cognitive Development and Functioning." *Educational Psychologist* 28, no.2 (1993): 117–148.

Bonanno, George A. "Resilience in the Face of Potential Trauma." *Current Directions in Psychological Science* 14, no. 3 (2005): 135.

Clohessy, Sue, and Anke Ehlers. "PTSD Symptoms, Response to Intrusive Memories and Coping in Ambulance Service Workers." *British Journal of Clinical Psychology/ British Psychological Society* 38, pt. 3 (September 1999): 251–265.

Dewane, Claudia J. "Posttraumatic Stress Disorder in Medical Personnel in Vietnam." *Hospital & Community Psychiatry* 35, no. 12 (1984): 1232–1234.

Folkman, Susan, Richard S Lazarus, Christina Dunkel-Schetter, Anita DeLongis, and Rand J Gruen. "Dynamics of a Stressful Encounter: Cognitive Appraisal, Coping, and Encounter Outcomes." *Journal of Personality and Social Psychology* 50, no. 5 (May 1986): 992–1003.

Folkman, Susan, Richard S Lazarus, Rand J Gruen, and Anita DeLongis. "Appraisal, Coping, Health Status, and Psychological Symptoms." *Journal of Personality and Social Psychology* 50, no. 3 (March 1986): 571–579.

Frank, Serena. "The Impact of Working with Trauma: Risk and Resilience Factors among Health Care Providers." *South African Journal of Psychiatry* 12, no. 4 (2006): 100–104.

Fuertes, Al B. "In Their Own Words: Contextualizing the Discourse of (War) Trauma and Healing." *Conflict Resolution Quarterly* 21, no. 4 (2004): 491–501.

Giacaman, Rita, Yoke Rabaia, Viet Nguyen-Gillham, Rajaie Batniji, Raija-Leena L Punamaki, and Derek Summerfield. "Mental Health, Social Distress and Political Oppression: The Case of the Occupied Palestinian Territory." *Global Public Health* (2010): 1–13. doi:10.1080/17441692.2010.528443.

González-Romá, Vicente, Wilmar B Schaufeli, Arnold B Bakker, and Susanna Lloret. "Burnout and Work Engagement: Independent Factors or Opposite Poles?" *Journal of Vocational Behavior* 68, no. 1 (2006): 165–174. doi:10.1016/j. jvb.2005.01.003.

Gravers, Mikael. "The Karen Making of a Nation." *Asian Forms of the Nation* (1996): 237–269.

Harel, Zev, Boaz Kahana, and John P Wilson. "War and Remembrance: The Legacy of Pearl Harbor." In *International Handbook of Traumatic Stress Syndromes*, edited by John P Wilson and Beverley Raphael, 263–275. New York: Plenum, 1993.

Harriden, Jessica. "'Making a Name for Themselves': Karen Identity and the Politicization of Ethnicity in Burma." *Journal of Burmese Studies* 7 (2002): 84–144.

Janoff-Bullman, Ronnie. *Shattered Assumptions.* New York: Free Press, 2002.

"Karen Department of Health and Welfare." *Karen Department of Health and Welfare,* 2012. http://kdhw.org/.

Karen Human Rights Group. "Attacks and Displacement in Nyaunglebin District" (2010). http://www.khrg.org/khrg2010/khrg10b6.html.

———. "Enduring Hunger and Repression: Food Scarcity, Internal Displacement, and the Continued Use of Forced Labour in Toungoo District" (2004). http://www.khrg.org/khrg2004/khrg0401d.html.

Laposa, Judith M, and Lynn E Alden. "Posttraumatic Stress Disorder in the Emergency Room: Exploration of a Cognitive Model." *Behaviour Research and Therapy* 41, no. 1 (2003): 49–65. doi: 10.1016/S0005-7967(01)00123-1.

Lazarus, Richard S. "On the Primacy of Cognition." *American Psychologist* 39, no. 2 (1984): 124–129. doi:10.1037/0003-066X.39.2.124.

Lim, Andrew George, Lawrence Stock, Eh Kalu Shwe Oo, and Douglas P Jutte. "Trauma and Mental Health of Medics in Eastern Myanmar's Conflict Zones: A Cross-Sectional and Mixed Methods Investigation." *Conflict and Health* 7, no. 1 (2013): 15. doi:10.1186/1752-1505-7-15.

Maslach, Christina, and Michael P Leiter. "Early Predictors of Job Burnout and Engagement." *Journal of Applied Psychology* 93, no. 3 (May 2008): 498–512. doi:10.1037/0021-9010.93.3.498.

McCann, I Lisa, and Laurie Anne Pearlman. "Vicarious Traumatization: A Framework for Understanding the Psychological Effects of Working with Victims." *Journal of Traumatic Stress* 3, no. 1 (January 1, 1990): 131–149. doi:10.1007/BF00975140.

North, Carol S, Laura Tivis, J Curtis McMillen, Betty Pfefferbaum, Edward L Spitznagel, Jann Cox, Sara Nixon, Kenneth P Bunch, and Elizabeth M Smith. "Psychiatric Disorders in Rescue Workers after the Oklahoma City Bombing." *American Journal of Psychiatry* 159, no. 5 (May 1, 2002): 857–859. doi:10.1176/appi.ajp.159.5.857.

Palm, Kathleen M, Melissa A Polusny, and Victoria M Follette. "Vicarious Traumatization: Potential Hazards and Interventions for Disaster and Trauma Workers." *Prehospital and Disaster Medicine* 19, no. 1 (March 2004): 73–78.

Pham, Phuong N, Patrick Vinck, Didine Kaba Kinkodi, and Harvey M Weinstein. "Sense of Coherence and Its Association with Exposure to Traumatic Events, Posttraumatic Stress Disorder, and Depression in Eastern Democratic Republic of Congo." *Journal of Traumatic Stress* 23, no. 3 (June 2010): 313–321. doi:10.1002/jts.20527.

Pines, Ayala, and Christina Maslach. "Characteristics of Staff Burnout in Mental Health Settings." *Hospital & Community Psychiatry* 29, no. 4 (April 1978): 233–237.

Rajah, Ananda. "A Nation of Intent in Burma: Karen Ethno-Nationalism, Nationalism and Narrations of Nation." *Pacific Review* 15, no. 4 (2002): 517–537.

Richard, Allison J, Catherine I Lee, Matthew G Richard, Eh KS Oo, Thomas Lee, and Lawrence Stock. "Essential Trauma Management Training: Addressing Service Delivery Needs in Active Conflict Zones in Eastern Myanmar." *Human Resources for Health* 7, no. 1 (March 3, 2009): 19. doi:10.1186/1478-4491-7-19.

Rutter, Michael. "Competence under Stress: Risk and Protective Factors." In *Risk and Protective Factors in the Development of Psychopathology*, edited by J Rolf, AS Masten, D Cicchetti, KH Nuechterlein, and S Weintraub, 181–214. New York: Cambridge University Press, 1990.

———. "Implications of Resilience Concepts for Scientific Understanding." *Annals of the New York Academy of Sciences* 1094 (2006): 1–12. doi:10.1196/annals.1376.002.

South, Ashley. "Karen Nationalist Communities: The 'Problem' of Diversity." *Contemporary Southeast Asia: A Journal of International and Strategic Affairs* 29, no. 1 (2007).

Vinck, Patrick, and Phuong N Pham. "Association of Exposure to Violence and Potential Traumatic Events with Self-Reported Physical and Mental Health Status in the Central African Republic." *JAMA* 304, no. 5 (2010): 544–552. doi:10.1001/jama.2010.1065.

Wilson, John P. "Traumatic Events and PTSD Prevention." In *The Handbook of Studies on Preventive Psychiatry*, edited by Graham D Burrows and Beverley Raphael, 281–296. Amsterdam, the Netherlands: Elsevier North-Holland, 1995.

Wilson, John P, and Boris Drozdek. *Broken Spirits: The Treatment of Traumatized Asylum Seekers, Refugees, War, and Torture Victims*. New York: Brunner-Routledge, 2004.

Chapter 10

Parallel Process as a Learning Tool in

Clinical Supervision within a Traumatized

Community

Case Examples from the Burma Border

Sarah Gundle

Introduction

In this chapter, I use case examples from my work as a supervisor working in a resource-poor, highly affected region of the world to demonstrate the challenges that people providing supervision in traumatized communities may encounter. The supervision takes place with counselors working with the estimated 140,000 displaced Burmese people living along the Thai-Burma border. In 1989 Dr. Cynthia Maung established the Mae Tao Clinic in Mae Sot, Thailand, to serve the needs of the activists fleeing the 1988 uprising. This clinic is now a comprehensive health care facility serving over 150,000 people a year from this community, in addition to Burmese who come across the border from Burma for care, and offers a wide variety of health services. Under Dr. Cynthia's leadership, the clinic has built a multidisciplinary treatment program that attracts volunteers from all over the world. Dr. Cynthia is the recipient of numerous awards, including the National Endowment for Democracy's 2012 Democracy Award, in recognition of her work in providing health care services and advocating for the rights of displaced people on the Thai-Burma border. The Mae Tao Clinic also has an active mental health center for children and adults. The Counseling Center was established in 2006 with the support of Burma Border Projects (BBP), the only nonprofit organization based in Mae Sot that specifically addresses the mental health of the displaced Burmese people on the Thai-Burma border. The Counseling Center was established to treat the mental health needs of this community, many of which are trauma-related. Among the issues addressed by the Counseling Center staff are the horrific experiences that the displaced Burmese have struggled with, including forced labor, child labor, torture, chronic illness, human trafficking, sexual violence, and exploitation of migrant workers, among other human rights abuses. The Child Recreation Center (CRC) was established in 2011, also with the support of BBP, to address the broad spectrum of developmental and psychosocial needs faced by children who have been through hardship and atrocity. Most of the children treated at the CRC have either witnessed or experienced violence themselves or been victimized by being forced to live under inhumane living conditions under an oppressive government.

BBP staff members are actively engaged with supporting the Counseling Center and Child Recreation Center at the Mae Tao Clinic. They provide support, training, and supervision to the Burmese staff of these two centers, in addition to conducting trauma and mental health trainings with other community-based organizations. The BBP clinical staff on the border is, in turn, supervised by an American-based clinical psychologist and clinical social worker. This supervision is provided remotely (via Skype) and by in-person training when these professionals visit the border.

Clinical supervision within a resource-poor, traumatized population looks very different than clinical supervision in the Western model. This is caused in part by the differing cultural expectations, experiences, and training of the supervisor and supervisee. These elements are key factors in why supervision approaches need to be adapted cross-culturally. There is a great deal of research on the necessity of and tools for adapting therapy and clinical supervision to make them culturally appropriate and coherent;[1] however, a culturally informed lens is not enough to enable understanding of what makes supervision effective in a refugee context. A deep understanding of the traumatic content of the material being discussed, and its consequences for both treatment and supervision, is also crucial. Within this already complicated matrix of cultural impact and trauma, an additional factor is that this work traverses both development and clinical work. In the period after colonialism, distinctions of power are marked not only by the lines dividing one country from another, but also by the ways difference is deployed across societies. In a postcolonial world, basic tenets of responsible development work need to be integrated into the clinical work, and there is no clear model for how to do this. At the macro level, this work involves postcolonial concepts of social justice and human rights; the meso, or intermediate, level involves community development work; and therapeutic work with the displaced Burmese and their families occurs at the micro level.[2]

In this chapter I focus specifically on an area that has not received much attention: the parallel process between the supervisees' experiences and the trauma reactions occurring for the displaced people they are working with. While an understanding of this process does not begin to adequately encompass the complex nature of supervision on the Burma border, it can be very helpful when used specifically to ground the supervisor-supervisee dyad in an understanding of the dynamics at play. It can help elucidate enactments that might become lost in the complexity of the work. Understanding and labeling it can create a bridge between the macro, meso, and micro levels the therapist is operating within. As in all treatment, but especially when dealing with victims of trauma, it is not uncommon for therapists to put themselves in the patients' shoes and experience what they experience. The therapist identifies with the patient and then enacts with the supervisor much of what the patient is feeling.[3] Understanding this process can be a starting place for understanding how the trauma symptoms of avoidance, splitting, dissociation, arousal, and projection are expressed at both individual and community levels. Case examples given below illustrate each of these symptoms.

Although the literature on vicarious traumatization describes the reactions of the therapist to trauma work, it largely does not focus on the specific parallel process that occurs, and on supervision's role.[4] Understanding parallel process can be a method for understanding vicarious trauma more specifically. This parallel process, when left unconscious, can lead to troubling, supervision-interfering results, ultimately making it difficult to support the supervisee and create a safe framework in which to discuss case material.

The specific context discussed here is the remote-based (Skype) supervision of Western clinical staff of Burma Border Projects. The supervision program started in 2009 as a result of the BBP staff tripling in size. The organization's growth precipitated a need to formally provide support to the new staff. The Western supervisees—social workers and counselors trained in Europe and the United States—were brought in to Mae Sot to be technical advisors. They have dual roles: in some cases they work directly with the displaced Burmese, and they also supervise the Burmese clinical staff treating clients in the Counseling Center in the Mae Tao Clinic and in several smaller local agencies. Because the local clinical staff members are all displaced Burmese, with their own trauma histories, sometimes severe, the boundary between the Western staff's supervision of and treatment of them can become at times diffuse.

Case material presented here illustrates the specific trauma-based parallel process that becomes apparent through supervision and ends up shaping the supervision relationship. Because the supervisees are doing both direct clinical as well as systemic work with agencies, clinics, and organizations, the parallel process themes discussed here illustrate both. The vignettes also briefly address (1) challenges in remote supervision, (2) direct interventions in supervision and training, and (3) navigating the interdisciplinary nature of the clinical team, including discipline differences between a psychologist supervisor and a social work clinician.

Trauma-Based Parallel Process

The fact that Mae Sot is a place filled with traumatized people touches all involved; no one is immune. A growing number of research studies suggest that a significant proportion of relief and development workers will eventually experience some version of traumatic-stress-related reactions.[5] These may include posttraumatic stress disorder (PTSD), depression, anxiety, or substance abuse. It is essential that people working within a severely traumatized community understand the dynamics of trauma and stress reactions, as well as how to care for themselves.

The concept of parallel process was put forward by Searles.[6] Put simply, the supervisee uses his or her own experience within supervision to help understand the patient's experience; the problems experienced in one relationship affect and are reflected by the other relationship. An unusual feature of this setting is that the mental health workers are dealing not only with their clients, but also with systems. In the context of supervision, therefore, the parallel process described here is not only within the supervision relationship, but also between the supervisees and the larger system of the organization they work for and the organizations they are engaged with on the border. A parallel process is at play wherein the supervisees' issues, both personally and systemically, become reflective of the trauma symptoms of the people they are helping. Supervisees then begin to develop similar affects and behaviors, expressing unconscious dynamics of their clients and themselves. Trauma-specific themes are reflected in both the supervisees' engagement with the community and the Burmese clients' experiences. Deconstructing and understanding these enactments through locating the parallel process can be critical to providing a therapeutic, corrective experience for clients and supervisees alike.

Treating victims of violence, torture, and displacement can lead to specific reactions such as burnout and vicarious traumatization for all involved: patient, supervisor, and supervisee.[7] People working within this severely traumatized population work under conditions of extreme stress, and the consequences of the work on individuals and group dynamics are intensified. Only through the lens of trauma, therefore, can we understand how various systems on the border interact: from individual clinical supervision to how organizations communicate, collaborate, and enter into conflict, the understanding of trauma is essential.[8] The clinical material presented here is organized around the major symptoms of trauma—avoidance, arousal, splitting, dissociation, and projection—all of which are defined below and elaborated on with case examples. Within these clusters of symptoms, specific themes emerge through an understanding of the parallel process.

Clinical Supervision on the Border

Clinical supervision is generally understood to be shared reflection of clinical work between an expert and another professional with the goal of helping the supervisee acquire deeper skills.[9] Clinical supervision is a distinct professional activity, with education and training facilitated through a collaborative interpersonal process. It involves observation, evaluation, feedback, facilitation of supervisee self-assessment, and acquisition of knowledge and skills by the supervisee via instruction, modeling, and mutual problem-solving. Building on the recognition of the strengths and talents of the supervisee, supervision promotes skill development.[10]

In the case of trauma-based clinical work, supervision serves the critically important role of helping the supervisee metabolize the traumatic content of the material being brought up.[11] The intensity of trauma-based work makes it essential that the clinician has a stable frame of support and care.[12] On the border, however, clinical supervision is not only about these things; it is also about helping supervisees navigate the incredibly complicated matrix of doing relational work within a postcolonial model. It is about helping them track their emotional responses and use that information constructively. It inevitably incorporates systems supervision because it is located within a system where, similar to the intergenerational transmission of trauma, the fear of repeating the colonial power differential is always present. These case examples illustrate how the supervision relationship can help locate and describe the parallel process at work, thereby making it possible to circumvent potential problems. Identifying the parallel process can transform the supervisee's trauma response into an empathic intervention.

Avoidance

Avoidance is a conscious or unconscious defense mechanism consisting of a refusal to encounter situations, activities, or objects that would produce anxiety or conflict.

CASE 1: IDENTIFICATION AND PASSIVITY

After working with Ms. B, a clinician I was supervising for over a year, I began to notice a type of passivity in her. Over time she became resistant to my suggestions. She appeared open to specific interventions I would suggest doing with the Counseling Center staff. But when I asked the next week whether she had attempted any of the interventions, she would reply that she had not and wasn't sure why. She also began canceling supervision or showing up to the prearranged Skype times late or not at all. Repeated attempts to empathically confront the supervisee's avoidance were not well received. I was surprised, as it seemed out of character for this formerly very responsible, competent, and smart clinician. I set limits on how many times she could miss. I began to feel that I was forcing the relationship. Ultimately, the supervision languished, and a previously positive supervisory relationship ended somewhat negatively for both of us. I wondered what went wrong and felt a sense of guilt for letting her down.

A year later, Ms. B, now living in the United States, and I were both involved in a trauma training in Mae Sot. One day she pulled me aside and, with great affect, told me that she had been considering how our supervision had ended and how bad she felt about it. She described how her identification with the Counseling Center staff began to precisely mirror her relationship with me. We both felt ineffectual. They too had stopped listening to her and showing up. She had not been able to change this process and, similar to my feeling, felt guilt and shame about it. As we discussed the parallel process at work, it became apparent that Counseling Center staff felt that by asking their clients to talk about their pasts they were re-traumatizing them. They therefore avoided asking their clients any probing questions and felt that my supervisee was asking them to delve more deeply into their clients' lives than they were comfortable doing. My supervisee felt a sense of shame at participating in re-traumatizing the staff.

I believe that if we had been able to locate this process at work before our supervision ended we might have been able to reverse its damaging course. By confronting the supervisee about her avoidance in a caring, empathic manner and labeling the identification we might have been able to model for the Counseling Center staff how they could work through similar issues with their clients. At least in hindsight my supervisee and I were able to understand what had happened between us.

CASE 2: ESTRANGEMENT AND FUTILITY

Not only the clients, but also the system, can have a profound effect on the therapist, supervisee, and supervisor. Another supervisee, Ms. Y, who was particularly talented at creating cohesive systems among people, began to scale back her involvement with the Counseling Center staff, focusing on other responsibilities more than she had previously. Around the same time, a volunteer psychologist had come to the Counseling Center from abroad to do time-limited skills-based training. As the outside volunteer's relationship with the staff became closer, Ms. Y began to feel a sense of estrangement and detachment from the staff. It was particularly jarring as she had worked very hard to build and maintain these relationships, and they had been hard-won. What felt odd was that she seemed to accept her new role as inevitable and did little to change it.

As Ms. Y, through supervision, began to unpack her estrangement, she realized that she was experiencing a parallel process to her staff members, who had similar feelings about their employer, the larger medical clinic. There had recently been a clinic reorganization at the very top level, and staff salaries had been cut across the board. Expectations had changed, people were reassigned to departments they did not choose, and benefits had been cut. Ms. Y had, similar to me, expressed surprise to them that they were not more upset about the changes. At the time she had noted a curious role acceptance in them, even of a perceived lesser role, as if it were inevitable; fighting it felt futile.

Once Ms. Y had used our supervision to locate her own feelings of estrangement as parallel to theirs, she was able to act more effectively. She was able to use supervision to discuss ways she could reassert herself and return to a sense of agency about her work. She was also able to discuss her experience with the staff members and encourage them to express their displeasure with the new clinic changes.

CASE 3: CONFLICTS OVER ENTITLEMENT

This case illustrates the process I went through of recognizing something in myself that shed light on what my supervisee, Ms. X, was struggling with. Entitlement can mean many things. A healthy sense of entitlement is necessary to fully articulate one's voice. In proper doses, it is a necessary ingredient in a person's mental health. In improper doses, it can lead to excessive narcissism. The Burma border presents an interesting example of the balance between healthy and unhealthy entitlement. Unlike my supervision relationships with fellows at a hospital finishing their psychology training, my supervision relationships on the Burma border are mostly remote. I am acutely aware of my status as a double outsider, remote both from Burmese culture and from the therapists actually working there. I am often aware of how tentative I feel when making suggestions or comments or offering interpretations. Often my language is couched, soft, and indirect, which is not my usual supervision style. Generally I have felt that my more timid approach is appropriate given my distance; it's respectful of what I don't know and haven't experienced. I tell myself I am being culturally sensitive. However, it may also impede the supervisory relationship. It might reflect my own guilt at not "actually" doing the clinical work.

When I brought up my feelings with my extremely talented and perceptive supervisee Ms. X, she suggested I "flip the script" and change that equation. My verbalization of my feelings of lack of entitlement in supervision with her opened up a space for her to address her own tentativeness with the Counseling Center staff. When you are well-versed in the politics of development and the insidious nature of colonialism, as all BBP staff members are, there is inevitable guilt about being brought in as an authority to talk about work with the Burmese when you are not Burmese. It is an inherent problem when we are the "experts" to people outside our culture; there is always a power differential. Ms. X realized that, in her desire not to re-create power structures (as much as is possible), she may have overstepped and become indecisive with the staff, creating confusion and misunderstanding. While appropriately respecting the inherent power dialectic, she had lost her own voice.

Verbalizing this parallel process has helped us both refine our clinical voices. In expressing her own lack of entitlement, she was able to address some of her own fears and get back to a place of trusting her own judgment. She has also been able to model trusting her own instincts and judgment for the Counseling Center staff.

Splitting

Splitting is a defense mechanism in which people or systems are perceived as "all good" or "all bad" rather than as a mix of the two. Splitting is inextricably related to safety; it makes an unsafe world or situation feel more manageable.

CASE 1: LACK OF POWER AS EXPRESSED
THROUGH MEDICATION MANAGEMENT

On the border, a place of great tension and instability, splitting is pervasive. People, grants, care centers, even reports are alternately devalued or idealized. The tenuousness of people's lives leads directly to instability in feelings of safety, which in turn leads to splitting. A significant example of splitting is medication. The use of medication in a Counseling Center on the border becomes representative of much more than alleviation of symptoms; it is inevitably related to power.

As in most medical facilities, mental health treatment tends to occupy a marginalized position. Mental illness and mental health counseling is not only stigmatized; its treatment is largely disparaged. This is also the case for the Counseling Center, and expresses itself though power relations between the staff members of the various medical departments. A pecking order appears to have established itself wherein senior medics have the most legitimacy, followed by other medics, medical department staff, then Counseling Center staff. This pecking order is further complicated by the fact that the Counseling Center staff members distribute medication, despite that being a medic-only task in the other departments. They distribute medication because the clinical interventions at the Counseling Center largely depend on the use of psychotropic medications and only one medic works there. Not only is dispensing medication the framework around which every therapeutic action in the Counseling Center revolves, the clinicians don't even report in the logbooks visits that don't involve medication. Their medication privileges foster resentment among the wider clinic staff and further alienate the Counseling Center staff from their peers. A complex picture emerges of a marginalized staff becoming even more marginalized because they are dispensing medication; and they are dispensing medication because they have internalized a worldview, corroborated by the clinic system as a whole, that only medication helps.

Within this complex picture, Ms. Y's contributions about relational therapy are inevitably devalued, just as the staff's contributions are in the clinic. Even after she has spent considerable time gaining a foothold of connection to the staff, working to impart an understanding of therapeutic options besides psychopharmacologic treatment, when any outsider comes into the Counseling Center who dispenses medication, the new member is idealized and she is devalued. This has occurred regularly across various supervisees from varying disciplines. Understanding this process as related to power, rather than as a personal rejection, has been useful. Mental illness is stigmatized, and there is no clear-cut way of treating it, particularly in a situation where the stressors have not been alleviated. It inevitably happens that staff members idealize the person who teaches them about medication, whether the person is a nurse, psychiatrist, or physician assistant, whether knowledgeable in approach or not. It is a method of gaining security in an insecure situation, a way of feeling not so marginalized in the wider medical community. In the larger perspective, the Counseling Center staff, coming from a profound lack of power in Burma and then experiencing a lack of power in the clinic, understandably grasp onto any method of taking back some of that power.

Working within an understanding of these power dynamics is essential when trying to introduce therapeutic options. For Ms. Y, identifying with the marginalized position of the staff and understanding the parallel process has allowed her to use her understanding of the splitting as a tool rather than experiencing it as an obstacle.

Dissociation

Dissociation is a psychological mechanism in which the mind splits off certain aspects of a traumatic event from conscious awareness. Dissociation can affect the patient's memory, sense of reality, and sense of identity.

CASE 1: ALIENATION/PLACELESSNESS

During her orientation, Ms. X expressed excitement about her new role in Mae Sot. Years earlier, she had lived in Mae Sot as a volunteer English teacher and computer tutor. Energized and excited by her job at the clinic, she wanted to do direct clinical work. She realized that she needed further training and went back to graduate school and became a social worker. She amassed experience in trauma-specific work, always with an eye toward one day returning to the clinic in Mae Sot to help with a different skill set. Armed with her degree, experience, and knowledge of trauma, she had triumphantly returned to her "dream job" and was driven and motivated. After her orientation was completed, she arranged an initial meeting with the Counseling Center staff she was to supervise. She asked what their goals were for their work together, anticipating that the work was so intense and overwhelming that their initial work together would be to scale back both expectations and goals. Unanimously, to her surprise, the group professed an interest in learning "English and computer skills."

Deflated, Ms. X came to supervision feeling alienated and alone. She felt that she had gone through all her training for naught; she could have just stayed, years ago, and offered them what they were asking for now. What role was she supposed to take now? Identifying with what she termed "placelessness," she felt powerless and hopeless.

Viewed through a certain lens, this situation indeed felt hopeless. Was this a Western construct of treatment being thrust on a group who didn't want it or value it? Was it a re-creation of colonial assumptions? Unsure how to understand this situation, we proceeded cautiously in supervision. I was aware of feeling responsible for maintaining her sense of excitement about the work, for helping her not lose sight of what she was there for. But the work felt strained, brittle.

It was only through identifying the parallel process of "placelessness" that she found a way back into the work and into developing a positive relationship with the staff. She found out that about half the Counseling Center staff had not chosen to work there; moreover, they had not wanted to work there. They felt, in fact, displaced. For all the staff, though, it was their only work option. Actively symptomatic, traumatized themselves, they were thrust into a situation where they had to listen to and actively process trauma stories. They felt victimized and re-traumatized by having to work there and, quite understandably, resented her insistence that they discuss trauma even further. Learning English and computer skills seemed to them a welcome respite from feeling so overwhelmed and flooded.

Once she was able to understand the parallel process at play, she was able to identify with the staff and use their mutual feelings of placelessness as a tool of engagement rather than estrangement.

CASE 2: FRAGMENTATION

My usually verbal and perceptive supervisee, Ms. X, experienced difficulty articulating to me the clinical process between her and one of the Counseling Center staff members. She reported feeling "tongue-tied." In addition, she reported helplessness and a general feeling of being unsure of herself professionally. She described feeling disconnected from her peers and her usual sources of support. She started having memory problems and described difficulty with managing her schedule. In supervision, this presented itself as frustration on the part of the supervisee that I wasn't rescuing her from her feelings of helplessness. She began to focus on ways in which I didn't disseminate information from the US-based board of BBP directly, ways in which she felt "left out."

Communication networks tend to break down when trauma is present. She experienced helplessness at her dissociative response, as her staff member had, followed by anger with me. In both cases, they began to focus on the deficits in the dissemination of information, resulting in increasing fragmentation at both levels. Frawley O'Dea wrote that "successful supervision of treatment of trauma survivors may require the supervisor to enter into the dissociative experiences of the supervisee in ways that invite symbolization and elaboration of the currently formless and unspeakable."[13] It was only through an understanding of the need to put feelings into words that we were able to understand her behavior as related to the staff member's dissociative trauma response. Understanding the origins of the fragmentation improved both the clinical as well as the supervisory relationship.

Arousal

Arousal is a cognitive and psychological activation in response to a traumatic situation leading to alertness and readiness to respond. It is a state of being responsive to sensory stimulation.

CASE 1: HYPERVIGILANCE: OPERATING
FROM A PLACE OF SCARCITY

Hypervigilance at a system level can resemble paranoia. Organizations on the Burma border largely do not collaborate. Different organizations working toward similar goals experience great difficulty sharing resources, credit, and information. People are secretive, hostility exists between organizations, and information is not widely shared. Even within the Mae Tao Clinic, where the different departments are all serving the same population, there can be difficulty communicating with one another. All the departments seem to operate from a place of fear that their resources may be taken from them. On the face of it, this approach does not appear to make sense. In such a resource-poor environment, one might understand the need to share resources as critically important. Therefore, understanding such responses as deriving from a place of trauma is useful.

One example of this type of hypervigilance playing itself out is at the Child Recreation Center at the Mae Tao Clinic. While BBP donates supplies to them for art projects, they also get donations from other places. Recently, one of the BBP Burmese staff, Ms. H, who works directly with children doing therapeutic play sessions at several different organizations, saw some interesting art supplies at the CRC that she thought she might use with one of her child cases. She asked one of the CRC staff whether she might take just a few of the supplies and was flatly denied. Ms. H was frustrated and disappointed by this denial. It was particularly surprising given that her organization, BBP, had donated a good percentage of the CRC's art supplies, had been instrumental in fact in creating the CRC, and that BBP's child director conducts weekly trainings and supervision for the CRC staff and is intimately involved with its daily operation. At the same time, Ms. H was experiencing frustration with one of her BBP colleagues, who felt that Ms. H wasn't giving her enough "credit" for her work helping conduct the psychosocial play sessions.

Understanding these two events as a parallel process was useful. Both Ms. H and the CRC staff member were clinicians who were guarding their resources, including their authority, carefully, despite external evidence that this wasn't required. They both work directly with children doing play therapy, and they have everything to gain by helping one another, yet the pull of feeling that someone was trying to take something from them contradicted these facts. It was only when we examined this parallel process through the lens of hypervigilance that we were able to understand why they were both having great difficulty sharing resources and credit.

Projection

Projection is an unconscious defense mechanism by which a person attributes to someone else unacknowledged ideas, thoughts, feelings, or impulses that they cannot accept as their own.

CASE 1: UNREMITTING STRESSORS

BBP staff on the border experience chronic, unremitting stress. BBP is a small, fledgling organization with a lack of resources, both financial and otherwise, and yet they have huge demands placed on them. Despite the lack of resources, the staff is expected to and in fact does run big programs. The staff clinicians, by design, have to stretch themselves very thin. There will never be time to accomplish all their goals. Similarly, the problems that arise within a horribly abused population, who then find themselves rootless and stateless, will never be fully addressed. Everyone on the border lives with this knowledge, and it informs the work ethic. Counseling Center staff members, as well as most staff clinicians in other organizations, have similar demands put on them. The results are the same: resentment, anger, and the feeling that they are not supported.

When the feeling of a lack of support was first expressed in supervision, it was unclear how to resolve it. Initially, I focused on my own limitations as a supervisor: my failings and how I could be more supportive. We focused on the different ways we were trained, as psychologist and social worker, and how our differing expectations of training might be getting in the way. We worked to elaborate the differences in our expectations of one another and how to find a common frame. Although it was helpful, after these changes were implemented the supervisee still felt overwhelmed and alone. We began to question whether she was engaged in an enactment that could be better understood through parallel process. There are always limitations; ways in which one can do better and improve. This is always true. However, the unremitting stressors on the border assure that there will almost never be a time when there will be a feeling of general ease and calm. As long as the work is unfinished and the very real stressors are present, it is invariably the case that the strain will be felt at both the individual, relational level and systemically. Recognizing this fact paradoxically eased the tension between us and helped increase her sense of agency with the staff.

CASE 2: IMPAIRED CRITICAL JUDGMENT
AND DISEMPOWERMENT

One day I noticed that Ms. B was increasingly critical of one of the Counseling Center staff members, who was in turn dismissive and judgmental toward his clients, occasionally calling them names and acting scornfully toward them. She tried to confront him in an empathic manner, but he became aggressive toward her, ultimately devaluing her to other staff members. She felt unsure how to proceed and began to dread being around him. Because the comments he made were so egregious, I too found myself being critical of him, wondering about his fitness for service. At the same time, he was being asked to conduct an ever-increasing array of clinical duties, within the Counseling Center and the wider clinic, including translation, which he hated. He didn't feel that he could set any boundaries on these requests and began working longer and longer hours.

Trauma survivors often lose critical judgment, with the result of increased conformity. At an individual level, this process can lead to a counter-aggressive response to aggression in clients; at the systems level, it can lead to hierarchical, punitive structures. As a situation feels increasingly out of control, organizational leaders can become more controlling. Sometimes they institute punitive measures in an attempt to forestall chaos. These attempts inevitably lead to disempowerment and helplessness.

In order to address his behavior, we had to address the strain he was under, as well as our own behavior. Realizing that his aggression was an attempt to gain control was a way into understanding our own aggression toward him.

CASE 3: UNRESOLVED GRIEF:
REPATRIATION AND RECONCILIATION

Ms. X was supervising a Counseling Center staff member treating a case of a person who was cautiously thinking about repatriation to Burma. Occasionally Ms. X met with both of them, as routinely happens in the Counseling Center. For this client, thinking about returning "home" was a source of stress and trauma. She began to be actively symptomatic again. Diagnosed with complex PTSD, she had been raped in her village and had lost several family members before fleeing. Once uprooted by trauma, she had rerooted herself in Thailand and made salient, supportive connections within the community. Ms. X began to have dreams of this patient and "couldn't get her out of her head." I too began to think about this patient at off hours; she entered my consciousness in a marked, unusual way. The client's counselor struggled with how to help her "forgive." The major work of supervision, between Ms. X and her supervisee and between me and my supervisee, was how to reframe repatriation as connected to reconciliation rather than forgiveness.[14] The client brought in to treatment her many intense nightmares, wanting to understand why they were starting again after a long period of not having them. The dreams were always about leaving her village.

As this client began to explore her connection to "home," Ms. X and I also began to explore our ideas of home. At the same time, Ms. X began to have regular conflicts with a German volunteer. The nature of the conflicts revolved around justice. There had been an issue between departments about the sharing of resources and, atypically for her, my supervisee took a very aggressive, protective stance. She sided firmly with her staff members and identified with them as beleaguered. It was only when I too began to be involved in the conflict between the departments, writing emails to various people, that I stepped back to question the parallel process at play. Generally our approach was to not take sides in internal clinic politics; it was inevitably ineffective and counterproductive. However, in this case we had both become activated in an unusual way.

As a grandchild of a German Holocaust survivor who was very important to me, the Holocaust figured heavily in my childhood. A legacy of this is that the unimaginable becomes real; it is not hard to believe that the worst can happen. It also left me with a residue of survivor guilt. I am fairly confident that if the volunteer had not been German I would not have responded as I had. As the client, her therapist, and Ms. X struggled with justice and reconciliation as related to repatriation and her trauma symptoms, I recognized that my uncharacteristic response to the German volunteer reflected their struggle as it intersected with my own. It was only through unpacking the parallel process at play that Ms. X and I were able to effectively withdraw our involvement in the clinic battle. Doing this completely changed the focus of the work from anger to grief, ultimately a far more productive way of understanding the client's reaction and worsening symptoms. Grief became an entry point for verbalizing her many losses as well as her ambivalence about returning "home."

Conclusion

Just as the lives of people exposed to violence, torture, abuse, and alienation can become organized around their traumatic experiences, so too can systems.[15] Without understanding the parallel process inherent in trauma work, we risk inadvertently recapitulating the very experiences that were so toxic. The complex interaction in Mae Sot between traumatized clients, overworked staff, pressured systems, and economic strain has the potential to collude in creating a system where staff and clients alike suffer psychologically.

The lens of supervision can be a useful tool in analyzing systemic and individual trauma reactions. As the case material illustrates, the willingness of both supervisor and supervisee to take risks and be vulnerable in the supervisory relationship is necessary to effectively explore parallel processes in supervision. Collaboration, trust, and mutuality in the supervision relationship assist in the unfolding development of the supervisee. They also contribute to the effect of the treatment on the clients being served. Supervision can thereby play a part in laying the groundwork for new ways of thinking and relating, wherein people do not become depleted or re-traumatized.

Notes

1 Neil Boothby, "Trauma and Violence among Refugee Children," in *Amidst Peril and Pain: The Mental Health and Well-Being of the World's Refugees*, ed. Anthony J Marsella et al. (Washington, DC: American Psychological Association, 1994), 239–259; Robyn L Trippany, Victoria E White Kress, and S Allen Wilcoxon, "Preventing Vicarious Trauma: What Counselors Should Know when Working with Trauma Survivors," *Journal of Counseling & Development* 82, no. 1 (2004): 31–37, doi:10.1002/j.1556-6678.2004.tb00283.x; Derald W Sue et al., *Multicultural Counseling Competencies: Individual and Organizational Development* (Thousand Oaks, CA: Sage, 1998); Guus van der Veer, Kaz de Jong, and Johan Lansen, "Clinical Supervision for Counsellors in Areas of Armed Conflict," *Intervention* (2004): 118–128.

2 Mary Nash, "Responding to Settlement Needs: Migrants and Refugees and Community Development," in *Social Work Theories in Action*, ed. Mary Nash, Kieran O'Donoghue, and Robyn Munford (London: Jessica Kingsley Publishers, 2005), 140–154.

3 Carol A Falender et al., "Defining Competencies in Psychology Supervision: A Consensus Statement," *Journal of Clinical Psychology* 60, no. 7 (July 2004): 771–785, doi:10.1002/jclp.20013.

4 Kelly R. Chrestman, "Secondary Exposure to Trauma and Self-Reported Distress among Therapists," in *Secondary Traumatic Stress: Self-Care Issues for Clinicians, Researchers, and Educators*, ed. B Hudnall Stamm, 2nd ed. (Lutherville, MD: Sidran Press, 1999), 29–36; Laurie Anne Pearlman and Paula S Mac Ian, "Vicarious Traumatization: An Empirical Study of the Effects of Trauma Work on Trauma Therapists," *Professional Psychology: Research and Practice* 26, no. 6 (1995): 558–565, doi:10.1037/0735-7028.26.6.558; Laura J Schauben and Patricia A Frazier, "Vicarious Trauma: The Effects on Female Counselors of Working with Sexual Violence Survivors," *Psychology of Women Quarterly* 19, no. 1 (1995): 64, doi:10.1111/j.1471-6402.1995.tb00278.x.

5 Charles R Figley, "Compassion Fatigue as Secondary Traumatic Stress Disorder: An Overview," in *Compassion Fatigue: Coping with Secondary Traumatic Stress Disorder in Those Who Treat the Traumatized*, ed. Charles R Figley (New York: Brunner/Mazel, 1995), 1–21.

6 Harold F Searles, "The Informational Value of the Supervisor's Emotional Experiences," *Psychiatry* 18, no. 2 (May 1955): 135–146.

7 Pearlman and Mac Ian, "Vicarious Traumatization."

8 James A Chu, "Ten Traps for Therapists in the Treatment of Trauma Survivors," *Dissociation* 1, no. 4 (December 1988): 24–32.

9 Susan W Gray and Mark S Smith, "The Influence of Diversity in Clinical Supervision: A Framework for Reflective Conversations and Questioning," *Clinical Supervisor* 28, no. 2 (2009): 155–179, doi:10.1080/07325220903324371.

10 Janine M Bernard and Rodney K Goodyear, *Fundamentals of Clinical Supervision*, 3rd ed. (Pearson, 2004); Falender et al., "Defining Competencies in Psychology Supervision."

11 Peter Hawkins and Robin Shohet, *Supervision in the Helping Professions: An Individual, Group and Organizational Approach* (Buckingham, UK: Open University, 2000).

12 Edna B Foa et al., eds., *Effective Treatments for PTSD: Practice Guidelines from the International Society for Traumatic Stress Studies* (New York: Guilford Press, 2009).

13 Mary Frawley-O'Dea, "Who's Doing What to Whom?," *Contemporary Psychoanalysis* 33 (1997): 5–18.

14 Mona S Macksoud and J Lawrence Aber, "The War Experiences and Psychosocial Development of Children in Lebanon," *Child Development* 67, no. 1 (February 1996): 70–88.

15 Kenwyn K Smith, Valerie M Simmons, and Terri B Thames, "'Fix the Women': An Intervention into an Organizational Conflict Based on Parallel Process Thinking," *Journal of Applied Behavioral Science* 25, no. 1 (February 1, 1989): 11–29, doi:10.1177/0021886389251002.

Bibliography

Bernard, Janine M., and Rodney K Goodyear. *Fundamentals of Clinical Supervision*. 3rd ed. Boston: Pearson Education, 2004.

Boothby, Neil. "Trauma and Violence among Refugee Children." In *Amidst Peril and Pain: The Mental Health and Well-Being of the World's Refugees*, edited by Anthony J Marsella, Thomas Bornemann, Solvig Ekblad, and John Orley, 239–259. Washington, DC: American Psychological Association, 1994.

Chrestman, Kelly R. "Secondary Exposure to Trauma and Self-Reported Distress among Therapists." In *Secondary Traumatic Stress: Self-Care Issues for Clinicians*,

Researchers, and Educators, edited by B Hudnall Stamm, 29–36. 2nd ed. Lutherville, MD: Sidran Press, 1999.

Chu, James A. "Ten Traps for Therapists in the Treatment of Trauma Survivors." *Dissociation* 1, no. 4 (December 1988): 24–32.

Falender, Carol A, Jennifer A Erickson Cornish, Rodney Goodyear, Robert Hatcher, Nadine J Kaslow, Gerald Leventhal, Edward Shafranske, Sandra T Sigmon, Cal Stoltenberg, and Catherine Grus. "Defining Competencies in Psychology Supervision: A Consensus Statement." *Journal of Clinical Psychology* 60, no. 7 (July 2004): 771–785. doi:10.1002/jclp.20013.

Figley, Charles R. "Compassion Fatigue as Secondary Traumatic Stress Disorder: An Overview." In *Compassion Fatigue: Coping with Secondary Traumatic Stress Disorder in Those Who Treat the Traumatized*, edited by Charles R Figley, 1–21. New York: Brunner/Mazel, 1995.

Foa, Edna B, Terence M Keane, Matthew J Friedman, and Judith A Cohen, eds. *Effective Treatments for PTSD: Practice Guidelines from the International Society for Traumatic Stress Studies*. New York: Guilford Press, 2009.

Frawley-O'Dea, Mary. "Who's Doing What to Whom?" *Contemporary Psychoanalysis* 33 (1997): 5–18.

Gray, Susan W, and Mark S Smith. "The Influence of Diversity in Clinical Supervision: A Framework for Reflective Conversations and Questioning." *Clinical Supervisor* 28, no. 2 (2009): 155–179. doi:10.1080/07325220903324371.

Hawkins, Peter, and Robin Shohet. *Supervision in the Helping Professions: An Individual, Group and Organizational Approach*. Buckingham, UK: Open University, 2000.

Macksoud, Mona S, and J Lawrence Aber. "The War Experiences and Psychosocial Development of Children in Lebanon." *Child Development* 67, no. 1 (February 1996): 70–88.

Nash, Mary. "Responding to Settlement Needs: Migrants and Refugees and Community Development." In *Social Work Theories in Action*, edited by Mary Nash, Kieran O'Donoghue, and Robyn Munford, 140–154. London: Jessica Kingsley Publishers, 2005.

Pearlman, Laurie Anne, and Paula S Mac Ian. "Vicarious Traumatization: An Empirical Study of the Effects of Trauma Work on Trauma Therapists." *Professional Psychology: Research and Practice* 26, no. 6 (1995): 558–565. doi:10.1037/0735-7028.26.6.558.

Schauben, Laura J, and Patricia A Frazier. "Vicarious Trauma: The Effects on Female Counselors of Working with Sexual Violence Survivors." *Psychology of Women Quarterly* 19, no. 1 (1995): 49–64. doi:10.1111/j.1471-6402.1995.tb00278.x.

Searles, Harold F. "The Informational Value of the Supervisor's Emotional Experiences." *Psychiatry* 18, no. 2 (May 1955): 135–146.

Smith, Kenwyn K, Valerie M Simmons, and Terri B Thames. " 'Fix the Women': An Intervention into an Organizational Conflict Based on Parallel Process Thinking." *Journal of Applied Behavioral Science* 25, no. 1 (February 1, 1989): 11–29. doi:10.1177/0021886389251002.

Sue, Derald W, Robert T Carter, J Manuel Casas, Nadya A Fouad, Allen E Ivey, Margaret Jensen, Teresa LaFromboise, Jeanne E Manese, Joseph G Ponterotto, and Ena Vazquez-Nuttall. *Multicultural Counseling Competencies: Individual and Organizational Development.* Thousand Oaks, CA: Sage, 1998.

Trippany, Robyn L, Victoria E White Kress, and S Allen Wilcoxon. "Preventing Vicarious Trauma: What Counselors Should Know when Working with Trauma Survivors." *Journal of Counseling & Development* 82, no. 1 (2004): 31–37. doi:10.1002/j.1556-6678.2004.tb00283.x.

Van der Veer, Guus, Kaz de Jong, and Johan Lansen. "Clinical Supervision for Counsellors in Areas of Armed Conflict." *Intervention* (2004): 118–128.

Chapter 11

Program Evaluation and Research

Catherine Lee, Courtland Robinson,

Kyaw Soe Win, and Paul Bolton

Introduction

Despite major advances in health research and technology, dramatic shortages in the health care workforce are a threat to health, development, and security around the world.[1] The critical shortage of human resources for health care is often underappreciated as a barrier to providing services, despite the fact that the primary component of a functional and equitable health system is the health workforce.[2] Increasing funding for programs and access to essential drugs will do little to reduce the burden of disease without sufficient attention paid to the people who deliver these services. Health systems face human resource challenges worldwide, but such challenges are most critical in developing countries and emergency settings.[3] In humanitarian emergency situations, the health workforce is underdeveloped and underutilized, particularly in relation to the employment of national staff and the involvement of beneficiaries as service providers for their communities.[4]

To overcome the above-stated obstacles, it is advised that health systems look to task shifting or to involving nontechnical workers in jobs that would otherwise have to be completed by highly-skilled health workers. Task shifting is important—for both short-term emergencies and as part of the long-term plan for improvement of health outcomes—because having health workers perform only those tasks for which their skills are absolutely necessary is one way to deliver health care with optimal efficiency.[5] In addition, task shifting that is implemented by training locally can have the double impact of increasing local capacity while also increasing the likelihood of keeping those human resources involved. Programs that engage beneficiaries directly in providing health care to their communities hold great promise for success. In the context of Burma, programs designed for refugees, migrants, internally displaced persons, and the general community can benefit from involving beneficiaries in direct service provision, which has several advantages, including overcoming language barriers, cultural issues, and barriers to access, because the providers themselves are from within each community.[6] Engaging service providers from the community is especially important in Burma because of issues of trust and acceptability for community members, and to ensure that service provision can continue even during times of displacement and movement.

The issues of a limited health workforce and the need for task shifting apply directly to community mental health programs. In light of current global shortages of psychiatrists, nonspecialist community health workers must be used to increase coverage of necessary mental health and psychosocial programs.[7] Evidence supports the use of task shifting in mental health programs in developing countries when appropriate training, support, and supervision are provided.[8]

Although task shifting has been identified as a feasible way to increase coverage for programs, questions still remain about which types of interventions are most effective for mental health programs. Randomized controlled trials (RCT) of interventions are an important step, but represent unique challenges to organizations and institutions interested in conducting them. RCTs, by randomizing participants into either a treatment or a control group to make comparisons between the groups, are the most rigorous way of determining whether a cause-effect relationship exists between the treatment and the measured outcome. However, trials of interventions increase the financial and time burdens on organizations and those participating in implementing the trials. In many cases, organizations are not able to allocate sufficient human resources and time to a long-term research study, despite recognizing the benefits of this work.

Low availability of funding to support trials is a major barrier, particularly for mental health research. In addition, in many cases the community reaction itself presents the greatest challenge, since mental health and counseling are sometimes not well understood or are stigmatized. If organizations and individuals can overcome these two challenges, trials still carry a great deal of additional burden. For trials of mental health interventions, rigorous data collection and additional activities such as focus-group discussions and exit interviews with clients add to the amount of work counselors and organization staff must conduct to better understand the effectiveness, acceptability, and appropriateness of the intervention being tested.

Many of the challenges faced in testing an intervention through an RCT can be overcome more easily through partnerships between local community-based organizations (CBOs), and between CBOs and other entities such as universities and research groups. When partnerships are formed, information exchange increases and the burden of work is more evenly distributed, with each party bringing specific talents to the project.

As an example, the partnership of local CBOs with a university to conduct a trial of an intervention enables the CBOs to receive training and support for study design and research practices, while the university gains a better understanding of actual implementation in the field and benefits from the extensive local knowledge of the CBO partners in tailoring the intervention to each community and context.

Theory

Research and evaluation of mental health interventions, particularly in humanitarian situations and developing countries, is an essential component of program design and implementation. Whereas concepts and structures of programs from evidence-based practices in Western countries can be adapted to various settings, research and properly documented evaluation ensure that programs in humanitarian situations and developing countries are designed with the local situation and culture in mind and can assist when changes are necessary for applicability to the community being served. As is often the case with research projects, the participants themselves may not receive direct benefits from being part of the research. Collectively, however, they create a base from which research is generated that can ultimately measure applicability of interventions to that population and aid in the adaptation of the intervention to increase acceptability and development of the program being researched.

An important element of research and evaluation is to communicate findings back to the community. This can be done in several ways and may involve reviewing findings with key stakeholders in the community or bringing together small groups of community members for discussion. Reviewing findings allows the community to remain part of the research process and allows individuals to provide further insights into the findings, to give clarifications on data collected, and to point out key areas that may have been missed during data collection.

A strong research base combined with community-level feedback throughout the process is an essential part of developing ownership of the program to ensure that, if the intervention is found to be appropriate, it can be carried forward and expanded. In cases where community-based organizations and individuals are not involved in the research and evaluation process, further expansion of the intervention can be impeded by lack of understanding of the program, low interest in an intervention that is not community-driven, and lack of individuals on the ground who have experience running the intervention and continuing proper measurement and evaluation.

Faculty of the Applied Mental Health Research (AMHR) group at Johns Hopkins University Bloomberg School of Public Health have developed and used a stepwise approach to help psychosocial programs evaluate the effect of their interventions. This approach has four elements: (1) Informing program design through the collection of data at the community level and using these (and other available data) to develop programs to treat psycho-social problems and enhance functioning and well-being; (2) Improving implementation through training and supervision in new interventions and expanding ability to identify those who need these interventions through improved assessment tools; (3) Monitoring program activities and addressing problems as they arise; and (4) Evaluating impact at the level of the individual, to determine whether interventions are effective. This approach, collectively referred to as DIME (design, implementation, monitoring, and evaluation), has been completed successfully with service organizations in multiple countries. An additional component of this approach is the involvement of community members and individuals from partner organizations to collectively conduct the research and analyze the findings through ongoing meetings and discussions. The findings from the DIME approach are continually reviewed by both the AMHR group research team and individuals in the community in order to ensure that data, particularly quantitative data, are appropriately interpreted and understood within the context of the actual situation at the research site.

Data collection at the community level is the first step toward cultural appropriateness using this approach. Given the need for local contextualization of mental health and psychosocial issues, as well as the importance of language in describing mental health problems, it is important to capture local idioms of distress and suffering before any interventions are developed. This allows for selection and adaptation of an intervention most likely to be an appropriate fit for the community in which it will be implemented.

For example, Johns Hopkins applied step one of the DIME approach in Democratic Republic of Congo to first determine whether or not depression syndrome exists among mothers in Kinshasa, prior to development of an intervention and testing via a trial setting.[9] Researchers conducted interviews with a convenience sample of eighty mothers who had given birth to a living child within the previous two years using a method called free listing, which produces a list of answers in response to one primary question. In this instance, each woman was asked two questions and asked to list as many responses as possible for each: "What are the main problems of women with babies less than 1 year of age?" and "What are the main problems of women that affect their babies and children?" In addition, each woman was asked four additional questions to generate lists of activities mothers with newly born babies are expected to engage in. Falling under four separate domains of responsibilities for taking care of self, family, baby, and community, these lists produced data later used to develop questions for assessing functional impairment in a culturally relevant manner. Responses deemed to represent the same concept, as decided by the local interviewers working in the local language, were grouped together. The local interviewers found that "worry, torment of the mind, and lack of peace" were grouped together and felt these were different ways women were describing mental distress. The research team found that these problems were frequently mentioned by women and, thus, concluded that this cluster of problems for mental distress was the most important mental health problem. Therefore, the symptoms of distress were understood as symptoms of "*maladi ya souci*," which, translated from the local language of Lingala, could be understood as a syndrome of worry. Researchers then reviewed the Diagnostic and Statistical Manual of Mental Disorders and found that the diagnosis most closely matching this local syndrome was major depressive disorder, because symptoms and presentation were similar. In addition, it was found that anxiety symptoms appear within the syndrome as well, similar to findings in Western populations where both depression and anxiety commonly occur at the same time, particularly for postpartum depression. These steps of uncovering the local language and understanding how individuals understand and present with symptoms of mental health problems was a key step in identifying an appropriate intervention within the context of salient problems identified from within the community.

As discussed above, cultural appropriateness toward the problems being addressed and the design of the intervention is critically important in conducting cross-cultural programs and research on mental health. In addition, two other key elements must be taken into consideration when conducting research in the field: consent and confidentiality.

Having proficiency in local language and a contextually appropriate consent process are major steps in making sure that research activities are ethical and well understood by individuals and organizations participating in the research process. In many cases, research projects must conform to the regulations of the institutional review boards of each respective institution involved, and in some cases, there may be a local ethics committee with terms of practice as well. In any case, the process for obtaining consent must ensure that the individuals from whom consent is being sought clearly understand the benefits and risks of participation, as well as other ethical considerations.

Confidentiality is important for the consent process, the actual implementation of services during the research process, and the maintenance of data collected. For the protection of individuals enrolled in the study, who may experience or perceive a stigma attached to seeking and receiving mental health services, the first step to ensuring confidentiality is to make sure that no identifying information is collected or stored with data collected, typically by using unique identification numbers for each individual. It is important that face-to-face meetings with study participants take place in a private space deemed acceptable by the participant. This poses a challenge in many settings in the field, where private space is difficult to come by, homes often are shared with multiple people, and it may be seen as unacceptable or be misunderstood for individuals to meet privately with someone, particularly someone of the opposite sex, over multiple sessions and an extended time. Maintaining confidentiality is a key step in developing trust with participants, especially important when providing mental health services. Those providing the services and participating in a research study should receive proper training on maintaining confidentiality, but training alone is not sufficient and should be combined with open discussions about possible situations where confidentiality might be challenged or broken. Open discussions allow research teams in the field to better understand the concerns of and context for those meeting with study participants and handling data, allowing for additional measures to be put in place as needed.

Examples from the Thailand-Burma Border

THE MENTAL HEALTH ASSESSMENT
PROJECT, MAE SOT, THAILAND

In response to a lack of systematic services and research on the effectiveness of mental health interventions for persons from Burma, three CBOs partnered with the Applied Mental Health Research group in 2010 to conduct a three-phase, twenty-five-month research project (with funding support from Victims of Torture Program, USAID). The community-based organizations Social Action for Women, Assistance Association for Political Prisoners–Burma, and Mae Tao Clinic worked on all phases of data collection, implementation, and data analysis. Burma Border Projects, an international organization, provided administrative support for the research.

In 2010, the research project collected data using qualitative methods of free listing and key informant interviews to explore the local terminology for mental health problems among the population of individuals from

Burma now living in Thailand who have experienced torture and violence. Following this, a quantitative instrument was developed to measure the salient mental health problems identified in the first phase. This instrument underwent validation and was used in the final intervention phase of the project. The intervention worked with local partner organizations to train and provide supervision support to a group of counselors and clinical supervisors who provide mental health outreach services to survivors of torture and systematic violence from Burma now living in Mae Sot, Thailand, a town located on the Thailand side of the active border crossing point between Thailand and Burma with a total population of approximately 120,000, of which 84,270 are registered migrant workers from Burma.[10]

QUALITATIVE RESEARCH: FREE LISTING
AND KEY INFORMANT INTERVIEWS
Free Listing

To better understand the problems and situations of persons from Burma who have experienced torture and systematic violence committed by organized groups, data were collected that focused on current problems of torture-affected persons and what constituted the most important aspects of normal functioning for people in this community.

The study began with a free listing exercise in which each of the forty-five respondents was asked to generate four lists, in response the following questions:

First List: What are the problems that Burmese displaced in Thailand experience?
Second List: How do these problems affect their families?
Third List: What are the routine activities that Burmese adults do for themselves?
Fourth List: What are the routine activities that Burmese adults do for their families?

The first two questions generated lists of problems and the remaining two questions generated lists related to local functioning. Respondents were identified through contacts at the three partner offices as individuals thought to be knowledgeable about the problems and situation of Burmese living in Thailand. Prior to the start of the free listing activities, the list of respondents was checked to make sure that both women and men and a variety of ages were represented.

In addition to asking general community members to answer these questions, the research team further investigated problems specific to persons who had experienced torture and systematic violence. Fifteen new respondents were selected in the same way as the original sample. These informants were asked the following questions:

> *First List*: What are the problems that affect Burmese who have
>   experienced torture or systematic violence?
> *Second List*: How do these problems affect their families?

The study team reviewed the problem lists and identified selected problems for more detailed exploration. Selected problems were those that were not well understood, could easily form a focus for an intervention provided by local workers without prior mental health experience using available program resources, were mentioned by many respondents, and appeared to be severe, based on the description of the problem and what was currently known about it.

Selection of the mental health/psychosocial problems for further exploration in the key informant interviews was based on the number of free-list respondents who mentioned the problems, their apparent severity, and the likelihood that these problems could be addressed by interventions that could be provided by the community mental health workers. The three main problems selected by the study team were worried/afraid (*mi ba sait bu/kyout dae*), disappointment (*sait nyit*), and disagreement (*sait wun gwe*).[11]

Key Informant Interviews

The issues selected from the free lists formed the basis for key informant interviewing. Key informant interviewing is an in-depth method of interviewing used to explore in greater detail the selected issues emerging from the free lists. Key informants are persons particularly knowledgeable about the topics being explored and willing and able to talk at length about these topics. These individuals were asked to tell all they know about each of the problems selected from the free-list data, including a description of symptoms, effects, and causes, and what people do about the problem or think could/should be done about it.

For this study, all key informants were part of the local community and were knowledgeable about the problems of torture survivors, but did not deal with these problems professionally (such as would health care workers, social workers, or counselors).

Most symptoms found in this community are linked to specific events/ concerns in ways that suggest that the symptoms themselves may be wholly appropriate and therefore normal reactions to abnormal situations rather than mental disorders. However, these symptoms also reflect additional feelings of being overwhelmed. In some cases they may lead to behaviors that are not appropriate, such as being overly vigilant. Many of the problems described by respondents are problems in the family (drinking, violence, and separation) that result from stressors in their current environment. Key informant qualitative data indicate that violence and drinking are linked and both may be exacerbated by economic problems.

Developing and Validating an Instrument Based on Qualitative Research Findings

Following completion of the qualitative research activities described above, a draft instrument (questionnaire) was developed reflecting the psychosocial problems that emerged among the same target population of adults from Burma now living in Mae Sot, Thailand. Testing consisted of assessing the instrument's local acceptability, clarity, validity, and reliability among the target population. The main problems addressed in this instrument are symptoms of depression and posttraumatic stress disorder (PTSD). Secondary measurements include anger and aggression, social support networks, anxiety, functioning, alcohol use, and coping.

To measure these problems, existing psychological instruments were identified that reflected the main and secondary salient issues that arose. All of these scales had been adapted and used in multiple countries and cultures. Both the functioning and coping scales were derived and created directly from the qualitative work. In addition to these scales, the final composite instrument included some demographic questions and some basic service utilization questions. The final composite instrument is referred to as the Mental Health Assessment Project Thai/Burma Questionnaire (MHAP Instrument).

Initial interviews constituting the pilot study found that the instrument and interview process were acceptable and understandable to the interviewees. A total of 165 torture and violence survivors were interviewed. Of this total, eighty-two were men and eighty-two were women. Most participants were between 25 and 45 years of age. In addition to these initial 165 interviews, thirty-one of these individuals were reinterviewed within four days of their initial interview. It was found that all scales measured the appropriate symptoms (good validity). In addition, consistent and strong results (reliability) were found for all the instrument scales, with the exception of the functioning and alcohol use scale.

To make adjustments to the alcohol use scale, visual aids were developed and the wording of the questions themselves revised based on feedback from interviewers and interviewees. For necessary revisions to the functioning section, further qualitative data were collected using male and female focus-group discussions, held to develop an expanded list of male and female function items following analysis of the validation study data. Items and wording were selected directly from the focus-group discussion data and the group decided to include items in the function section for male and female tasks/activities based on frequency mentioned and applicability to the community.

A great deal of emphasis is given to locally defined measure of daily functioning because of the effect that mental health problems can have on daily functioning and the need for locally relevant questions about this. For example, questions typically asked in Western countries are difficult to ask in situations where one may not face difficulty because the activity does not exist. For example, asking someone whether they have difficulty climbing stairs is difficult to adapt to situations where stairs don't exist. In addition, even less culture-specific questions may not have applicability across populations with varying levels of physical requirements or where men and women have distinctly different roles, as is the case in most developing countries. Therefore, developing the MHAP Instrument focused on creating locally relevant measures of function for both men and women.

The MHAP Instrument can now be used to assess the impact of a community-based psychosocial intervention on PTSD and depression symptoms among displaced Burmese in Mae Sot, Thailand. The methods used in this project—qualitative methods resulting in instrument selection and adaptation, followed by instrument piloting and validity/reliability testing—have been used with success in other areas of the world (Southern Iraq and Kurdistan) under the same overarching grant. These methods are particularly useful in situations where need has not been well measured and the effect of interventions has not been demonstrated.

Selection of the Intervention

The intervention selected, based on the qualitative research in the study, was a psychotherapeutic intervention aimed at treating mood and anxiety problems in adults, named Components Based Intervention (CBI). CBI is based on similar transdiagnostic psychotherapeutic interventions in the United States, but was specifically adapted for low-resource settings that rely on task shifting or the use of community mental health workers (CMHWs) or lay counselors. The differences of CBI from high-income transdiagnostic models include: (1) a more limited number of elements, (2) simplified language, (3) step-by-step guides for each element, and (4) training and supervision designed to ultimately place the decisions about element selection, sequencing, and dosing in the hands of CMHWs.

In transdiagnostic approaches, counselors are trained to implement the common elements (or components) that are effective and piece multiple components together depending on the presenting problem of the client. CBI was designed to treat a range of symptoms within common mental health problems, such as symptoms related to traumatic experiences, depression, anxiety, and substance use. This then allows for a single training, while giving counselors the ability to treat a range of problems. CBI consists of ten evidence-based elements, such as "getting active" or gradual exposure, that can be combined into different flows to meet the most pressing mental health need of the client. A typical CBI course of treatment involves eight to ten sessions, but is flexible to go longer if the client needs more time. CBI was determined to be a particularly useful approach in the study setting, because data from the qualitative study and the validity study, as well as local input, indicated that there were multiple psychosocial and mental health problems within the target population. Given its flexibility to treat different presenting problems, CBI was chosen by the AMHR group and the implementing partners as the most appropriate intervention for use in Mae Sot, Thailand.

Training and Selection Process for
Counselors and Clinical Supervisors

Counselors and clinical supervisors were nominated by their respective organizations and ranged in age from 22 to 61. Of the counselors and clinical supervisors working on the research project, only two counselors had previous training in counseling and concurrently held a position as counselors at their organization, and one clinical supervisor was a physician with counseling experience. Counselors had to be over the age of 18, be available to attend all training days, work either part-time or full-time in the trial, be able to read and write Burmese, have done previous work providing social support, and have an interest in mental health and counseling. Clinical supervisors had to be significantly older than 18, have a high school education and at least some advanced training, be bilingual in English and Burmese, work full-time, and have some previous counseling experience.

Counselors and clinical supervisors both received a two-week initial training, with clinical supervisors receiving additional training at that time toward their duties as supervisors. The primary responsibilities for counselors included holding community awareness campaigns/workshops, recruiting clients into the research study, providing weekly counseling sessions for clients, and attending a weekly supervision meeting with their clinical supervisors. While clinical supervisors assisted counselors in their recruitment activities in the community and occasionally counseled clients of their own, their primary tasks were to conduct the weekly supervision meetings, provide clinical advice directly to counselors, and maintain regular communication with the clinical trainers for supervision, using both e-mail and phone calls.

Counselors commonly reported that this training was extremely beneficial because they received instruction in a systematic method whereby they were given steps to follow and the means to set up a treatment plan for individual clients. Prior to the start of the research project, no organizations in the research setting were providing systematic counseling services with monitoring and evaluation components. Instead, many organizations provided general training on mental health, psychosocial activities, and general counseling skills. The training provided by the research project, and the overall approach to standardized monitoring and evaluation of both individual CMHW skills and client outcomes, were well-received by counselors, particularly because this new approach was felt to provide a more efficient system in which to carry out services.

The initial training was designed to be short, to take into account the reality for many low- and middle-income or developing areas where clinical trainers are in short supply or have limited time. Continued ongoing supervision and small-group work were believed to be sufficient to develop the skills of the CMHWs, and while data from the research project indicate that the CMHWs can maintain fidelity to the intervention, it is important to note that CMHW motivation might be maintained or improved through more systematic, regularly scheduled refresher trainings.

Supervision
For the research project, counselors were put into one of three groups, with each group led by a clinical supervisor. The clinical supervisors were responsible for bringing the group together for weekly meetings to review the counseling provided to clients, discuss recruitment and enrollment of clients, and organize the information from the counselors to share with the project research team and clinical trainers. Group size ranged from six to seven counselors, and two of the groups had a mixture of part-time and full-time counselors.

Although the initial plan was to have only weekly supervision meetings, clinical supervisors found that they had difficulty providing supervision to each person in the large group, particularly when caseloads were full. In response, the clinical supervisors took time outside the weekly group meeting to meet individually with counselors. In addition, they also met with counselors just before and just after their sessions with clients to prepare them and correct mistakes or answer questions as needed.

Recruitment for the Study and Enrollment into the Study: Lessons Learned

One of the greatest challenges faced by the counselors in this research project was the community's lack of understanding and familiarity with both mental health and research on this topic, particularly regarding understanding and acceptance of the research and intervention processes. In addition, the counselors in the research project were the first group to attempt to systematically conduct counseling activities in the community.

Early on in the study, after receiving training on the counseling method, counselors were tasked with going into the community to recruit potential clients for the research study. At that time, they were faced with community members who generally did not want to cooperate with or listen to the counselors. The community believed that "mental health is just for crazy people . . . and avoided these types of services and the [people] providing the services because they did not have a clear understanding of counseling."

Compounding the fact that the community in general had a low level of understanding of counseling, it was also felt that community recognition of the counselors as service providers had not been established. One counselor explained "the community does not believe in the counselors because they recognize each other since they are living in the same area. They don't want to receive counseling from these counselors." This indicates that community-based mental health service providers potentially face additional challenges because of their dual role as a community member and counselor. Particularly in this setting, where the community believes only highly trained physicians deal with mental health issues, the counselors were met with the obstacle of starting work without community recognition of their abilities and roles as service providers, as can often be the case when task shifting occurs with new levels of workers.

The counselors developed new strategies for approaching the community to explain their work. Culturally appropriate posters and flyers were created that also incorporated pictures to assist with explaining their work to individuals with low literacy. In addition, the counselors created a short program in cooperation with a radio station commonly listened to by people from Burma living in Thailand. While these were useful approaches, counselors explained a key change in their approach to the community that helped increase community acceptance: going as a group to approach potential clients rather than as an individual.

Later in the research project, through these community-based awareness-raising efforts, the community response slowly shifted, becoming more positive. Counselors saw a marked increase in community understanding and acceptance since the start of their work in the research project. Counselors also widened their network of contacts by working together with current clients who were willing to introduce them to others who might be interested in receiving services.

Counselors also faced challenges because clients did not want to talk about their past history, often explaining to the counselors that they had put the past behind them and were more focused on problems in the current situation. Counselors explained that this disconnect between clients' interest and counselors' aim in the project made it difficult to meet research project goals, since the clients wanted to talk about one thing and counselors were tasked with providing counseling for another.

Individual client availability was also a challenge for counselors. The clients for whom these counselors were providing services were migrants living in an unstable situation in which they moved all the time to other areas, sometimes unexpectedly. In general, counselors empathized with the situation of their clients and understood the reasons they were not available, as well as acknowledging that this was a minor problem compared to other challenges faced.

Related to client availability on a weekly basis was the issue of availability for the duration of counseling sessions. Availability for the duration of the sessions was a combination of overall availability and level of interest on the part of the clients. Although the intervention was designed to provide complete treatment in eight to ten one-hour sessions of counseling per client, a total duration shorter than initially planned, the length of time was still problematic. Counselors often made extra efforts to travel to the clients, were flexible in rescheduling appointments, and would make adjustments to the number of sessions per week or length of a given session to better accommodate the clients' availability.

Ongoing Data Collection during the Trial

As stated earlier, trials of interventions include rigorous collection of multiple forms of data. This is often seen as a burden put on the service providers and organizations, but in this research project these data were found to be instrumental in motivating counselors as well.

The role of data collection, either for trials such as this or for regular program implementation, should not be viewed solely as an added burden for service providers. Instead, data collection should be integrated into their regular work, since it was commonly reported as a source of positive motivation.

Case Stories
CHALLENGES OF RESEARCH AND PROGRAMS IN THE FIELD

Because counselors in this program came from Burma to work in Thailand, most individuals did not have official legal status in Thailand. Some of the counselors had papers or identification cards provided by their organization, which afforded some protection from arrest and detention by Thai authorities, but did not appear to do enough to alleviate their worries regarding security. The research project responded to the concern regarding security by putting a security plan into action whereby all counselors and clinical supervisors could access support if arrested by the Thai police.

Counselors also reported that their general work as a counselor sometimes caused them to experience negative consequences of additional stress and emotions. Counselors explained this in terms of "being emotionally tired" and said that even though the work is not physical in nature, their minds became tired. The research project team took steps to alleviate the negative emotional consequences of this work by limiting the caseload of each counselor to a manageable number (one to two clients if part time and three to five clients if full time), asking clinical supervisors to meet with individuals as often as possible to ask about their emotional states, and including sessions in their training and supervision specifically focused on self-care.

All the CMHWs had experienced an array of traumatic events in their past. This was cause for concern for the research project's team because it was unclear what the implications would be for the counselors' own well-being after listening to and counseling other individuals through their past events and problems. In general, counselors reported that they were able to learn to separate themselves from the stories of their clients and professionally provide them with counseling without carrying too much of the stress from that session away with them. This developed over time, though, and counselors often discussed how they felt at the start of their work compared with their feelings after several months of experience. They found that their work involved more emotions, compared with being a general health worker (a position that some had experience with prior to the research project), and explained that when they first started they had difficulty sleeping, cried, and carried emotions from a session with them. After some time, however, counselors explained that they used skills learned from their training and other positive coping strategies to deal with the emotional aspect of the work.

An additional problem faced by counselors was that their clients were all migrant workers living in unstable conditions. These clients often expressed facing current problems in addition to their past traumatic events, while the counselors were trained to provide counseling for the latter. During sessions with clients and their work as counselors, however, they found that the majority of clients' current problems were related to food and housing. In addition, they felt that the clients expected some financial support from the counselors to help with their daily expenses despite a lack of funds to provide this.

An additional negative consequence for many counselors was lack of time because of other work or commitments. For those with other responsibilities in their organizations, it was often expressed that they hold multiple positions and feel pressure from their organizations to prioritize the other jobs over that of being a counselor. Management of the workload caused stress for counselors personally, but stress was also caused by lack of time and support for counselors for their counseling sessions and for managing non-counseling support requests. It was often explained that counselors felt their work was more difficult than that of health workers working on general physical health of clients because counseling work takes more time, particularly to build trust with the client. Many counselors commented that the additional time needed to build trust, listen to long stories from the clients, assist clients with non-counseling support requests, and the need for repeated visits was difficult to manage, not because of the emotions involved, but because of the necessity of taking time for these activities.

COPING

To deal with the negative effects experienced during their work, many counselors reported individually initiated, positive coping strategies. Most accomplished this by applying skills learned from the counseling training to themselves. For example, counselors explained that they would look at negative or problematic thoughts they had and change the thought to be more positive, a method employed with their clients. In general, counselors found the techniques applied during counseling beneficial for them and practiced on themselves on a regular basis to cope with the frustrations and stress of their job. In some cases, counselors acknowledged that stress was present mainly during the time of the counseling session, but they were able to "leave all the stress, . . . [not] take that stress home," and "relax within a short time." Relaxation often came from activities such as playing guitar, singing, watching television or spending time with friends and family; however, it was also mentioned that counselors would benefit from support for their coping by having someone they could talk to. Counselors recommended that organizations and research projects take steps to have some individuals from outside regular project positions provide counseling and emotional support to them. Although clinical supervisors were in a position to watch for warning signs of emotional problems and stress among the counselors in their groups, it was often reported that counselors felt the clinical supervisors were too busy to provide sufficient support. Therefore, counselors expressed a desire for a designated person or persons from whom they could receive counseling and support. This highlights the importance not only of teaching coping and self-care, but also of the role of supervisors in monitoring the well-being of their counselors. While supervisors cannot be expected to provide all support that might be needed, the level of contact they have with the counselors means they are in a unique position to notice the need for a response and work with counselors to get the support they need.

HOW BENEFICIARIES VIEW THIS TYPE OF PROGRAM

Between August and September 2012, four interviewers worked in pairs to conduct in-depth interviews with treatment clients and wait control clients from the study to improve the ongoing use of CBI with persons from Burma and inform the application of CBI counseling in other settings. A random sample of forty clients who had completed their participation in the RCT was interviewed. The feedback survey consisted of a total of thirty-four questions. Treatment clients were asked to respond to all thirty-four questions, while wait control clients were asked only the seven questions that applied to them.

From the feedback provided by this sample, it was determined that most clients who participated in the study were recruited directly from project counselors or other acquaintances. In general, though many clients were initially unfamiliar with counseling, they had few negative perceptions prior to starting treatment and believed that participating in the project would help them feel better. It is possible that these findings are linked, and that this trust of the project is related to the close personal relationships between the project counselors, as members of their community, and their clients.

Few obstacles were reported as barriers to receiving counseling. Transportation concerns were addressed by allowing clients and counselors to agree on a meeting location that best suited their needs, sometimes having the counselor travel to meet the client and sometimes arranging transportation with another person. Security and privacy were also not major concerns. The most frequently noted obstacle was scheduling, which was often overcome by making appointments in advance and allowing the timing of sessions to be flexible.

In general, the duration and quality of services were reported to be good or acceptable. The most useful skills clients mentioned acquiring were techniques for managing feelings and reframing thoughts. Clients reported few difficulties; those most commonly reported were the emotional difficulty of recounting personal stories/memories. Clients also mentioned that the first session was the most difficult because they were not yet comfortable with the counseling methods.

Feedback on individual counselors was almost exclusively positive, including reports that counselors were both friendly and knowledgeable. All clients said they would recommend this counseling method to others, except one client who said he or she did not have anyone to make the recommendation to. Benefits clients mentioned included improved mental health, acquisition of skills related to maintaining personal mental health, empowerment such as confidence and mental strength, and having a safe environment to share their feelings.

SUPERVISION

Clinical supervisors often spoke of taking more time to work one-on-one with CMHWs, particularly those without much prior experience, to encourage them and increase their confidence. Clinical supervisors also stepped in for some situations in which they noticed their counselors having difficulty managing their workload. In one case, clinical supervisors felt they noticed that counselors were too busy, often working as teachers or caregivers in boardinghouses, and took action to report this to the counselors' managers for their other work. They explained that this work as a counselor is also part of the organization's overall work and asked the managers to reduce the overall amount of work for the counselors. In most cases, this was understood by the managers, who were able to work out a better system for the counselors' workloads, such as the managers approving regularly scheduled time off for counselor to have supervision meetings and to see clients.

POSITIVE EFFECTS

Beyond financial remuneration, many counselors found that they learned new skills, experienced positive self-development, created relationships with others, and developed personal coping skills as a result of the project. The majority of counselors commented on gaining personal and professional skills such as communication, listening, and observation skills. Counselors also expressed experiencing changes related to their emotions and feeling more mature and crying less. Self-development was particularly striking for the former political prisoners working as counselors. At the start of the project, team members were concerned about the potential for negative effects on these counselors in particular; however, they all expressed in some way that they felt the benefits for themselves as individuals outweighed the challenges they faced working with clients and the emotions experienced from the work.

Furthermore, counselors found that their relationships with others improved as a result of this work. Counselors explained that they experienced less fighting and more understanding within their families as a result of learning to be more patient and understanding through their work. Each counselor explained some way that this work had allowed him or her to develop as an individual, and many talked about being able to connect more with others. Despite the fact that the research project did not explicitly aim to have the work influence the personal lives of the counselors, it is interesting to see that they were able to find ways to connect the work to their lives and make improvements based on their experiences as a counselors for others. For many, it was not only a way to develop personally, but also a way to create a network of friends and acquaintances in the community.

Notes

1   Lincoln Chen et al., "Human Resources for Health: Overcoming the Crisis," *Lancet* 364, no. 9449 (December 27, 2004): 1984–1990, doi:10.1016/S0140-6736(04)17482-5; International Organization for Migration, *Assessment of Mobility and HIV Vulnerability among Myanmar Migrant Sex Workers and Factory Workers in Mae Sot District, Tak Province, Thailand* (Bangkok, Thailand: International Organization for Migration, 2007).

2   Hani Mowafi et al., "Facing the Challenges in Human Resources for Humanitarian Health," *Prehospital and Disaster Medicine* 22, no. 5 (October 2007): 351–359.

3   International Organization for Migration, *Assessment of Mobility and HIV Vulnerability.*

4   Ibid.

5   Mowafi et al., "Facing the Challenges in Human Resources."

6   Catherine I Lee et al., "Internally Displaced Human Resources for Health: Villager Health Worker Partnerships to Scale Up a Malaria Control Programme in Active Conflict Areas of Eastern Burma," *Global Public Health* 4, no. 3 (2009): 229–241, doi:10.1080/17441690802676360; Luke C Mullany et al., "Impact of Community-Based Maternal Health Workers on Coverage of Essential Maternal Health Interventions among Internally Displaced Communities in Eastern Burma: The MOM Project," *PLoS Med* 7, no. 8 (August 3, 2010): e1000317, doi:10.1371/journal.pmed.1000317.

7   Laura Janneck et al., "Human Resources in Humanitarian Health Working Group Report," *Prehospital and Disaster Medicine* 24, suppl. 2 (August 2009): s184–193.

8   Ibid.; Vikram Patel, "The Future of Psychiatry in Low- and Middle-income Countries," *Psychological Medicine* 39, no. 11 (November 2009): 1759–1762; Sudipto Chatterjee et al., "Evaluation of a Community-Based Rehabilitation Model for Chronic Schizophrenia in Rural India," *British Journal of Psychiatry: Journal of Mental Science* 182 (January 2003): 57–62; Amit Dias et al., "The Effectiveness of a Home Care Program for Supporting Caregivers of Persons with Dementia in Developing Countries: A Randomised Controlled Trial from Goa, India," *PLoS ONE* 3, no. 6 (June 4, 2008): e2333, doi:10.1371/journal.pone.0002333.

9   Judith K Bass et al., "Post-Partum Depression in Kinshasa, Democratic Republic of Congo: Validation of a Concept Using a Mixed-Methods Cross-Cultural Approach," *Tropical Medicine & International Health: TM & IH* 13, no. 12 (December 2008): 1534–1542, doi:10.1111/j.1365-3156.2008.02160.x.

10   International Organization for Migration, *Assessment of Mobility and HIV Vulnerability.*

11   The terms "worried" and "afraid" (*mi ba sait bu/kyout dae*) were combined by the interviewers during analysis because these phrases were considered to have the same meaning.

Bibliography

Bass, Judith K, Robert W Ryder, Marie-Christine Lammers, Thibaut N Mukaba, and Paul A Bolton. "Post-Partum Depression in Kinshasa, Democratic Republic of Congo: Validation of a Concept Using a Mixed-Methods Cross-Cultural Approach." *Tropical Medicine & International Health: TM & IH* 13, no. 12 (December 2008): 1534–1542. doi:10.1111/j.1365-3156.2008.02160.x.

Chatterjee, Sudipto, Vikram Patel, Achira Chatterjee, and Helen A Weiss. "Evaluation of a Community-Based Rehabilitation Model for Chronic Schizophrenia in Rural India." *British Journal of Psychiatry: Journal of Mental Science* 182 (January 2003): 57–62.

Chen, Lincoln, Timothy Evans, Sudhir Anand, Jo Ivey Boufford, Hilary Brown, Mushtaque Chowdhury, Marcos Cueto, et al. "Human Resources for Health:

Overcoming the Crisis." *Lancet* 364, no. 9449 (December 27, 2004): 1984–1990.
doi:10.1016/S0140-6736(04)17482-5.

Dias, Amit, Michael E Dewey, Jean D'Souza, Rajesh Dhume, Dilip D Motghare, KS
Shaji, Rajiv Menon, Martin Prince, and Vikram Patel. "The Effectiveness of a Home
Care Program for Supporting Caregivers of Persons with Dementia in Developing
Countries: A Randomised Controlled Trial from Goa, India." *PLoS ONE* 3, no. 6
(June 4, 2008): e2333. doi:10.1371/journal.pone.0002333.

International Organization for Migration. *Assessment of Mobility and HIV
Vulnerability among Myanmar Migrant Sex Workers and Factory Workers in Mae
Sot District, Tak Province, Thailand.* Bangkok, Thailand: International Organiza-
tion for Migration, 2007.

Janneck, Laura, Nicholas Cooper, Seble Frehywot, Hani Mowafi, and Karen Hein.
"Human Resources in Humanitarian Health Working Group Report." *Prehospital
and Disaster Medicine* 24, suppl. 2 (August 2009): s184–193.

Lee, Catherine I, Linda S Smith, Eh Kalu Shwe Oo, Brent C Scharschmidt, Emily
Whichard, Thart Kler, Thomas J. Lee, and Adam K Richards. "Internally Displaced
Human Resources for Health: Villager Health Worker Partnerships to Scale Up a
Malaria Control Programme in Active Conflict Areas of Eastern Burma." *Global
Public Health* 4, no. 3 (2009): 229–241. doi:10.1080/17441690802676360.

Mowafi, Hani, Kristin Nowak, Karen Hein, and Human Resources Working Group.
"Facing the Challenges in Human Resources for Humanitarian Health."
Prehospital and Disaster Medicine 22, no. 5 (October 2007): 351–359.

Mullany, Luke C, Thomas J Lee, Lin Yone, Catherine I Lee, Katherine C Teela, Palae
Paw, Eh Kalu Shwe Oo, et al. "Impact of Community-Based Maternal Health
Workers on Coverage of Essential Maternal Health Interventions among Internally
Displaced Communities in Eastern Burma: The MOM Project." *PLoS Med* 7, no. 8
(August 3, 2010): e1000317. doi:10.1371/journal.pmed.1000317.

Patel, Vikram. "The Future of Psychiatry in Low- and Middle-Income Countries."
Psychological Medicine 39, no. 11 (November 2009): 1759–1762.

Part V.

Looking to Peace in the Future

Chapter 12

The Other Side of Political Trauma

Protest, Empowerment, and Transformation

Khin Ohmar and Mary O'Kane

Introduction

Burma's people have enacted rich forms of protest against state oppression throughout their turbulent modern history, including this current transition period from military dictatorship to "military-guided" democracy. Among the significant sites of protest against Burma's military regime that took state power in 1962 are Burma's interstate borderlands with Thailand, Bangladesh, India, and China. In 1988, the regime's violent suppression of nationwide popular protests brought more than 10,000 prodemocratic activists to join allied ethno-nationalist groups in border regions, just as global Cold War political structures unexpectedly began disintegrating. Since then, the types of political resistance undertaken in the borderlands have proliferated and transformed in ways not possible in space dominated by the military regime. Burma's border-based civil society movement has emerged over the past fifteen years in these politically marginalized spaces and comprises an estimated five hundred human rights–oriented organizations, though actual numbers are fluid because of localized political and international funding contingencies. These activist organizations focus on political advocacy, human rights advocacy and education, and welfare services in areas such as women's and children's rights, refugee rights, internally displaced persons rights, migrant and labor rights, health, media, education, community development, and the environment.

Burma's civil society organizations based in the interstate borderlands work in a complex environment that includes local and displaced communities from Burma and other states, other groups from Burma's opposition movement, multiple types of officials from multiple states, secular and faith-based international nongovernmental organizations (NGOs), intergovernmental agencies, globalized media, and advocacy, solidarity, and research actors. However, they frequently face exclusion pressures from some actors they could and should be working alongside. Unfortunately this is often the case in the context of international humanitarian responses to traumatized communities, where activist groups are usually viewed by international humanitarian organizations as unrelated to trauma and outside their range of appropriate responses to it. This is even though activists are part of, not different from, the community that is going through a traumatic experience such as civil war or military dictatorship. Karen, Ta'ang, and Kachin activists, for example, are living through the same civil war and oppression as others in their Karen, Ta'ang, and Kachin communities. From our perspective, this conceptual oversight prevents some important questions from being asked about the effects of trauma in conflict-affected communities. For instance, where does this undying commitment of activists in the community to struggle for justice and peace in Burma come from? Given Burma's protracted political problems, how is this commitment being carried from generation to generation? If some activists have never been to the front lines of armed conflict or to their homeland, how does their commitment to bringing about political and social change stay with them?

Trauma in and around Burma can be understood as political either because it is caused directly by armed conflict and oppression or by discrimination compounded by Burma's political problems. This chapter starts from the position that responses to political trauma by those who experience the trauma are not limited to victimhood but also include protest.[1] Victimhood is broadly understood here as a state of being wherein a person and/or community not only incurs grievous, debilitating harm but also lacks, or is perceived to lack, adequate agency to recover and act for themselves without external (to the community as well as the individual) intervention and representation. As a concept, victimhood commonly denotes a combined sense of suffering, helplessness, and passiveness. While it is widely recognized that trauma can induce a victim response, it is less recognized that it can also engender a protest response. A protest response is understood broadly here as a mobilizing effect, a positive political agency wherein community members organize to change their harmful situations. Understanding protest as a response to political trauma stems from recognizing that political trauma is caused by problematic sociopolitical and economic *systems*.[2] Therefore, these systems need to be changed to heal and move forward, and systemic change requires organized community activism. Accordingly, people in Burma's traumatized communities have responded to the systemic nature of their political trauma with this fiery spirit of outrage, duty, and determination that "we have to do something about this!"

It is our observation that the recognition of protest as a dimension of political trauma responses is largely missing from conventional medical approaches, including as they are applied in international humanitarian contexts. This becomes the case when, in the course of implementing their programs, humanitarian approaches abstract peoples' trauma from its systemic (i.e., broader political) context and treat only the individual. That is, humanitarian responses are directed at individual-level trauma, particularly as an illness, without recognizing that it is also related to community-level trauma. When international humanitarian organizations look at activist movements emerging from conflict-affected communities, they generally fail to see the relationship between protest and trauma, or they separate protest from trauma. Thus, they conceptualize activists and traumatized individuals as two separate groups: one to be engaged and the other outside their range of professional concern.

To the contrary, we argue that protest and victimhood are part of the same community response to political trauma and that protest responses need recognition, respect, and support as much as victim responses do. Protest and victimhood are two sides of the same coin, so to speak. This positive and productive link between trauma and protest, we argue, must be fostered to support community recovery, empowerment, and the possibility of working toward a peaceful and potential-filled future. A broader conceptualization of trauma that recognizes protest would encourage international actors to develop a more in-depth and historically and geographically contextualized—that is, a more comprehensive—understanding of community responses to political trauma, including diverse forms of political and social activism. This would illuminate spaces of policy and program overlap and open up options for new, more inclusive, holistic, and effective program and policy options for responding to the needs of trauma-affected communities.

Even though nearly all Burma's border-based activists live with effects of trauma, our purpose is not to describe their trauma experiences, analyze their effects, or identify differences in resilience to traumatic symptoms between activists and non-activists. It is to highlight some main activities and methods of operation of Burma's border-based civil society movement that are context-specific protest responses to the political trauma inflicted on and in their communities. In doing so we aim to promote recognition of, and respect for, the activism and other forms of positive political agency of people suffering in this way. We acknowledge that the opinions expressed here are ours and should not be assumed to represent others in Burma's heterogeneous border-based movement. Also, we acknowledge our privileged position, enabling us to express our opinions through this English-language, academic, and professionally focused publication and the asymmetrical power relations that this engenders in relation to the still-silenced voices in

Burma's resistance movement and communities unable to participate directly in this or other globalized public spheres.

This chapter is structured into three sections. The first section discusses the relationship between trauma and activism and the relationship between activists and international humanitarian actors to explain why autonomous protest responses of traumatized communities are marginalized. The second section, the main focus of the chapter, discusses five areas of activism undertaken by Burma's border-based activists: movement-building, welfare, social and political critique, advocacy, and articulating a vision of a future Burma. Exploring all dimensions of activism is beyond this chapter's scope; therefore, only some aspects are discussed to provide an overview. The third section briefly discusses Burma's current political transition and its implications for border-based activism.

Trauma, Activism, and Political Borders

The relationship between politics, trauma, and protest is seemingly obvious but has attracted little empirical or theoretical attention in any field. From Khin Ohmar's experience as an activist since 1988, work in Burma's border-based movement, and over two hundred research interviews O'Kane has participated in with border-based activists, we know that accumulative and ongoing experiences of personal and community trauma feature predominantly as motivation for why activists do what they do. Poststructuralist international relations theorist Jenny Edkins has made some observations of the relationship between political trauma and protest that resonate with Burma's border-based activist experiences. She suggests that a key aspect of the psychological impact of political trauma is a deep sense of betrayal that comes with realizing that the state and community, which we are socialized to believe from an early age will ensure protection and security, are in fact sources of violence and insecurity.[3] That is, political trauma involves a realization by individuals of a profound disconnect between the promises of protection made by state leaders and community and actual practices of violence in their world. This schism forces an attempt to come to terms with this injustice, to make sense of it.

People in trauma-affected communities can thus face a dilemma: do they bury their truth, deny their reality, and swallow their words, or do they resist and fight for justice and change? There appears a choice between a victim and a protest response. Political and social crises are precisely the moments when agency—the human capacity to change one's conditions—is most urgently needed and the political and ethical agent in each of us is called upon to respond.[4] Protest is not exerted "against all odds" in times of political trauma but is part of the range of human responses to it. However, the urge to respond occurs along with the effects of serious psychological and often also physical injury and in the face of attracting more harm. In this way, as Edkins argues, "the concept of trauma oscillates between victimhood and protest and can be linked with or articulated to either."[5]

In and around Burma, protest takes myriad forms, not all readily recognizable by those outside the situation. Kevin Heppner has shown that Karen villagers' facing human rights abuses from patrolling Burma Army battalions hide in jungle areas near their villages not because they are victims but as a strategy of refusing to surrender their homes and fields to military control.[6] Karen Human Rights Group reports document the ongoing positive agency exerted by children, women, and village groups facing militarization and conflict.[7] Forced migration across Burma's borders is also a form of resistance; it is a refusal to live under the terms of the military regime and a survival strategy. Women, children, non-Burman ethnic people, and lesbian, gay, bisexual, transgender, and intersex people who experience trauma rooted in discrimination compounded by pressures of authoritarian conditions and displacement also exert positive agency in many ways.[8]

As members of Burma's trauma-affected communities became more empowered, they wanted to do more to bring about positive change. They organized more systematic responses to their community's needs wherever they were located. Their commitment to their work continued despite remaining psychologically vulnerable, though many relate how the richness and complexity of friendship and solidarity in their organizations contributed to trauma healing over time. The need to respond effectively pushed activists to seek financial, material, and knowledge resources to improve their capacity and organize into groups among themselves as well as with regional and international groups. They began establishing offices, strategizing activities and programs, and building solidarity networks. Their ability to organize autonomously has been increasingly facilitated by post-Cold War factors such as intensifying globalization processes moving into and across state borderlands, including human rights norms.

Interestingly, however, as border-based activists became more autonomously organized and empowered, the international humanitarian aid community working in the area largely responded to them with suspicion: "These activities are political, these activists are political. We don't associate with them because we only deliver humanitarian services." Activists saw a line being drawn through their community by international actors, dividing those perceived to be acting as victims from those enacting protest responses. This conceptual division categorizing members of the traumatized community shapes international approaches to the community as a whole.

The categorical distinction between victim and activist in international humanitarian settings has its roots in dominant accounts of the modern nation-state system. These accounts articulate and work to perpetuate specific understandings of politics/international relations and related concepts such as forced displacement and humanitarianism.[9] Critical analysis of international humanitarian regimes—regimes that emerged around the United Nations High Commissioner for Refugees (UNHCR), whose norms, values, and practices set standards for all international humanitarian settings—reveal their role not only as providing relief assistance, but also as participating with states in the ordering and disciplining of displacement through mechanisms of social and political control (e. g., the rules determining who is eligible for assistance and under what conditions).[10] These mechanisms include the prohibiting or excluding of autonomous (political) activity by people in displaced communities in humanitarian spaces such as refugee camps. An outcome of this logic is to bring into being a binary opposition between the humanitarian and the political.[11]

Critical world politics theorist, Peter Nyers, analyzes how the humanitarian realm in these dominant accounts of international relations is granted positive attributes and becomes understood as the sphere of ethical behavior while, as its opposite, the political realm is cast negatively as the domain of cynical, self-interested and "devilish" behavior.[12] From this perspective, humanitarian action and political action are cast as two distinct fields and separate modes of acting while being accorded moral weighting in oppositional relation to each other. Thus, a perceived encroachment of politics into a humanitarian sphere is seen as threatening to the "neutral" status of humanitarian action.[13]

Operating according to the rules of the international relations/politics frame set by states, international NGOs' approaches define the limits of humanitarian spaces by respecting lines distinguishing what states define as political from what they define as nonpolitical; lines that cut through trauma-affected communities. These lines take multiple forms; spatial boundaries such as interstate borders or camp fences; identity borders such as the distinction between refugees and forced migrants without state travel documents, and behavioral borders such as the distinction between displaced people who don't engage in activism and those who do. Border-based activists, however, approach the community as a whole, regardless of where state borders lie.

The dominance of statist world views undermines the political and social complexity and ambiguity inherent in humanitarianism and activism by overlooking the political grounding of humanitarianism while obscuring the social grounding of border-based activism. This permits activists and their activism to be framed first and foremost as something other than humanitarian activities. The binary opposition between the humanitarian and the political manifests as a tension between humanitarian actors and border-based activists, undermining respect and communication while engendering suspicion and distance between the two types of actors—both of whom are responding to the community's trauma. It is important to recognize that there are individual humanitarian actors who do not subscribe to this tension and work collaboratively with community-based activists. Unfortunately, their approach does not reach an institutional level and their influence fades after they leave, as they almost always do when displacement is protracted and placements last for an average of two years.

At stake here is the marginalization of important dimensions of communities' own responses to their trauma. Recognizing protest as a response to trauma, the issue thus becomes one of how to take a more holistic and inclusive approach to trauma in situations of displacement. One place to begin is to examine the asymmetrical power relationships that structure life in humanitarian situations that position international humanitarian actors as rescuers who know and are in charge of what needs to be done and members of traumatized communities as helpless, lacking expert knowledge, and in need of rescue and instruction. Instead, we could ask how can we build relationships that are genuinely and self-reflectively based on equality and partnership? What do such relationships look like in practice? What opportunities are revealed by such an approach? A way forward, we suggest, is to explore the diverse, rich, and complex forms of social and political activism already engaged in by activists, appreciate the agency and expertise they manifest, and look for opportunities to collaborate.

Civil Society Activism in the Borderlands

Burma's border-based civil society has been made possible because its activists remain embedded in their communities and the interstate borderlands at the same time. They do not perceive their communities as split into separate political categories by state borders and camps but negotiate state borders to access their community members where they are located. As their communities span state borders, so too does the activist movement, making it difficult to place them and their communities as a whole clearly inside or outside Burma. In fact, a significant part of their success comes from their ability to traverse Burma's territorial borders. From this position on the very edges of the modern nation-state system, activists and their communities struggle against strong marginalizing forces. With the state/citizen bond nonexistent and with denial of the state protection citizens would normally expect to receive, activists are forced to pursue their activism outside any state institutional framework.

While an absolute distinction between violent and nonviolent forms of protest is impossible in conflict and politically oppressive situations, border-based activists play a unique role in the peaceful struggle for justice and federal democracy in Burma. Some borderland towns and cities have emerged as hubs where organizations' offices are based and activists conduct much of their work. These include Mae Sot, Sangklaburi, Mae Sariang, Mae Hong Son, Chiang Mai, Bangkok (Thailand); Ruili (China); Aizawl, Imphal, and New Delhi (India); and Dhaka (Bangladesh). The movement's reach is determined by connections activists have with people and places throughout the country, primarily following ethnic networks: Karen to Karen, Shan to Shan, Mon to Mon, Burman to Burman, and so forth. The advantage they have created through this borderland position is to be connected simultaneously with their communities in Burma and in displacement, with globalized actors who support their activism, and—this is vital—with each other. Being able to work together across ethnic lines in politically and socially organized ways at this level of exposure, intensity, and consistency is something that has been extremely difficult in Burma under the military dictatorship.

DEVELOPING A BORDER-BASED RESISTANCE MOVEMENT

Reflecting back, Burma's border-based civil society activism emerged ad hoc; its growth was not premeditated or strategically planned. As various organizations' capacities developed over time, the advantages of collaboration and coalition-building within and across issue areas became apparent. In the beginning, however, these possibilities were yet to be envisioned, and advancements were made through trial and error and by reacting to opportunities that presented themselves. Of the multiple processes that various activists embarked on to develop the border-based civil society movement, three are discussed here: self-education, national reconciliation within the movement, and the women-led democratizing of the border-based resistance movement leadership.

First, activists are situated in positions of effective statelessness outside a state institutional frame in which formal educational institutions and systems operate and are supported. Thus, they have undertaken for themselves the enormous task of self-education to acquire the knowledge and skills requisite for human rights–oriented activism. Their activism demands the skills to work across multiple cultural, knowledge, and linguistic sites and in multiethnic, multilingual, multicultural, and constantly changing environments. They must be able to translate grassroots problems and political opinions into English, frame them in human rights discourse, communicate them to people in positions of high institutional authority, and address various publics through global media. Additionally, they must be able to translate human rights concepts and political opinions and processes into local vernaculars and communicate with people more isolated from global processes and the types of knowledge, norms, and values they carry. Likewise, they must be proficient in the use of a range of communication methods and technologies, from the internet to oral traditional. In short, they must comprehend multiple world views and engage them in culturally appropriate ways and with confidence.

Their education methods involved a combination of "learning by doing," through implementing projects and programs, and more formalized training, workshops, conferences, and seminars with invited local and global knowledgeable experts. As activists became known beyond the border, opportunities arose to attend training on democracy and rights-related issues provided by global civil society organizations that bring together activists from prodemocracy struggles and democratizing countries around the world. With growing capacity, activists implemented "training of trainers" programs, first for themselves and then for community members and next-generation activists. Six-month to one-year education opportunities were developed within the movement by organizations and alliance groups for groups of up to twenty students per intake, and most civil society organizations have now developed their own small internship programs. The time and resources spent on training and workshops over the years to build the skills indicates the difficulty and complexity of educating a movement of activists outside formal education systems and institutional support.

Second, the placement of national reconciliation at the heart of their political strategies by many, including all the major border-based political and civil society organizations, demonstrates their commitment to tackling the root causes of Burma's political instability. Further, it has provided them with a foundational basis for growth. In addition to being an aspiration, national reconciliation provides the movement with the principles of equality and human rights to guide the day-to-day practices of intra-movement engagement to sort out differences, address distrust, and build relationships across ethnic divides within and across organizations. This reflects the movement's "planning in action" approach to political and social struggle.

National reconciliation processes within the border-based movement were instigated by leaders of ethnic nationality groups, student groups, elected members of parliament, and political parties in the borderlands after the 1988 uprising and 1990 elections with the formation of the Democratic Alliance of Burma in 1988 and the National Council of the Union of Burma in 1992. However, emerging civil society groups broadened and solidified the role of the principles of national reconciliation within the movement by forming alliances and networks across social issues and identity categories such as women, youth, the environment, health care, education, human rights documentation, and media. In 2000, international funding was secured to form the National Reconciliation Program (NRP), which more systematically supported initiatives promoting and strengthening interethnic relations at all levels of the movement and through federal and state constitution drafting processes and community work. Through layers of consultations, the constitution drafting processes arrived at a set of basic principles for the formation of a federal union agreed on by groups from all sectors of the movement. While there remains a range of political opinions within the movement on these issues, promoting these broadly supported principles of national reconciliation has enhanced the movement's legitimacy internationally and strengthened the movement politically vis-à-vis the military regime/current form of government.

Third, democratizing dimensions of the traditional, male-dominated leadership of the border-based resistance movement is an important area of relative achievement and an ongoing key aspiration of civil society groups, in particularly women's and youth organizations. There are two main areas of progress. First, women and youth leaders have introduced human rights and grassroots community concerns into the movement's top policy positions and cease-fire negotiation demands. Second, they have instigated intra-movement debate on the need for women and next-generation leaders. In the case of women's political representation, women activists have worked hard learning the international conventions and instruments on women's rights and gender equality, researching women's experiences in other countries, understanding complex global debates around women's leadership and quota systems, articulating principles of gender equality in relation to culture, and strategic lobbying. For example, a clause that guarantees at least a 30 percent quota for women's participation in political leadership and decision-making bodies was enshrined in the draft federal constitution.[14] Their efforts are supported by international donors, who raise the issue of women's and youth representation with male leaders. While there is still some way to go, women are achieving increasing representation in policy and strategy forums at the movement's top levels, predominantly through the Women's League of Burma (WLB). Women are also making some progress in taking leadership positions in male-dominated alliance groups and organizations. Youth-based alliances such as the Student and Youth Congress of Burma have done similar work in relation to youth and women's representation and are also more included in these forums. While there is still much to achieve, women and youth activists are creating opportunities for younger generation leaders to emerge in a movement where established male leaders have dominated powerful positions for decades.

The emergence and capacity development of Burma's civil society movement is slow, laborious, challenging, and uneven, leaving it open at times to harsh criticism. Some organizations have developed significant capacity to provide services and influence in international debate on Burma and attract international recognition for their achievements. For example, highly respected international human rights awards have been presented to Dr. Cynthia and Mae Tao Clinic, the WLB, the Shan Women's Action Group, and the Assistance Association for Political Prisoners (Burma) (AAPPB) to name a few. Others continue to struggle from positions of less advantage and visibility.

WELFARE SERVICE RESPONSES

Many activists began their work responding to suffering in their communities on both sides of Burma's borders because so many community members are denied state protection and/or international assistance or, if in camps, assistance is partial. Estimating the number of people of Burma in this situation of effective statelessness is difficult, though it is in the several millions. While there are credible counts of people from Burma in camps or registered with either a "host" state or the UNHCR in Thailand (142,600), Malaysia (97,000), and Bangladesh (30,000), there are only rough or no estimates of the number of migrants without state travel documents in Thailand (2–3 million), Bangladesh (200,000–500,000), Malaysia, China, and India, and, further afield, in Pakistan, Singapore, and other countries. There are estimates of people displaced in eastern Burma (500,000), Kachin State (100,000) and Rakhine State (115,000); however, little is known of numbers in other parts of Burma. This forces the large majority of migrants to exist in an institutional protection gap and survive however they can.

Among the world's most isolated and vulnerable, particularly to Burma's west, community members are forced to live as migrants with no or little access to crisis or social services. Though it is beyond border-based organizations' capacity to reach but a small percentage, it is to these community members in neighboring countries and borderlands that they direct their welfare programs.

In conflict, aggressors target and destroy not only people and material possessions, but also, as psychiatrist Derek Summerfield highlights, the institutions constituting the social fabric and coping mechanisms of a community: family, schools, religious places, and health care services.[15] Forced migration caused by extreme poverty and lack of opportunity contributes to damaging the social fabric of communities at home. In places migrants move to there are no community structures, intensifying their vulnerability to abuse and exploitation. Therefore, welfare programs of border-based activist groups focus not only on individuals, but also on re/building coping mechanisms and community structures responsive to these conditions.

The largest and most well-known of these initiatives, the Mae Tao Clinic (MTC), is featured in this book. However, there are many remarkable programs of varying scale developed by activists around Burma's borders. Connected to but independent from the MTC is the Back Pack Health Worker Program, which trains and coordinates teams of medics around all Burma's borders to travel on foot through conflict and militarized areas providing emergency and basic health care, health education, and recording vital data about health conditions in these areas. There are now ninety-five teams working in twenty field areas targeting a population of approximately 206,000, and a further 1,500 medics locally trained.[16] Another example is the Karen Women's Organization, which, among its range of programs, has activities addressing gender and sex-based violence in the Karen community.[17] They not only campaign against state perpetrated rape as a weapon of war[18] but support survivors of gender-based violence in the community through running safe houses, advocating for improved justice mechanisms, and educating to transform societal values and norms that sustain gender inequality.[19]

It is important to note that the development of welfare programs has not occurred evenly around Burma's borderlands. The largest and most effective programs occur along the Thai-Burma border because of relative advantages in communications technologies, travel, resource access, and Thailand government policy. Very few resources, comparatively, are directed toward Burma's western borderlands, including for activist capacity-building to initiate and run programs. Contributing to this imbalance are the much higher costs and challenges of working in lesser developed areas—costs that, despite urgings from activists on Burma's east and west, international funding agencies find difficult to justify given their financial constraints. Another factor contributing to silence around welfare programs in the west, in particular for the Rohingya, is the tension between Rakhaine and Rohingya, which unfortunately also resonates through much of Burma, including some, not all, of the border-based resistance movement.

POLITICAL AND SOCIAL CRITIQUE

Making sense of the gap between the way the world is and the way it should be forces those affected by political trauma to engage in social and political critique; to assess what should be done about trauma and the factors contributing to it. Survivors and their communities, therefore, have things to say that are very compelling.[20] The problem is that inside Burma, the military regime closed, with violent force, all channels through which to speak publicly and, therefore, public spaces in which to speak. In Burma's borderlands activists created spaces and methods through which to undertake the task of political and social critique of the Burmese regime and publicly disseminate their information. We discuss three modes of critique: human rights documentation, media, and community educative deliberation processes.

First, human rights organizations began researching, documenting, writing, and publishing international standard human rights reports in the late 1990s, and an opus of around two hundred reports has accumulated. These reports not only document specific human rights and environmental problems at points in time, but now also analyze the emergence and transformation of issues over the past fifteen to twenty years. Organizations have trained networks of human rights documenters in their constituent areas to collect information and record human rights violations and problems as they occur, sending that information to border-based offices. The Network for Human Rights Documentation—Burma formed in 2004 to facilitate the coordination of its twelve organizational members on human rights documentation processes.[21] Their activities are many and include inputting documented cases of rights violations into a common database using Martus, an open-source software that encrypts the information and allows for its analysis and storage. This database provides nationwide information for current campaigns and will be useful for future processes of transitional justice, including the possibility of a United Nations–led commission of inquiry into war crimes and crimes against humanity in Burma.

Second, in Burma's borderlands, activists established their own media groups. Initially they were intended to provide a voice for the opposition movement; however, with increased media and journalist training, over time they forged and defend their independence from political groups. Global communications scholar Lisa Brooten observed that border-based media groups developed along three trajectories: to provide a means of international outreach, to improve communication within the Burmese opposition movement, and to serve each of the country's major ethnic communities.[22] Media groups publish predominantly on websites but also in print, and translate their content into multiple languages, including Burmese, English, ethnic nationalities languages of their main constituencies, and, increasingly, languages of neighboring countries.

Higher-profile media organizations, such as *Irrawaddy*, the *Democratic Voice of Burma*, and *Mizzima*, report on events and political developments in Burma and provide vital public space for Burmese- and English-language debate through research articles, commentary, and analysis. The latter two organizations connect with, provide training for, and coordinate teams of inside journalists—working underground until recently—in Burma. The formation in 2003 of Burma News International (BNI), a coalition of media organizations, is described as a milestone in the emergence of Burma's border-based media.[23] BNI raises the profile of news from ethnic areas and from local perspectives to increase knowledge, both inside Burma and globally, of its rich and complex ethnic diversity.[24] Nine of the eleven partners are run by and targeted toward ethnic communities, giving BNI as a collective unparalleled reach into rural areas and enabling them to offer the most comprehensive coverage of any Burma media.[25]

The third way activists produce social and political critique is through engaging in educative deliberative processes as a mode of education, inquiry, and decision-making from the grassroots level up through the movement. Educative deliberation, explains critical feminist political theorist Brooke Ackerly, is a means of inquiry and "the skeptical scrutiny of elitist, coercive, exclusionary, and potentially exploitative values, practices, and norms and the development of a set of criteria for evaluating values, practices, and norms."[26] In the absence of a public sphere, it is very difficult for communities to engage in debates to shape and articulate shared norms, values, and aspirations. Moreover, there are no preexisting, institutionalized, political and social mechanisms to systematically and democratically establish representation to advocate policy positions reflecting these common understandings. Border-based activists approach this dual task of identifying community opinion and building legitimate representation through educative deliberative methods of facilitating workshops, seminars, and training. Based on the principles of equality, inclusiveness, and listening to silenced voices, it is a democratizing process that dovetails with the movement's national reconciliation agenda, wherein groups discuss common problems, learn from each other's experiences and perspectives, and devise practical approaches to bring change.[27]

Educative deliberation contrasts dramatically with the hierarchical, coerced, and gendered decision-making practices dominant in militarized society in Burma. Learning to participate in educative deliberative processes involves a cultural shift for participants, to unfamiliar but liberating ways of relating, and requires cultural sensitivity to facilitate well. In this way, communities develop and become aware of their common norms and values and activists gain legitimacy as representatives in political spheres. An example of this process is the Women Exchange meetings facilitated by MAP Foundation, through which the *Automatic Response Mechanism (ARM): What to Do in Case of Sexual Violence for Migrant and Refugee Women* was produced. In this book, women from Burma in Thailand developed, through extensive discussion, detailed appropriate responses to sexual violence for their situations.[28] Activists in turn have used this resource to lobby for appropriate policy with states and international agencies.

INTERNATIONAL ADVOCACY

In spite of the dangers of speaking out in Burma, brave activists constantly push the barriers of public expression and protest, under military rule and now during this transitional political phase. However, without free and global media, their messages are stifled. A primary aim of border-based activism has been mobilizing international support for communities and activists inside Burma and keeping Burma issues highlighted on the international stage. Border-based activists engage in international advocacy in partnership with a range of international and regional actors and have devoted great energy over the past two decades to building solidarity networks around the globe. Through these channels, they bring their human rights cases and reports to the attention of policy makers at the UN level, to individual governments, and to solidarity activists in other countries who advocate their respective governments. The success of these advocacy strategies over the years is reflected in the supportive policies of many countries on Burma, which inform not only bilateral relations but also feed into UN resolutions on Burma, and European Union and International Labour Organization positions on Burma.

A primary focus of border-based international advocacy is the UN system, including states' UN diplomatic missions: the General Assembly

(UNGA); the Security Council (UNSC); the Human Rights Commission/ Council (UNCHR); the Commission on the Status of Women; the Convention on the Elimination of All Forms of Discrimination against Women; the Convention on the Rights of the Child; issue-based world conferences; special envoys, and rapporteurs. In collaboration with key Burma activists and UN-registered international NGOs, border-based activists organize and participate in delegations at each relevant UN forum as they are scheduled throughout the year.

A major achievement of UN-level advocacy has been the adoption of consecutive annual resolutions on Burma by the UNGA since 1991[29] and by the UNCHR from 1992 to 2005 and by the UNCHR from 2005 to present.[30] UNGA and UNCHR resolutions afford international recognition of Burma's problems and recommendations to the regime to follow international human rights and humanitarian laws but not the legal basis for international action. As resolutions accumulated over the 1990s and 2000s, key Burma advocates, both international and border-based, strategized a campaign to have the UNSC pass a resolution on Burma that would carry the weight of enforceable international law. The January 2007 draft resolution sponsored by the United States and United Kingdom was vetoed, but the campaign did succeed in having Burma put on the UNSC agenda, significantly raising international pressure on the regime.[31]

International advocacy also involves networking with key global human rights organizations such as Amnesty International and Human Rights Watch, academics, and media groups. Working with Burma solidarity groups in North America, Europe, Australia, New Zealand, Japan, South Korea, and India, and civil society organizations in the Southeast Asian region, is particularly important, and their lobbying credibility has been bolstered by reports from the border. Issues-based campaigns implemented over the years include the forced labor and anti-tourism campaigns of the 1990s; the free Burma/Aung San Suu Kyi/political prisoners campaigns through the 2000s; the UNSC campaign of the mid-2000s, and current calls for the UN to establish a commission of inquiry. Increasingly close global connections developed through collaborating on campaigns, study tours to the border, and hosting border-based activists in various countries has grown support, capacity, and legitimacy for participants in diverse networking sites. Hence, campaigns raising public awareness about Burma issues are strengthened and solidarity groups' capacity to influence their government's Burma policy has been amplified. Indeed, all these facets and threads of international advocacy undertaken by various activists on different issues across diverse sites complement and reinforce each other with synergetic effect.

For example, the Free Burma's Political Prisoners campaign was initiated in early 2009 by the AAPPB and Forum for Democracy in Burma and included the participation of all border-based, international, and regional solidarity groups, as well as Avaaz, a globally focused online activist campaign group. With the slogan, "Free Burma's Pro-Democracy Prisoners," the campaign petition secured approximately 700,000 signatures from more than sixty-five countries within three months. The petition called for Ban Ki-moon and the UN to commit to working for the release of all Burma's political prisoners. As a result of the collective efforts of activist groups globally, the call was included in the 2009 UNGA resolution on Burma and was adopted by states as a key benchmark to measure Burma's reform progress before, throughout, and after the military regime's 2010 elections and up to the present.

ARTICULATING A COMMON VISION OF A FUTURE BURMA

Protesting against an abusive political regime or harmful social practices cannot alone bring about desired change. Resistance must involve articulating a shared vision of a common future and identifying the different political, social, cultural, and economic elements constituting that future. Without this, it is very difficult if not impossible to move forward in a positive direction. Further, realizing this future requires its advocates to embody and promote the values and practices their visions are built on. This point has been reflected in the activities of the NRP and educative and deliberative democratic practices described above. However, this also is not enough; a shared vision of the future also needs more formal articulation.

The most significant articulation of a vision of a future Burma that is alternative to the 2008 constitution produced by the military regime is the border-based movement's draft federal democratic constitution. The resistance movement's constitution drafting process commenced shortly after the 1990 elections in Burma's eastern borderlands with the participation of all major ethno-political and prodemocratic groups. However, the process stalled when cease-fire negotiations of the mid to late 1990s caused the withdrawal of some key groups, the movement's headquarters in Manerplaw in Karen State was captured by the military regime in December 1994, and because of funding shortages. With NRP-channeled funding, the process was revived in 2000 and a Federal Constitution Drafting and Coordination Committee was formed in 2005 to oversee the process. By this time, civil society organizations had emerged in the borderlands and negotiated their inclusion in the constitution drafting process. Around this time, a second level to the process commenced, with ethnic groups drafting state- and division-level constitutions in line with the federal-union level drafting process. A second draft of the federal democratic constitution, adopted in 2008 by more than ninety organizations and 120 individuals, rests on eight basic principles: popular sovereignty; equality; self-determination; federalism; minority rights; democracy, human rights, and gender rights; multiparty democratic system and secularism.[32]

This extensive and inclusive drafting process lasted more than a decade and a half and fostered a broad understanding of the national- and state/ division-level constitutions. This understanding also extended into the broader community via community projects and border-based media. A shared understanding and vision has informed activists' various advocacy processes and enabled them to quickly and effectively critique the military regime's constitution drafting process and the 2008 constitution from a united position. This is one area where a more common movement-wide policy position has been possible. The commitment and effort given to the constitution drafting process is starting to pay off in other ways also. Information about the process has filtered into Burma over the years via networks and border-based media and international radio programs promoting recognition of ethnic equality issues. A younger generation of Burmese activists inside Burma—for whom ethnic concerns have always been surrounded by silence—is taking up ethnic equality as a core issue. The post-2010 military-dominated government can no longer hide this issue behind a veil of silence.

Border-Based Activism and Burma's Political Transition

The current reform processes have demonstrated some positive steps toward change at the policy level, providing opportunities but also enormous challenges. These challenges have included the problematic nature of many new laws, policies, and institutional structures currently being put into place that facilitate less-than-genuine reform and that could possibly reinforce another authoritarian governing regime, albeit in a different form. The changes in Burma are affecting border-based activism significantly and in diverse and uneven ways. Here we consider activists' responses, contributions, and challenges in relation to transition processes, as well as new pressures undermining border-based activism.

Border-based activists are aware of, and sensitive to, existing resistances to their participation in the current reform process, not least because—after two decades of state media vilification and the outlawing of all border-based organizations by the military regime—many in Burmese society have grown to view them with apprehension. Further, the Unlawful Association Act used to incarcerate many political activists remains in force. The wall of fear erected by the military regime between inside and the border remains barely touched by reform processes. At the same time, the experiences of the border-based civil society grounded in its rights-based approach can provide a key contribution to achieving genuine democratic reform.

There are many valuable attributes border-based activists can contribute to new partnerships with activists inside as they work to develop a robust civil society. First, they continue through their monitoring activities to act as government watchdogs and rights advocates internationally and as agents for capacity-building of communities and activists. When engaging directly inside, they can encourage civil society activists to practice freedom of expression where silence has been a safety shield and can call for the inclusion of marginalized voices in various forums. In doing so, they can support civil society actors to foster a culture of autonomous action and independent space while defusing the existing culture of fear and shifting expectations of having to take orders and look above for instruction. Additionally, there are organizational, program, and project management skills they can share, as well as knowledge of and experience with international discourses on human rights and democracy they have already translated and adapted for local contexts. They bring rich national, regional, and global networks across a range of sectors and established relationships to draw on network contacts to bolster their position vis-à-vis state institutions. Vitally, it is at the organizational level that border-based activists exert the strongest agency as they provide independent voice and examples of Burma organizations operating in democratic ways without the fear engendered by a culture of top-down governance.

Border-based activists have already begun to respond to Burma's changing conditions in a variety of ways. Some organizations have unofficially opened branches in their respective constituencies inside Burma under new names to expand their internal networks and activities while avoiding the repercussions of the barriers discussed above. Though it provides some advantages, this strategy is also not without drawbacks, as they must work under a low profile and have little space to play a significant role. Like all other civil society groups in Burma, they are concerned with security, their voice is restricted, and in some cases their independence compromised. It is difficult under these conditions to support other groups operating in a culture of fear to be independent if they are compromised themselves. Their priority at this stage, however, is to establish a stronger foothold back in their constituent areas.

Second, activists continue their work on the border. Inside civil society groups are not yet ready to take up the "check and balance" role, monitor the trajectory of change in human rights conditions, and provide a critical public voice in a risk-free way. At the same time, the conditions of the vulnerable and displaced communities with whom they work have not changed, and their services continue to be urgently needed. However, providing these services is getting increasingly harder as international donors are withdrawing their assistance. Further, the human insecurity conditions of Kachin, Shan, Rohingya, and Rakhine communities in particular have drastically deteriorated during this reform phase and need international advocacy.

Third, ethnic-based civil society groups actively lobby for community and human rights perspectives to be included in cease-fire negotiations with the government. Of particular concern for civil society groups with community members in refugee camps in Thailand and Bangladesh is their exclusion from decision-making processes determining the timing, processes, and outcomes of future repatriations. Nevertheless, they continue to vocally strain against the glass walls that surround, in practice, the principle of including all affected in decision-making processes—a principle featuring in international community rhetoric on displacement. Activists of some ethnic communities whose political leadership spans the border are working to rebuild a more united leadership to represent their ethnic demands.

Fourth, some activists have begun to travel between the border and inside to work strategically with their existing and expanding networks. They support the capacity-building and empowerment activities of inside activists and negotiate for independent space for civil society. They are introducing inside actors to their international resource and solidarity networks so this weight of support can increase the leverage of civil society. One aim is to foster a mutually reinforcing dynamic between border-based and inside activists and groups. Traversing back and forth, these activists are able to retain their freedom and, thus, take unique advantage of emerging opportunities to benefit civil society across these locations. At the same time, there is the possibility that their future access to the country can be blocked.

Activists are also facing new barriers to their inclusion. First, the government has signaled its recognition of the significance of border-based political actors by holding informal meetings with key activists. After several discussions, there remain no avenues for activists' dignified return, as there are no official policies or procedures guaranteeing their safety, freedom to continue their activism, or legal recognition of their organizations. Rather, activists are expected to simply slip back and return to society. They are then, of course, subject to the same depoliticizing conditions as all other citizens, and the critical voice of the border-based movement will be muted. Their risk of arrest for their activist past also leaves them vulnerable, adding another layer of silencing through self-censorship. Second, the government has attempted to deflate critical voices by courting key activists with offers of attractive conditions, advisory roles, and/or promises it lacks the capacity to deliver—offers that most activists have rejected. Third, the reduction and withdrawal of international donor funding from border-based programs to inside Burma is increasing pressure on activists, who remain compelled to continue regardless. This increased funding squeeze and its consequences weakens the contribution border-based activists can make to shaping a genuine reform process.

These depoliticizing pressures are indicative of the contradictory, complex, and fragile character of Burma's reform process. If Burma is undergoing democratic reform, why is the border-based civil society movement, which works for that very democratic change, facing amplified pressure to cease? Significant political struggle still needs to occur to progressively win vital freedoms inside Burma, thus signaling a continued need for border-based activism at this time.

Conclusion

At times, activists feel closer to achieving progress with their social and political goals, including national reconciliation, and at other times further away. What is undeniable is that they started with very few resources and built themselves into a political and social force promoting democracy, responding to their communities' needs, advocating on their behalf, and shaping global opinion on Burma. This nonstop commitment from communities, groups, and individuals of Burma is inspiring and needs recognition.

It is important not to lose sight of the core driving force of border-based activism: that it is a manifestation of the protest response of Burma's traumatized communities. Failure to recognize it as such not only sidelines this key component, which is a part of the catalyst for change and recovery for these communities, but ignores the kind of change communities want to happen and how they want it to happen. Recognizing protest as a part of trauma responses means harnessing a source of strength for change; if traumatized communities cannot exert their own agency, how can they seek the truth and justice to heal their trauma? Both sides of the trauma response need to be nurtured and strengthened together so that the community can move forward.

Notes

1 Jenny Edkins, *Trauma and the Memory of Politics* (Cambridge: Cambridge University Press, 2003), 9.

2 Victorian Foundation for Survivors of Torture, *Rebuilding Shattered Lives* (Melbourne: Victorian Foundation for Survivors of Torture, 1998), 9, http://www.foundationhouse.org.au/LiteratureRetreive.aspx?ID=25045.

3 Edkins, *Trauma and the Memory of Politics*, 9.

4 Slavoj Žižek, *A Ticklish Subject* (New York: Verso, 1999), 191–194; Engin F Isin, "Theorizing Acts of Citizenship," in *Acts of Citizenship*, ed. Engin F Isin and Greg M Neilson (London: Zed Books, 2008), 28–35.

5 Edkins, *Trauma and the Memory of Politics*, 9.

6 Kevin Heppner, "We Have Hands the Same as Them: Struggles for Local Sovereignty and Livelihoods by Internally Displaced Karen Villagers in Burma," Karen Human Rights Group, 2006, http://www.khrg.org/papers/wp2006w1.htm.

7 Karen Human Rights Group, *Dignity in the Shadow of Oppression* (Mae Sot, Thailand: Karen Human Rights Group, 2006), http://www.khrg.org/khrg2006/khrg0605.pdf; Karen Human Rights Group, *Village Agency* (Mae Sot, Thailand: Karen Human Rights Group, 2008), http://www.khrg.org/khrg2008/khrg0803.pdf; Karen Human Rights Group, *Self Protection under Strain: Targeting of Civilians and Local Responses in Northern Karen State* (Mae Sot, Thailand: Karen Human Rights Group, 2010), http://www.khrg.org/khrg2010/khrg1004.pdf.

8 For example, see MAP Foundation, *Migrant Movements 1996–2010* (Chiang Mai, Thailand: MAP Foundation, 2010), http://www.mapfoundationcm.org/pdf/eng/MigrantMovements_1996-2010.pdf; "LGBT Rights," Human Rights Education Institute of Burma, http://www.hreib.com/index.php?option=com_content&view=article&id=605&Itemid=591.

9 Richard Devetak, "Post-Structuralism," in *Theories of International Relations*, ed. Scott Burchill et al. (New York: Palgrave, 2009), 184–187; Richard K Ashley, "Living on Border Lines: Man, Poststructuralism, and War," in *International/Intertextual Relations: Postmodern Readings of World Politics*, ed. James Der Derian and Michael J Shapiro (Lexington, MA: Lexington Books, 1989).

10 For further reading on the discursive and material production of the humanitarian/political divide see Jennifer Hyndman, *Managing Displacement: Refugees and the Politics of Humanitarianism* (Minneapolis: University of Minnesota Press, 2000); Nevzat Soguk, *States and Strangers: Refugees and*

Displacements of Statecraft (Minneapolis: University of Minnesota Press, 1999); Peter Nyers, *Rethinking Refugees* (New York: Routledge, 2006); David Campbell, "Why Fight? Humanitarianism, Principles and Post-Structuralism," *Millennium* 27 (1998).

11 Nyers, *Rethinking Refugees*, 26.

12 Ibid.

13 Ibid.

14 "The Constitution of the Federal Republic of the Union of Burma (Second Draft)," media.wix.com/ugd/30e5a3_2c4fdob4f1e3e9ce8749cb50d348f9b5.pdf.

15 Derek Summerfield, "Sociocultural Dimensions of War, Conflict and Displacement," in *Refugees: Perspectives on the Experience of Forced Migration*," ed. Alastair Ager (London: Pinter, 1998).

16 "BPHWT Mid-Year Report 2012," Backpack Health Worker Team, http://www.backpackteam.org/wp-content/uploads/reports/2012%20Mid%20Year %20Report%20final-0409122.pdf.

17 Karen Women's Organization, "Home," http://karenwomen.org/.

18 Karen Women's Organization, "Reports," http://karenwomen.org/reports/.

19 "SGBV," DVD, 2006, http://www.youtube.com/playlist?list=PL28465F822ED18ACF.

20 Edkins, *Trauma and the Memory of Politics*, 9.

21 Network for Human Rights Documentation—Burma, "About Us," http://www.nd-burma.org/.

22 Lisa Brooten, "Beyond State-Centric Frameworks: Transversal Media and the Stateless in the Burmese Borderlands," in *Global Communication: New Agendas in Communication*, ed. Karen Wilkins, Joe Straubhaar, and Shanti Kumar (New York: Routledge, 2014), 142–162.

23 Brooten, "Beyond State-Centric Frameworks."

24 "Home," *Burma News International*, http://www.bnionline.net/.

25 Brooten, "Beyond State-Centric Frameworks."

26 Brooke Ackerly, *Political Theory and Feminist Social Criticism* (Cambridge: Cambridge University Press, 2008), 18.

27 Ibid., 18.

28 MAP Foundation Thailand, *Automatic Response Mechanism* (Chiang Mai, Thailand: MAP Foundation, 2003), http://www.mapfoundationcm.org/pdf/eng/english_arm1.pdf.

29 "UN General Assembly Resolutions on Burma," Altsean-Burma, http://www.altsean.org/Research/UN%20Dossier/UNGA.htm.

30 "Commission on Human Rights Resolutions: Myanmar," Office of the High Commission for Human Rights, http://www.ohchr.org/en/countries/asiaregion/pages/mmindex.aspx.

31 "UN Security Council Draft Resolution/Statements on Burma," Altsean-Burma,
    http://www.altsean.org/Research/UN%20Dossier/UNSC.htm.

32 "Federal Constitution Drafting Process," Ethnic Nationalities Council,
    http://www.encburma.net/index.php/constitutions-drafting/68-constitution
    -drafting/173-federal-constitution-drafting-process-.html; Mungpi, "Burmese
    Opposition Groups Challenge Junta's Constitution," *Mizzima*, February 14, 2008,
    www.mizzima.com/news/regional/226-burmese-opposition-groups-challenge
    -junta's-constitution.pdf.

Bibliography

Ackerly, Brooke. *Political Theory and Feminist Social Criticism.* Cambridge:
    Cambridge University Press, 2008.

Altsean-Burma. "UN General Assembly Resolutions on Burma."
    http://www.altsean.org/Research/UN%20Dossier/UNGA.htm.

———. "UN Security Council Draft Resolution/Statements on Burma."
    http://www.altsean.org/Research/UN%20Dossier/UNSC.htm.

Ashley, Richard K. "Living on Border Lines: Man, Poststructuralism, and War." In
    International/Intertextual Relations: Postmodern Readings of World Politics, edited
    by James Der Derian and Michael J Shapiro, 259–321. Lexington, MA: Lexington
    Books, 1989.

Backpack Health Worker Team. "BPHWT Mid-Year Report 2012."
    http://www.backpackteam.org/wp-content/uploads/reports/2012%20Mid%20Year
    %20Report%20final-0409122.pdf.

Brooten, Lisa. "Beyond State-Centric Frameworks: Transversal Media and the Stateless
    in the Burmese Borderlands." In *Global Communication: New Agendas in
    Communication*, edited by Karen Wilkins, Joe Straubhaar, and Shanti Kumar,
    142–162. New York: Routledge, 2014.

Campbell, David. "Why Fight? Humanitarianism, Principles and Post-Structuralism."
    Millennium 27 (1998): 497–521.

"The Constitution of the Federal Republic of the Union of Burma (Second Draft)."
    February 2008. media.wix.com/ugd/30e5a3_2c4fd0b4f1e3e9ce8749cb50d348f9b5.pdf.

Devetak, Richard. "Post-Structuralism." In *Theories of International Relations*, Scott
    Burchill, Andrew Linklater, Richard Devetak, Jack Donnelly, Terry Nardin, Matthew
    Paterson, Christian Reus-Smit, and Jacqui True, 183–211. New York: Palgrave, 2009.

Edkins, Jenny. *Trauma and the Memory of Politics.* Cambridge: Cambridge University
    Press, 2003.

Ethnic Nationalities Council. "Federal Constitution Drafting Process."
    http://www.encburma.net/index.php/constitutions-drafting/68-constitution
    -drafting/173-federal-constitution-drafting-process-.html.

Heppner, Kevin. "We Have Hands the Same as Them: Struggles for Local Sovereignty and Livelihoods by Internally Displaced Karen Villagers in Burma." Karen Human Rights Group, 2006. http://www.khrg.org/papers/wp2006w1.htm.

"Home." *Burma News International*, May 29, 2006. http://www.bnionline.net/.

Human Rights Education Institute of Burma. "LGBT Rights." http://www.hreib.com/index.php?option=com_content&view=article&id=605&Itemid=591.

Hyndman, Jennifer. *Managing Displacement: Refugees and the Politics of Humanitarianism*. Minneapolis: University of Minnesota Press, 2000.

Isin, Engin F. "Theorizing Acts of Citizenship." In *Acts of Citizenship*, edited by Engin F Isin and Greg M Neilson, 15–43. London: Zed Books, 2008.

Karen Human Rights Group. *Dignity in the Shadow of Oppression*. Mae Sot, Thailand: Karen Human Rights Group, 2006. http://www.khrg.org/khrg2006/khrg0605.pdf.

———. "Reports." http://www.khrg.org/index.php.

———. *Self-Protection under Strain: Targeting of Civilians and Local Responses in Northern Karen State*. Mae Sot, Thailand: Karen Human Rights Group, 2010. http://www.khrg.org/khrg2010/khrg1004.pdf.

———. *Village Agency*. Mae Sot, Thailand: Karen Human Rights Group, 2008. http://www.khrg.org/khrg2008/khrg0803.pdf.

Karen Women's Organization. "Home." http://karenwomen.org/.

———. "Reports." http://karenwomen.org/reports/.

MAP Foundation. *Automatic Response Mechanism*. Chiang Mai, Thailand: MAP Foundation, 2003. http://www.mapfoundationcm.org/pdf/eng/english_arm1.pdf.

———. *Migrant Movements 1996–2010*. Chiang Mai, Thailand: MAP Foundation, 2010. http://www.mapfoundationcm.org/pdf/eng/MigrantMovements_1996-2010.pdf.

Mungpi. "Burmese Opposition Groups Challenge Junta's Constitution." *Mizzima*, February 14, 2008. www.mizzima.com/news/regional/226-burmese-opposition-groups-challenge-junta's-constitution.pdf.

Network for Human Rights Documentation—Burma. "About Us." http://www.nd-burma.org/.

Nyers, Peter. *Rethinking Refugees*. New York: Routledge, 2006.

Office of the High Commission for Human Rights. "Commission on Human Rights Resolutions: Myanmar." http://www.ohchr.org/en/countries/asiaregion/pages/mmindex.aspx.

"SGBV." Video, Directed by Kawlah Films, Thailand-Burma Border: Kawlah Films and Karen Women's Organization, 2006, http://www.youtube.com/playlist?list=PL28465F822ED18ACF.

Soguk, Nevzat. *States and Strangers: Refugees and Displacements of Statecraft.* Minneapolis: University of Minnesota Press, 1999.

Summerfield, Derek. "Sociocultural Dimensions of War, Conflict and Displacement." In *Refugees: Perspectives on the Experience of Forced Migration*, edited by Alastair Ager. London: Pinter, 1998.

Thein Sein. "Address to the UN General Assembly." Address given at the 67th Session of the United Nations General Assembly, United Nations, September 27, 2012. http://www.mizzima.com/research/8126-text-of-thein-seins-un-speech.html.

Victorian Foundation for Survivors of Torture. *Rebuilding Shattered Lives.* Melbourne: Victorian Foundation for Survivors of Torture, 1998. http://www.foundationhouse.org.au/LiteratureRetreive.aspx?ID=25045.

Žižek, Slavoj. *A Ticklish Subject.* New York: Verso, 1999.

Contributors

Kathleen Allden: Dr. Allden is a faculty member of the Department of Psychiatry of Geisel School of Medicine at Dartmouth. She is an expert in the psychosocial and neuropsychiatric consequences of war, forced displacement, and torture, in a career bridging the fields of humanitarian assistance, clinical intervention, and human rights. She has worked in multiple refugee, postconflict, and natural disaster settings in Asia, Africa, Europe, North America, and Haiti. Dr. Allden has over twenty-five years of experience working with war-affected Southeast Asian communities and has helped develop, since its inception in 1999, Burma Border Projects, an organization dedicated to the mental health of displaced people from Burma. She has provided mental health services, training, technical assistance, and consultation for numerous nongovernmental, governmental, health care, and academic organizations, including the International Rescue Committee, the International Committee of the Red Cross, Physicians for Human Rights, Partners in Health, UN High Commissioner for Refugees, UN High Commissioner for Human Rights, and the US, Mexican, and Danish governments. She was medical director of the Harvard Program in Refugee Trauma and directed two clinical programs for refugees, asylum seekers, and survivors of torture in Boston, the Indochinese Psychiatry Clinic, and the International Survivors Center. She was program director for the Peter C. Alderman Foundation and cochaired Harvard Humanitarian Initiative's working group on mental health and psychosocial support. Dr. Allden is coauthor of the UN protocol on medical-legal documentation of torture and other cruel and degrading treatment, called the Istanbul Protocol, and has provided training and expert medical-legal testimony on this topic. During her career, Dr. Allden has written extensively on the psychological consequences of war and human rights abuse, and on developing effective psychosocial humanitarian responses. She has trained a broad range of health and mental health providers around the world including community health workers, indigenous medics, mental health professionals, physicians, and students.

Nancy Murakami: Ms. Murakami is currently the director of social services at the Bellevue/NYU Program for Survivors of Torture (PSOT), the first and most comprehensive torture treatment center in the New York City area addressing the complex needs of torture survivors. She received her master's degree in social work from Columbia University, with a concentration in international social welfare and program development and evaluation. She received specialized clinical training in therapeutic methods of addressing the impact of psychological trauma on children, adults, and families while at the Anti-Trafficking Program and Counseling Center of Safe Horizon, a New York City advocacy and assistance agency for victims of crime and abuse. Prior to joining PSOT, Nancy was the director of counseling training for the nonprofit organization Burma Border Projects, based on the Thai-Burma border at Dr. Cynthia Maung's Mae Tao Clinic in Mae Sot, Thailand. She provided clinical and administrative training and supervision, program and resource development, and capacity-building to Mae Tao Clinic and to other community-based organizations providing services to the displaced Burmese communities inside Burma and in Thailand. Prior to becoming a licensed clinical social worker, Nancy taught secondary school and led health and gender-based initiatives as a Peace Corps volunteer in rural communities in Malawi, Africa. Nancy currently serves on the board of directors for Burma Border Projects.

Aung Khaing Min: In 1997, "AK" was 24 years old, in his senior year of studying International Relations at Rangoon University, when he was arrested and imprisoned for seven years as a political prisoner in Burma. He was released in 2002. One year later, AK fled across the border to Mae Sot, Thailand, and joined the Assistance Association for Political Prisoners (Burma), eventually becoming chief of staff. In 2005, AK was awarded a scholarship to attend Indiana University, where he pursued a double major in political science and international studies. After graduation, AK went back to the Thai-Burma border to continue work with the Assistance Association of Political Prisoners. He has a master's degree in public administration at Northeastern University in Boston.

Kristin Kim Bart: Ms. Bart is dedicated to addressing inequality and violence in the lives of women and girls in developing and humanitarian contexts around the world. For the past decade, she has worked for the International Rescue Committee (IRC), both in the field programs and at headquarters. Currently she is the senior technical advisor for Women's Protection and Empowerment (WPE) programs and oversees a team of six advisors who provide technical support and ensure high quality WPE programming in Africa, Asia, and the Middle East. With the IRC, Kristin has led programs in Liberia, Pakistan, Thailand, and Uganda and provided onsite and remote technical support to a range of others including Iraq, Sierra Leone, and the Democratic Republic of Congo. She has designed and implemented programs to address a range of types of violence against women and girls in emergency settings, built the capacity of local organizations to address women's rights violations, and managed and supervised technical and nontechnical staff. She holds a master's degree from Columbia University's School for International and Public Affairs.

Paul Bolton: Dr. Bolton's main areas of expertise are program design, implementation, monitoring, and evaluation. His work treats all four elements as part of an integrated whole in which applied research methods play a core role. He uses this approach to conduct needs assessments and to plan and evaluate programs with service providers including major NGOs. This work has encompassed programs dealing with physical health (including infectious diseases) and, more recently, psychosocial problems in North America, Latin America, Sub-Saharan Africa, Central and Southeast Asia, Eastern Europe, and the Caribbean. Much of this work has been with refugees and internally displaced persons during the disaster post-emergency phase, persons affected by violence, and other adults and children living in difficult circumstances. Dr. Bolton has also conducted program evaluations of psychosocial interventions in Africa and Asia in the form of randomized clinical trials.

Jessica Bowes: Jessica Bowes is former director of adult mental health and psychosocial services for Burma Border Projects, a nonprofit organization in Mae Sot, Thailand, that provides psychosocial and mental health support to Burmese refugees and migrant workers. In her work, she provided training, supervision, curriculum and program development, and capacity-building to the Mental Health Department at the Mae Tao Clinic and the Mental Health Program at the Karen Department of Health and Welfare, in addition to other community-based organizations. She received her BS in psychology and master's in social work from the University of Washington. In Seattle, Jessica worked within the Native American community and other underserved populations, counseling in the areas of domestic violence, historical trauma, substance abuse, posttraumatic stress disorder, and mindfulness. It was her experiences as a volunteer with the Burmese community in Mae Sot in 2007 that inspired her decision to seek out an education with a focus on culturally sensitive mental health.

Kenneth Curry: Dr. Curry is an addiction medicine physician based in Sydney, Australia. He works as medical director of two hospital-based drug and alcohol services and in private practice. He has developed teaching for Sydney Medical School students in addiction medicine and in spirituality in medicine and is a clinical senior lecturer in the discipline of addiction medicine. He has taken teams to the Burma border since 2004 to teach about mental health and drug and alcohol problems to Karen primary health workers.

Eh Kalu Shwe Oo: Eh Kalu is a founding member of the Backpack Health Worker Team and director of the Karen Department of Health and Welfare (KDHW). He trained as a medic in eastern Burma and has worked over four decades as a community health leader for the Karen. As head of KDHW, he spearheads programs that have reduced malaria by more than 80 percent; increased access to reproductive health, tuberculosis, and trauma care; and provided critical data on disease trends and the health impact of human rights violations in eastern Burma. He has spoken on behalf of the Karen people around the United States and has partnered with universities such as Johns Hopkins and the University of California, Berkeley, to develop innovative community health programs. His public health interventions, such as the mobile obstetric medic program and mobile health clinics, have been recognized and replicated in other low-resource settings worldwide.

Abigail Erikson: Abigail Erikson is a licensed clinical social worker who has dedicated her professional career to improving the lives of women and girls. For more than fifteen years, Abigail has focused on women's reproductive health and rights and gender-based violence response and prevention programming. Abigail lived and worked in northern Thailand for several years, including three years on the Thai-Burma border, where she directed the International Rescue Committee's (IRC) sector to address violence against women and girls in the Karenni refugee camps. Abigail is the principal author of the joint IRC/UNICEF psychosocial guidelines *Caring for Child Survivors of Sexual Abuse in Humanitarian Settings*. Abigail is currently a Senior Technical Advisor with the IRC's Women's Protection and Empowerment Technical Unit, where she oversees the development of new program models to better empower and protect women and girls in humanitarian contexts.

Christina Fink: Professor Fink is Professor of Practice of International Affairs at George Washington University. She joined the Elliott School in 2011. She is a cultural anthropologist who has combined teaching, research, and development work throughout her career. She received her BA in international relations from Stanford University and her MA and PhD in social/cultural anthropology from the University of California at Berkeley. She served as a visiting lecturer at the Pacific and Asian

Studies Department at the University of Victoria in 1995, and from 2001 to 2010, she was a lecturer and program associate at the International Sustainable Development Studies Institute in Thailand. During the same period, she also ran a biannual capacity-building training and internship program that she developed for members of Burmese civil society organizations, including women's groups. In addition, she has worked as a coordinator for the Open Society Institute's Burma Project, a trainer and project consultant for an Internews oral history project, and a program evaluation consultant for the Canadian International Development Agency, the National Endowment for Democracy, and the Dag Hammarskjold Foundation. Her current research interests include the challenges of development in repressive states, gender issues in development, the development of civil society in ethnically diverse societies, and the use of oral history to document and understand social and political change. She is the author of *Living Silence in Burma: Surviving Under Military Rule* (Zed Books, 2nd edition, 2009), "Relieving Burma's Humanitarian Crisis," in *Burma's Search for National Identity* (World Scientific 2010), "Burma 2007: The Moment of the Monks," in *Civil Resistance and Power Politics* (Oxford University Press, 2009) and "Ongoing Militarization in Burma's Ethnic States: Causes and Consequences," in *Contemporary Politics* (2008). She is the coeditor of *Converging Interests: Traders, Travelers, and Tourists in Southeast Asia* (University of California Press, 1999).

Sarah Gundle: Dr. Gundle is a clinical psychologist in private practice in New York specializing in trauma. She holds a doctorate in clinical psychology from the Wright Institute and a master's degree in international affairs from Columbia University, with a concentration in human rights. Dr. Gundle lectures on trauma and international mental health at St. Luke's–Roosevelt Hospital, where she is adjunct faculty and is on the supervisory staff. She serves as a trauma consultant to various nonprofits in Manhattan and is credentialed through both St. Luke's–Roosevelt Hospital and Columbia University. She is a member of the 9-11 Trauma Commission therapist network, APA Disaster Relief Network, New York State Psychological Association Disaster/Crisis Response Network, the International Red Cross Disaster Team, the Cornell School of Medicine Women's Mental Health Consortium, and the NYC Medical Reserve Corps. In addition, she is a member of Physicians for Human Rights (PHR) and a volunteer in their Asylum network, where she evaluates the mental health of torture and persecution survivors seeking asylum in the United States. Dr. Gundle has worked in the past at the UN, the

International Center for Peace and Democracy Training (Tel Aviv), and Defense for Children International (Jerusalem), where she focused on issues related to children's rights, torture, and refugee mental health. She was the founder and director of Images for Peace, a nonprofit devoted to coexistence between Arab and Jewish children through photography in Jaffa, Israel. Dr. Gundle currently supervises the Adult Clinical Director of Burma Border Projects in Mae Sot, Thailand.

Whitney Haruf: Ms. Haruf is a somatic psychotherapist from Colorado. She worked for SalusWorld and Burma Border Projects for two years throughout northern, central, and southern Thailand. She is currently the family stabilization specialist for the Refugee and Asylee Programs at Lutheran Family Services Rocky Mountains. She is indebted to the staff from Fortune, Mae Tao Clinic's Counseling Center, and Foundation for Education and Development for all their kind consideration and support.

Hay Mar San: Hay Mar San was born and raised in Karen State. Her interest in community development began while she was a student of physics at Dagon University and volunteered for a year with Save the Children as a community health worker. In 2005, she moved to Mae Sot, Thailand, passed the high school equivalency test, and began working for Aide Médicale Internationale as a psychosocial worker in Mae La refugee camp. In 2011, she started her current role as a child and youth psychosocial officer with Burma Border Projects (BBP). She is responsible for developing and delivering BBP's child psychosocial play session programs, staff trainings, and child activities at Mae Tao Clinic's Child Recreation Centre, as well as individual counseling/mentoring for select cases. She is also a parent and family trainer for the Happy Families Program (a local adaptation of the Strengthening Families Program). Hay Mar San finds her work enriching because she enjoys working with children, both watching and participating in their growth.

Derina Johnson: Originally from County Wicklow, Ireland, Derina Johnson spent three years living on the Thai-Burma border as the founding director of child and psychosocial services for Burma Border Projects. She collaborated with local staff, including teachers and child protection advocates, to develop culturally appropriate, accessible, and sustainable approaches to psychosocial care for children and youth. Her projects included the establishment of a psychosocial care center for children at the renowned Mae Tao Clinic. Derina also acted as deputy chair for Asia Pacific Refugee Rights Network's Right to Health working group, developing and delivering mental health training to refugee groups, advocates, and legal representatives. Derina studied psychology at University College Dublin, and play therapy and psychotherapy at the Children's Therapy Centre, Westmeath. She began her professional career in social care with young people and established her own play therapy practice in inner-city Dublin for children and families affected by violence, substance abuse, and other family and societal difficulties. Currently Derina is a PhD student at Trinity College Dublin's School of Social Work and Social Policy, where she is researching the lived experiences of displaced children and how they navigate their personal and social worlds.

Khin Ohmar: Khin Ohmar came to the Thai-Burma border after organizing and participating in the 1988 democracy uprising in Burma. She joined the All Burma Student's Democratic Front before resettling in the US in 1990 to advocate nationally and internationally on Burma as well as complete a degree at Simon's Rock College. Returning to the Thai-Burma border in 1998, she joined the Burmese Women's Union and the Women's League of Burma. Today, she chairs the Network for Democracy and Development (Burma) and is foreign affairs secretary of the Forum for Democracy in Burma. She is coordinator of Burma Partnership, a network of Burma-concerned civil society organizations in the Asia-Pacific region. In 2012, Khin Ohmar's name was removed from Burma's blacklist, and she has since been able to travel frequently to Rangoon and beyond to collaborate with civil society organizations there, all the while continuing—and building bridges with—her border-based work.

Kyaw Soe Win: Kyaw Soe Win is a former political prisoner and current staff at Assistance Association for Political Prisoners–Burma (AAPP). He received training in common elements treatment approach in 2010 and became AAPP's clinical supervisor, overseeing the work of all their counselors. He was promoted in 2013 and currently works as the chief clinical supervisor for their program. His interest is in increasing access to evidence-based counseling treatments in Burma as part of the larger reconciliation process.

Lucinda Lai: Ms. Lai began working on the Thai-Burma border in 2011 with an international public service fellowship from Stanford University, where she had completed her undergraduate degree in human biology. Working on issues of mental health has provided her with unique insights into medicine, protracted humanitarian crises, community-based health care, and cultural differences, through the indelible form of human narratives. To expand her understanding of how political and economic transitions affect the health of vulnerable populations, she went on to earn a master's degree in sociology as a Gates Scholar at the University of Cambridge. She is currently studying medicine at Harvard Medical School and hopes to become a global health doctor for health and human rights in Southeast Asia.

Catherine Lee: Dr. Lee has worked on public health programs for rural communities, internally displaced persons, and migrants in Burma and Thailand for ten years. Working specifically with local health officials and local community-based organizations, she has experience with issues related to health and human rights, maternal health and child health, population-based survey methodology, and conducting randomized controlled trials of counseling interventions for torture and trauma survivors. She has also played a role in the development and expansion of community-based malaria control programs, reproductive health programs, and health information systems in these areas. Currently, she works as a research associate in the International Health Department at the Johns Hopkins Bloomberg School of Public Health based in Mae Sot, Thailand, in addition to being faculty at the Thammasat University School of Global Studies in Rangsit. Her current research work includes a situational analysis of young people in Thailand at higher risk for HIV, a qualitative and quantitative study on very young adolescents' transitions to healthy adulthood (sexual and reproductive health) in refugee camps and migrant communities in Thailand, Ethiopia, and Lebanon, and continued research on the implementation of community-based counseling programs for survivors of torture and systematic violence for adults from Burma and Iraq.

Andrew George Lim: Dr. Lim is an emergency medicine resident physician at the University of Washington–Harborview Medical Center and a research fellow of health and human rights at the University of California, Berkeley. Through Community Partners International and their Thai-Burmese border affiliate Global Health Access Program, he has led trainings in public health information systems and village-level infectious disease prevention for community health workers in eastern Burma. He has also coordinated advanced trauma management education and mental health seminars for mobile medics in Burma's conflict areas. His research focuses on the psychological traumatization of health providers in low-resource conflict settings and interventions to improve their mental resilience. He served for three years on the board of directors for the US Campaign for Burma and currently writes about Burma's social and political issues as a *Huffington Post World* blog contributor. An alumnus of Brown University, Andrew completed his graduate education at the UC San Francisco School of Medicine and the UC Berkeley School of Public Health.

Moe Moe Aung: Moe Moe is a member of the Karenni Women's Organization (KNWO). She works for the International Rescue Committee's (IRC) Women's Protection and Empowerment, focusing on capacity-building for the Karenni women's community response to gender-based violence. She is also responsible for the Peaceful Family Initiative, a violence prevention program for married couples. She played an instrumental role in a law reform project in the Karenni refugee community that aims to rewrite and standardize the rules and regulations and dispute-resolution mechanisms in the camps to bring the camp justice administration system in line with Thai and international standards. Previously, she worked as a coordinator for the Karenni Development Research Group, a forum of Karenni civil society organizations that documents environmental and human rights violations occurring as result of development projects in the Karenni State (inside Burma). She is a strong advocate for the Karenni people, both domestically and internationally, and has conducted meetings and trainings for cease-fire and civil society organizations and has participated in UN and government meetings in Geneva, Washington, DC, and Colombo, and hosted a press conference in Bangkok. In 2007, she was one of the Ethnic Nationalities Council delegates to represent the Karenni women's community at a US congressional meeting and visited First Lady Laura Bush at the White House. During that period, she was KNWO's advocate at the Women League of Burma. She has extensive training on mental health, psychosocial care, and gender-based violence response. In 2003–2004, she was an intern with the Burma Lawyers' Council. In 2005–2006, she received a one-year special training on diplomacy and advocacy by the National Council of the Union of Burma.

Naw Dah Pachara Sura: Pachara Sura is her Thai name; her Karen name is Naw Dah. She was born in Kyaw Ki Hta village in Pa Ah district of Myanmar. She came to Thailand to study from elementary school to university and graduated with a degree in political science from Kamphaeng Phet Rajabhat University. After finishing at a Thai high school in Tak province, Naw Dah entered Eden Valley Academy in Mae La refugee camp to improve her English. She was a volunteer teacher at a Thai primary school in Mae La Klo village near Mae La camp for two years before taking a job with the Karen Department of Health and Welfare (KDHW). With KDHW, Naw Dah works as the mental health officer and logistics and budget manager.

Mary O'Kane: Mary O'Kane has been working with organizations of Burma on the Thai-Burma border since 1999 and living in northwestern Thailand on and off since 1990. In particular, she has volunteered with women's organizations during the emergence of the border-based women's movement, based first with the Burmese Women's Union and later with the Women's League of Burma. She is completing a PhD in international relations at Monash University, Australia, on the politics of Burma's border-based activists, who mostly work from positions of effective statelessness. She has taught subjects on Burma at the Australian National University. Her academic publications include *Borderlands and Women: Transversal Political Agency on the Burma-Thailand Border* (Monash Asia Institute, 2005), and "Sweat and Tears: The Political Agency of Women Activist-Refugees of Burma" (*Intersections: Gender, History and Culture in the Asian Context,* May 15, 2007).

Courtland Robinson: Dr. Robinson is an associate professor in the Johns Hopkins Bloomberg School of Public Health, Department of International Health, Health Systems Program, and also serves as deputy director of the Center for Refugee and Disaster Response. He has been involved in migrant and refugee research and practice since 1979, with a particular focus on Asia. His current research and teaching activities focus on populations in migration, whether displaced by conflict and natural disaster or in the context of migrant labor and human trafficking.

Saw Ku Thay: Saw Ku Thay was born in Mon State, Burma. Saw Ku Thay worked with Médecins Sans Frontières in Mae La Refugee camp in Thailand, as a home visitor and counselor providing health education and prevention services and HIV/AIDS pre- and post-test counseling from 2000 to 2004. Starting in 2004, Saw Ku Thay began working at Mae Tao Clinic in Mae Sot, Thailand, and he received training in a range of specialized services, including nursing and medic care, reproductive and child health, basic mental health and counseling, and advanced mental health and treatment. At Mae Tao Clinic, Saw Ku Thay worked as a Voluntary Counseling and Testing Department counselor, a mental health counselor, and as Counseling Center program manager. In 2012, Saw Ku Thay resettled in the United States, where he currently resides.

Saw Than Lwin: Saw Than Lwin was born in Karen State, Burma/Myanmar. He graduated with a degree in mechanical engineering from Yangon Institute of Technology, Myanmar, in 2002. He crossed into Thailand and joined Mae Tao Clinic, where he currently serves as program manager of community health outreach. Previous roles at Mae Tao Clinic include manager of HIV voluntary counseling and testing and manager of the

Mental Health Counseling Center. He also worked with HIV/AIDS and psychosocial clients outside Mae Tao Clinic by collaborating with other organizations and communities. He participated in counseling for psychosocial clients, HIV voluntary counseling and testing, home-based care, and antiretroviral therapy. He organized monthly self-help group discussions for HIV clients, the homeless, and shelter residents with severe social problems. He supervised monthly nutrition distribution to more than three hundred HIV families. He is responsible for school health, reproductive health outreach, and health promotion and disease control among migrant workers in Mae Sot and surrounding areas. Saw Than Lwin says he is happy to be a staff member of Mae Tao Clinic because he can help vulnerable migrant communities by providing free health and social services. He plans to continue working at Mae Tao Clinic even as funding is reduced.

Sid Mone Thwe: Sid Mone was born in Chaung Sone Township and grew up in Paung Township of Mon State inside Burma/Myanmar. After attending government primary school, he entered Be Lu Ma monastery and then Kan Oo Zay Ta Wan monastery for further education. Pursuing an interest in international language skills, Sid Mone Thwe transferred to Sitagu International Buddhist Academy in Sagaing for another four years of study. Sid Mone Thwe came to Thailand in January 2004 and worked for the community-based organization Social Action for Women for six years as teacher, boardinghouse master, child protection focal point, and project supervisor of the Johns Hopkins University Mental Health Assessment Project. During this time, he attended Wide Horizon School's higher learning program, receiving a diploma in community development. In 2011, he moved to the International Rescue Committee (IRC) and worked on their child protection project (IMPACT). He is currently a training officer for IRC's Project for Local Empowerment/ Women's Protection and Empowerment program. He says, "Mostly I work for children, which I am very pleased to do because I believe that children are our future."

Thandar Shwe: Thandar Shwe studied history at the Mawlamyine University in Myanmar, and holds a certificate of midwifery from the School of Nursing and Midwifery in Mawlamyine, Myanmar. She worked as a midwife inside Myanmar for more than a decade. Thandar Shwe then relocated to Mae Sot, Thailand, where she worked as a supervisor at the Mae Tao Clinic Mental Health Counseling Center and as a counselor for the Mental Health Assessment Project, a collaborative research initiative led by Johns Hopkins University's Bloomberg School of Public

Health. Thandar Shwe is currently a primary health care field officer for the nongovernmental organization NICCO, in Pha-an, Myanmar.

Liberty Thawda: Ms. Thawda was born in Thaketa Township near Yangon, Burma. She obtained her BA and MA degrees at Spicer Memorial College in India, where she focused on child and youth education, child development, and psychology. After completing her education, she moved to Mae La Refugee Camp on the Thai-Burma border to work as a math teacher for middle and high school students. In a subsequent role with a UNICEF-sponsored NGO, she received intensive psychosocial training that led her to become a psychosocial trainer to refugee teachers. This experience gave Ms. Thawda a rich understanding of psychosocial matters and children's needs, and resulted in her involvement in the development of the in-camp child protection referral system. Since 2007, she has been working with Burmese migrant communities around Mae Sot, Thailand, developing and delivering psychosocial and training programs for teachers, community leaders, and child protection workers. Ms. Thawda is currently the deputy director of child protection and education at Mae Tao Clinic.

Meredith Walsh: Ms. Walsh is an independent consultant working on the Thai-Burma border for seven years. She has served as technical advisor for reproductive health at Mae Tao Clinic, Burma Medical Association, and the Adolescent Reproductive Health Network. Her current work involves conducting translational research and applying evidence-based outcomes to improve the quality of facilities-based and community-based health care for displaced people from Burma on the Thai-Burma border. She is cofounder of a nonprofit that assists refugees from Burma newly resettled in Worcester, Massachusetts. She received her master of public health with a focus on international health and development from Tulane University and her advance practice nursing degree from the University of Massachusetts. She currently works in primary care as a family nurse practitioner at a community health center in Massachusetts.

Index

Note: Page numbers in *italics* refer to the illustrations.

groups in, 4–5, 25, 26, 31–34, 38, 41–42, 99, 164, 189, 292; forced labor used for infrastructure projects, 33–34; health care infrastructure in, 188–89; historical background, 25–26; independence, 25–26; map of, x; military rule (1963–2011), 26–29; Millennium Development Goals, 113; name of country, 3–4, 42n1; political transition in, 302–5; religious groups in, 25, 27; repatriation to, 28–29, 72, 154–55, 255–56; restoring wellbeing to population of, 41–42; torture, interrogation, and imprisonment in, 29–31; Unlawful Association, Emergency, and Immigration Acts, 210, 303; war and violence in, 4–5. *See also* mental health and psychosocial issues on Burma border

Burma News International (BNI), 298

burnout, 226–27, 245

Cambodia, 6, 36, 39, 148

Chiang Mai, Thailand, 97, 292

child abuse, 122

child labor, 115–16

Child Protection Act (2003), Thailand, 115

child protection referral system (CPRS), 122, 124

Child Recreation Center (CRC), MTC, 109, 125–26, 242–43, 253

children and young people, 109–30; abandonment of, 109, 119–20; basic safety and security issues, 114–15, 121–22; boardinghouses for, 112, 119–22, 125, 127–29, 278; in Burma border context, 113–20; CBOs and, 111, 122–25; culturally sensitive treatment of, 111–13, 122–23; education of, 117–20; family and community support systems, 122–25; health care for, 117; international best practices regarding treatment of, 109–13; mentoring programs for, 127–29; in migrant communities, 113–14, 114–15; nonspecialized support programs for,

125–27; parenting of, 116, 123; political activism, youth involvement in, 294–95; psychosocial programs for, 120–29; registration of births to migrant parents, 40, 114–15; repatriation of, 72; in workforce, 115–16

China, 24, 25, 26–27, 285, 292, 295

chronic illness, 188, 191–95. *See also* HIV/ AIDS; malaria; tuberculosis

Civil Registration Act (2008), Thailand, 115

civil society organizations. *See* political activism

clinical supervision, 246, 271–73, 278. *See also* parallel process and clinical supervision

cognitive appraisal, 230

Committee for the Promotion and Protection of Child Rights (CPPCR), Mae Sot, Thailand, 114, 115, 122

community and family, separation of service providers from, 229–30, 235

community-based organizations (CBOs), 85–103; assessing community needs, 74; for children and young people, 111, 122–25; domestic violence and, 149–50; education and awareness-raising at community level, 77; FED, 98–103; feedback to, 263; Fortune (Shan organization), 92–98, 99, 103; IASC *Guidelines* and, 85–86; importance of community role in its own healing, 51; individualized curative interventions, 91–92, 97–98, 103; KDHW, 86–92; outreach, support groups, training, and education, 89–91, 93–96, 100–102; partnerships, 86–87, 99–100, 101, 199, 262–63; preventive interventions, 96–97, 102–3; providers of services, 59–60; service providers in Karen State and Burma border, 220–21

community [mental] health workers (C[M] HWs), 100, 102, 270–71, 272, 275, 278

complex emergencies, 85–86

Karen: female village heads, treatment of, 31–32; refugee camps in Thailand, 36–37, 38; service providers in Karen State (*see* service providers); substance abuse and, 171

Karen Department of Health and Welfare (KDHW), 65, 86–92, 99, 220–21, 235

Karen Human Rights Group (KHRG), 114, 289

Karen National Union (KNU), 73, 191, 220, 231

Karenni refugee camps in Thailand, 36–37, 38, 148–49. *See also* gender-based violence

Karenni Women's Organization, 158

Karen Women's Organization, 32, 296

Karls, James, 56

key informant interviews, 266, 268–69

Khin Ohmar, 285, 288, 317

Khmer Rouge, 6

Kleinman, Arthur, 9, 10

Kumpfer, Karol, 122

Kyaw Soe Win, 261, 317

Lai, Lucinda, 163, 317–18

land mine injuries, 189, 205–10

Lang, Hazel J., 31

Laos, 36, 39, 163

Lazarus, Richard S., 230

Lee, Catherine, 261, 318

Lim, Andrew George, 219, 318–19

Lopes Cardozo, Barbara, 74–75

Mae Hong Son, Thailand, 75, 148, 292

Mae La camp, Thailand, 73, 74, 168–69, 171–74

Mae Ra Ma Luang, Thailand, 73

Mae Sariang, Thailand, 292

Mae Sot, Thailand: burning of refugee camp near, 37; CBOs in, 67, 86, 99; children and young people in (*see* children and young people); General Hospital, 191, 204–5, 206; parallel process and clinical supervision in,

242, 244, 245, 247, 251, 256; political activism in, 292; program evaluation and research in, 266, 267, 269, 270, 271; vulnerable populations in, 190, 191, 195, 200, 204–6, 211

Mae Tao Clinic (MTC), viii, 66–72; assessments and interventions at, 65, 66–72, 78; CBOs and, 101; children and young people, caring for, 109, 117, 120, 121, 123; chronic illnesses, 191–94; CRC, 109, 125–26, 242–43, 253; HIV/AIDS at, 195–200; land mine injuries at, 205–10; parallel process and clinical supervision at, 242–43, 244, 253; political activism and, 295, 296; program evaluation and research by, 266; reproductive health services, 189, 201–4; vulnerable populations served by, 190–91

malaria, vii, 73, 88, 91, 92, 102, 117, 228

Malaysia, 295

MAP Foundation, 299

Maung, Cynthia, 66, 101, 190–91, 205, 242, 295

Maw Ker, 205–6, 207–8

Mayadas, Nazneen S., 54

Médecins Sans Frontieres (MSF), 196–97

mediation of domestic violence cases, 156–58

medical anthropology, 9–11

medical care. *See* health care; service providers

medication management, 249–51

meditation, 24, 31, 41, 76, 112, 124, 195, 209, 231

Men's Health Center, 199

mental health and psychosocial issues on Burma border, vii–viii, 3–17; cultural and social dimensions of, 9–11; defining psychosocial and mental health, 52–53; global mental health and, 8–9; guidelines and resources, 11–16; historical context, 25–34; human rights issue, mental health as,

Segal, Uma A., 54

service providers, 219–36; anxiety and depression of, 228–30, 232; assessment and intervention, 59–60; burnout of, 226–27, 245; in CBOs in Karen State and Burma border, 220–21; clinical supervision of, 246, 271–73, 278; C[M]HWs, 100, 102, 270–71, 272, 275, 278; coping mechanisms of, 230–33, 235, 276–77; domestic violence and support for, 158–59; education and training of, 221, 271–73; family and community, separation from, 229–30, 235; HIV/AIDS services staff, 201; legal status and security of, 275; local idioms of distress used by, 221–22, 222; at MTC, 70–71; positive effects of counseling on, 279; resilience of, 233–36; substance abuse by, 231–32, 235; task shifting, 261–62; traumatic stress experienced by, 223–25, 275–76; vicarious traumatization of, 225–26, 244, 245, 276. *See also* parallel process and clinical supervision

services. *See* assessment and intervention

sexual trafficking and sexual abuse. *See* gender-based violence

Shan: Fortune (psychosocial organization), 92–98, 99, 103; Women's Action Group, 295

Shoklo Malaria Research Unit, 117

Sid Mone Thwe, 109, 321

Singapore, 295

Social Action for Women, 123, 199, 266

social and cultural dimensions. *See* cultural and social dimensions

somatoform disorder, 7

Somwong,Pranom, 41

South, Ashley, 33

Sphere Project: *Humanitarian Charter and Minimum Standards of Humanitarian Response*, 11–12, 51, 60–61, 77, 166; people-centered humanitarian focus of, 53

splitting, 249–51

staff. *See* service providers

Standards for Privacy of Individually Identifi able Health Information, U.S., 61

statelessness, 5, 115, 254, 292–93, 295

stigma associated with mental disorders, 9, 41, 76, 193, 249–50

strength-based approach, 53–54

Strengthening Families Program, 122

substance abuse, 163–78; assessment and intervention, 174–77; in Burma border camps, 167–70; by Burmese activists in Thailand, 36; conflict-affected populations and, 164–66, 168–69; DARE Network, 177; diagnosing and classifying, 166–67; domestic violence and, 148, 158; by former political prisoners, 212; GBV and, 148, 158, 168, 169; gender differences in, 36, 169, 171–72; global mental health and, 8; "Golden Triangle" drug trade and, 163–64; HIV/AIDS and, 165–66, 168; at MTC, 70; PU-AMI and, 78; in refugee camps in Thailand, 38; by service providers, 231–32, 235; "social disease," alcoholism as, 170–74; traditional drug and alcohol use, 170–71; withdrawal, 167

Substance Abuse, Drugs and Addictions Guidebook (AMI), 169–70

suicide, 15–16, 45, 57, 62–65, 69–71, 99, 165, 169, 198, 232, 233

Summerfield, Derek, 296

systems theories, 55–56

task shifting, 261–62

tatmadaw, 26, 28, 31–32, 34, 37, 114

Thailand, 24–25, 34–42; activists, policies toward, 34–36; attitudes toward Burmese in, 40; Burma border refugee camps in, *xi*; Child Protection Act (2003), 115; Civil Registration Act